Worldwide Successful Pediatric Nurse-Led Models of Care

Cecily L. Betz

Editor

Worldwide Successful Pediatric Nurse-Led Models of Care

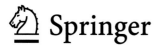 Springer

Editor
Cecily L. Betz
Center for Excellence in Developmental Disabilities
University of Southern California
Los Angeles, CA, USA

ISBN 978-3-031-22151-4   ISBN 978-3-031-22152-1   (eBook)
https://doi.org/10.1007/978-3-031-22152-1

This Springer imprint is published by the registered company Springer Nature Switzerland AG
The registered company address is: Gewerbestrasse 11, 6330 Cham, Switzerland

Preface

This text is unlike other pediatric and child health nursing texts previously published. Typically, many of the texts published for pediatric/child health nurses are focused on nursing education texts for undergraduate and graduate level students. Other nursing-related texts published for nurses who provide care to infants, children, and adolescents and their families center on specialized areas of clinical practice such as pain, family-centered care, and developmental care. This text addresses an area of practice that has not been addressed before—nurse-led models of care for infants, children, adolescents, and families. This text provides readers with new perspectives and insights about models of care that our international colleagues from seven countries, Australia, Brazil, Canada, Sierra Leone, Singapore, South Africa, and the United States, have developed, implemented, and tested.

As the reader will note, these models of care have been developed by nurses with differing practice backgrounds and levels of education as well as in collaboration with interdisciplinary colleagues. As evidenced throughout this text, the regulatory practice requirements differ internationally. In the United States, independent nursing practice referred to as full practice authority (FPA) is being implemented throughout the country. FPA enables advanced practice nurses to enhance their scope of practice to function independently to its fullest extent (ANA 2020; Bosse et al. 2017; Stucky et al. 2020). The reader will find mention of independent practice in some of the chapters. As the array of chapters in this text demonstrate, pervasive and widespread opportunities exist for our colleagues who recognize service needs of the infants, children, adolescents, and families that can be addressed uniquely based upon a nursing model of care.

The models of care presented in this text share the commonality of being nurse-led. However, each and every model presented in this text is uniquely different and is representative of the diversity of care models possible for nursing development and implementation. These models demonstrate the infinite possibilities that exist for our nursing colleagues to move forward to think and act boldly to extend the boundaries of accepted nursing practice. The presentations of the models of care described in this text indicate the vision, creativity, determination, and professionalism of the nursing colleagues who undertook these efforts to create new and unique nurse-led services for service populations in need.

Each of the nurse-led service model chapters is organized in a similar format for readers to provide a thorough understanding and insights about each of these programs. The *Introduction* provides an overview of the content that will be covered in the chapter. In the section on *Background Information*, authors provide readers with an overview of the need for the model. To do so, the authors describe the target population and setting of the service model, which provide interesting details of the uniqueness of each of the programs, particularly since this text has an international focus. The authors share the impetus for development of their models and the process undertaken to develop and implement the model/service. These are important details to share as the reader will find that each nurse-led program undertook a uniquely different approach that was influenced to a great deal by the population served, the setting, resources, and culture. The theoretical frameworks of each of these nurse-led programs are described as they shaped its development and implementation.

One of the primary intents of this text was to provide readers with sufficient detail about each of the nurse-led service models that would enhance program development of other nurse-led models of care for the pediatric and adolescent population and their families. In the chapter section entitled, *Description of the Nurse-Led Model*, these descriptions are shared with the purpose of inspiring other pediatric/child health nursing colleagues to develop, implement, and test similar and/or new models of nurse-led services. To that end, the authors provide descriptions of the organizational components of the service model, detailed descriptions of the services provided, and the setting wherein these services are provided. As described in this text, the service models are located in a variety of clinical and community-based settings that demonstrate the fluidity of nursing practice. Descriptions of the nursing and interdisciplinary team members involved with the provision of services and support are identified as well as their roles and responsibilities as well as the position requirements for staffing support. Readers will find useful information about the methods of evaluation that were used as depending on the service purposes, population served, setting, staffing and resources available; there is a wide variety of methods used for evaluation.

These nursing experts provide their unique expertise and experience with implementing these nurse-led services in the section entitled, *Challenges and Facilitators*. Authors share candidly with readers the challenges faced in the development and implementation of this nurse-led model. Facilitators that enabled this program to be implemented are presented as well, which are relevant and important considerations for service model development (i.e., administrative support). Issues of sustainability are addressed that include the issues associated with financing and reimbursement.

In the sections, *Service Adjustments* and *Lessons Learned*, the authors share their candid appraisal of their program development efforts. That is, the modifications that were needed to make the program more effective are presented. The authors provide advice to colleagues as to what was learned to make the program more effective and feasible. Based upon their service model development, the authors share their future plans in the section entitled, *Future Implications for Clinical Practice and Research*. Each of the chapters conclude with a presentation of *Useful Resources* that include websites, social media, and educational materials.

Other chapters in the text intersect with the descriptions of the nurse-led model of care chapters. One of the chapters, authored by Dr. Eanes, provides a theoretical lens, based on the Urie Bronfenbrenner Social-Ecological Theory (1977) upon which nurse-led initiatives can be developed that are focused on the needs of disadvantaged pediatric and adolescent populations. One of the chapters provides decades-long perspectives pertaining to the lessons learned with the involvement of nurse-led service models focused on the needs of adolescents and young adults with long-term conditions. The introductory chapter provides an overview of all the chapters in the text. The concluding chapter presents a summary and analyses of the nurse-led programs found in this text.

It is hoped that nurses and our interdisciplinary colleagues who read this text will be inspired to create new nurse-led models of care in their own practice settings whether in traditional clinical sites or in community-based settings. The worldwide nurse-led models of care demonstrate the robustness of innovative nursing practice that exists and will continue to evolve and grow to address healthcare needs of infants, children, adolescents, and their families.

Los Angeles, CA, USA   Cecily L. Betz

References

American Nurses Association (2020). ANA's principles for advanced practice registered nurse (APRN): Full practice authority. Retrieved on November 12, 2020 from: https://www.nursing-world.org/~49f695/globalassets/docs/ana/ethics/principles-aprnfullpracticeauthority.pdf.

Bosse J, Simmonds K, Hanson C, Pulcini J, Dunphy L, Vanhook P, Poghosyan L. Position statement: full practice authority for advanced practice registered nurses is necessary to transform primary care. Nurs Outlook. 2017;65(6):761–5.

Bronfenbrenner U. Toward an experimental ecology of human development. Am Psychol. 1977;32:513–31.

Stucky CH, Brown WJ, Stucky MG. COVID 19: an unprecedented opportunity for nurse practitioners to reform healthcare and advocate for permanent full practice authority. Nurs Forum. 2020;56:1–6. https://doi.org/10.1111/nuf.12515.

Contents

Nurse-Led Models of Care for Infants, Children, Youth, and Families: Introduction and Overview

Cecily L. Betz

Introduction

This text offers the reader with a unique and often overlooked perspective on nurse-led services and programs that have been developed for infants, children, youth, and their families. Most clinically focused nursing texts, particularly those who that are written for pediatric/paediatric and child health nurses and practitioners focus on health-care issues based upon more well-known traditional models of nursing care. This text is different from traditional perspectives of pediatric/paediatric and child health nursing practice. The chapters of this text offer a diverse range of nurse-led clinical programs and services in hospital-based and community-based settings. As the reader will note, these models of care are representative of the scope of nursing practice worldwide, which varies based upon institutional, regulatory, community, and cultural needs.

This text is focused on providing readers with international exemplars of nurse-led/nurse-directed pediatric/paediatric and child health models of care. These models are representative of the broad scope of pediatric/paediatric and child health nursing practice that exists in clinical and community-based settings. The nurse-led models of care featured in this textbook address the divergent needs of infants, children, youth, and their families across the health-illness continuum of care. The nurse-led models presented in this text focus on approaches developed and implemented by pediatric/paediatric and child health nurses for infants, children, and youth who have health-care needs ranging from preventive to acute care.

The purpose of this text is to provide exemplars of innovative and forward-thinking models of nursing care that can be adapted/replicated in other clinical and

C. L. Betz (✉)
Center for Excellence in Developmental Disabilities, University of Southern California, Los Angeles, CA, USA
e-mail: CBetz@chla.usc.edu

© The Author(s), under exclusive license to Springer Nature Switzerland AG 2023
C. L. Betz (ed.), *Worldwide Successful Pediatric Nurse-Led Models of Care*, https://doi.org/10.1007/978-3-031-22152-1_1

community-based settings worldwide. An aspect of interest to readers is to showcase innovative models that are practiced in countries that are not necessarily known in the field of pediatric/paediatric and child health nursing. These are models of care that provide readers with new information and insights that have been developed, implemented, and evaluated. Typically, models of care are written about those from high-resource countries. This textbook contains chapters about the models of care that have been in practice in low-resourced countries and in other parts of the world that are not well known in high-resource countries. A major intent of this textbook is to inform readers of these nurse-led models and to facilitate worldwide linkages with colleagues internationally from areas/continents worldwide not typically featured in pediatric/paediatric and child health textbooks that include Africa, Asia, and South America. Nurse-led models of care described in this text provide readers with incentives and opportunities to replicate similar nurse-led models of care in their own clinical/community-based settings. The remaining portion of this chapter provide readers with a synopsis of the nurse-led models of care featured in this textbook that have been developed and implemented by nursing practice innovators. The chapter descriptions are organized by age groups, theory-driven approaches to care and staff initiative. Table 1 provides a listing of these practice exemplars by name, population served and country.

Table 1 Country, population focus, and settings of nurse-led services/programs

Nurse-led service/ program	Country	Population focus	Setting
Leading a Nurse Practitioner-designed Newborn Circumcision Clinic	USA	Newborns	Outpatient Service of Major Pediatric Medical Center located at a suburban satellite setting
Baby Steps: Improving the Transition from Hospital to Home for Neonatal Patients and Caregivers through Nurse-Led Telehealth	USA	Neonates	Transfer of Care Model: Neonatal Intensive Care Unit to Home implemented at major Pediatric Medical Center
Breatheasy: A Nurse-Led "Care Through Family" Service Model,	South Africa	Infants	Transfer of Care Model: in-patient setting to home implemented at Children's Hospital
Evolution of a Complex and Home Care Program for Children with Chronic Diseases	Singapore	Children with Medical Complex (CMC)	Children's Complex and Home Care Services (CCHS) are provided to children and youth who are medically stable but require long-term medical technology support to be discharged from KK Women's and Children's Hospital (KKH) to home

Table 1 (continued)

Nurse-led service/ program	Country	Population focus	Setting
Caring for Patient on Extracorporeal Membrane Oxygenation (ECMO) in the Pediatric Intensive Care Setting	Singapore	Critically ill neonates and children with severe respiratory and/or cardiac failure	Pediatric Intensive Care Unit of KK Women's and Children's Hospital (KKH)
Canadian Nurse Practitioner-Led Paediatric Rehabilitation Complex Care Program	Canada	Children and Youth with Medical Complexity	Holland Bloorview Kids Rehabilitation Hospital (HBKRH), children's rehabilitation hospital with academic affiliation with the University of Toronto
Affirming and Empowering Kids: Creating an Independent and Comprehensive Gender-affirming Healthcare Center.	USA	Transgender and gender-diverse Children, Youth and Adults	Transhealth Northampton, an independent and comprehensive, nurse-led, health-care center in a community-based setting
From Patient Studies to a Hospital-Wide Initiative: A Mindfulness Journey	USA	Nurses and Interdisciplinary Health Care Professionals	Pediatric Medical Center
Transitioning from Pediatric to Adult Care in Sickle Cell Disease: An innovative nurse-led service model.	USA	Youth and Young Adults with Sickle Cell Disease	Outpatient Setting of Pediatric Medical Center
Nurse-Led Service Models: Lessons Learned Over 25 Years	USA	Adolescents and Emerging Adults	Community-based setting; Outpatient Setting of Pediatric Medical Center
Leveraging a Professional Nursing Organization to Create an Anti-Trafficking Care Model	USA	Children at risk for, exploited and abused in human trafficking	National Initiative, *NAPNAP Partners for Vulnerable Youth* created by National Association of Pediatric Nurse Practitioners (NAPNAP)
Interactional Model of Caring for Families of Children with Chronic Conditions	Brazil	Families of Children with Chronic Conditions	Clinic located on University Campus

(continued)

Table 1 (continued)

Nurse-led service/ program	Country	Population focus	Setting
A Pediatric Eczema Shared Care Model	Australia	Children and Youth with Eczema	Multidisciplinary eczema shared care model implemented to improve provision of eczema care comprised of NP-led pediatric eczema service, training and resource materials distributed nationally, and Collaborative Pharmacy Eczema Model of Care
The Social-Ecological Theory of Child Development: A Framework For Nurse-Led Initiatives And Models of Care	USA	Children, Youth and Families	Framework of Care
The Sierra Leone National ETAT+ Programme: Delivering Nurse-Led Emergency Paediatric Care	Sierra Leone	Acutely Unwell Children	Implementation of National Emergency Services Model throughout hospitals in Sierra Leone

Neonates, Infants, and Early Childhood

Authors Drs. Natasha North and Minette Coetzee describe a pediatric nurse practitioner-led service model in South Africa to facilitate the discharge of children with tracheostomies or requiring home ventilation to their homes, many of whom will live in low-resourced environments. In this chapter, *Breatheasy: A Nurse-Led 'Care Through Family' Service Model*, authors describe this innovative and as authors describe "resourceful" model of care that has enabled nearly 1000 infants to be discharged and managed at home since its inception in 1989. A key component of this program is the promotion and on-going support of the mother-infant bonding and attachment, whether the infant is hospitalized or discharged to home management. In the *Breatheasy* program, intensive training is provided to the primary caregiver (mother/family relative) to enable the infant's home management. The team approach to teaching also involves experienced parents who have faced similar circumstances with their own children and provide unique role modeling and mentorship to these new mothers. The community-based services and supports offered through *Breatheasy* may include addressing issues of water, sanitation, or electricity that are nonexistent in informal settlements that exist on municipal properties not designated for housing purposes. The challenges addressed in this program demonstrate that seemingly formidable obstacles can be, as this well-established nurse-led program has demonstrated, to be feasible. The achievements of this program in addressing the needs of infants with complex medical needs in low-resourced environments are long-standing.

Authors Williams, Wood, and Lajoie describe in the chapter entitled, *Leading a Nurse Practitioner-Designed Newborn Circumcision Clinic* the development, implementation and evaluation of this nurse-led model of care. This innovative nurse-led *Newborn Circumcision Clinic (NCC)* in collaboration with physician colleagues provides services to infants who were not circumcised during the immediate newborn period. The authors provide extensive detail on the extensive planning that was required to develop and implement this clinic as there were few models available for replication. With the support of institutional and interdisciplinary leaders, this nurse-led model of care was established. As well, which was influential as well with the establishment of NCC, Full Practice Authority was enacted in Massachusetts on January 1, 2021, that enabled nurse practitioners to engage in prescriptive practice without supervision according to state regulatory requirements. Authors provide a thorough description of the functional and structural components of this innovative NCC. Program evaluation is an essential component of clinic services, which provides the necessary data to closely monitor the processes and outcomes of care. As reported, data are gathered on family satisfaction, cost–benefit analysis, and clinical outcomes, which have demonstrative positive outcomes. The excellence and programmatic innovations of NCC have been recognized by the American Academy of Nursing (AAN) as an Edge Runner model of care.

Drs. Sarik and Matsuda, research nurse scientists of Nicklaus Children's Hospital in Coral Terrace Florida, describe the telehealth program developed for infants and their caregivers following their discharge from the Neonatal Intensive Care Unit (NICU) in the chapter, *Baby Steps: Improving the Transition from Hospital to Home for Neonatal Patients and Caregivers Through a Nurse-Led Telehealth Program.* This nurse-led program is composed of an interprofessional team that includes NICU service professionals, telehealth specialists, and researchers. Through the *Baby Steps* program, telehealth services that include clinical assistance, assessment of postdischarge needs/concerns, and anticipatory guidance are provided following NICU discharge for an interval of 24–48 h. Additional services as needed are provided for the next 2 weeks.

The authors detail for the reader the process undertaken to develop *Baby Steps* that involved a collaborative research and leadership partnership between Nicklaus Children's Hospital and the University of Miami School of Nursing and Health Studies. Through this partnership, the nurse researchers collaborated on the acquisition of extramural grant funding for *Baby Steps*, development and implementation of research, project oversight, and project dissemination efforts. A wide range of dissemination products have been generated that include manuscripts, poster, and podium presentations at professional meetings, informal in-house communications, and podcasts. The programmatic efforts of this interprofessional team that involve a prominent use of telehealth are described providing the reader with a clear understanding of the services available through *Baby Steps*. Authors detail the program-specific challenges, opportunities, and service adjustments this team encountered with the implementation of *Baby Steps*. As the author share, the success and feasibility of this extramurally-funded program have been demonstrated; they are hopeful that *Baby Steps* will continue with future funding.

A nurse-led model of emergency pediatric care based on the World Health Organization validated Emergency Triage Assessment and Treatment+ (ETAT+) framework is presented in the chapter *The Sierra Leone National ETAT+ Programme: Delivering Nurse-Led Emergency Paediatric Care.* The impetus for the development of this nurse-led program was to create new models of care designed to improve the mortality rates of newborns and children under 5 years of age caused by preventable deaths associated with malnutrition, malaria, tuberculosis, and pneumonia. Furthermore, as presented in this chapter, Sierra Leone has been ravaged by an ongoing civil war that ended just over 20 years ago, the Ebola epidemic in 2014–2015, and the COVID-19 pandemic. These cataclysmic events caused irretrievable consequences for the population of Sierra Leone.

Dr. Christopher Hands and the authoring team provide a description of the alternative model of care that was implemented to assess and provide treatment to acutely unwell children in an underresourced system of health care. As evidence of the challenges to provide care under these circumstances, of the 13 government hospitals near Freetown in 2016, only four hospitals had access to a reliable source of electricity and to running water on the pediatric wards. None of the hospitals had a triage program to determine clinical acuity and treatment needs of the children who presented at the hospital. The elaborate process of the implementation of the nurse-led emergency pediatric care in several institutional settings, which involved staff training and ongoing-mentorship, is described. As the authors describe, the challenges with implementation reflect the cultural norms and lack of resources evident in Sierra Leone. As revealed, the feasibility of this innovative nurse-led service was found to be initially promising.

Jemma Weidinger, Eczema Nurse Practitioner, Perth Children's Hospital, who is the lead author of the writing team, describes strategies that were implemented to improve access to care for infants and children with eczema in Western Australia (WA) in the chapter, *A Paediatric Eczema Shared Care Model.* Authors describe a multifaceted approach to improve the provision of services and supports for infants and children with eczema and their families. The National Allergy Strategy (NAS) Shared Care Model for Eczema provided the theoretical framework for the development of the Eczema Model described in this chapter. Through intramural funding support from Perth Children's Hospital, two clinics were established and resource materials for the community and health-care professionals were developed. The two clinical models, although similar in mission, were differently focused.

The goals of the nurse-practitioner-led pediatric eczema was to improve access to care as families had previously experienced prolonged wait times for specialty care appointments as well as to improve home home-care management. Problems with treatment adherence were noted with the former model of care as limited time for family education was available that were contributory to the limitations with eczema treatments at home. Another eczema/allergy clinic that was based on a multidisciplinary model of care was established as well for optimal eczema management and treatment of common food allergies. In addition to establishing these service models, educational partnerships for eczema management were developed with two national partner organizations—the National Allergy Strategy (NAS) and

Allergy & Anaphylaxis Australia (A&AA). Another component of the NAS that is under development is the collaborative Pharmacy Eczema Model of Care (CPEM) in partnership with the School of Allied Health/Discipline of Pharmacy at The University of Western Australia. The CPEM is envisioned to provide pharmacists with guidance with the treatment of children with eczema and allergic food conditions.

Broad Range of Children, Youth and Young Adults

In this chapter, *Affirming and Empowering Kids: Creating an Independent and Comprehensive Gender-Affirming Healthcare Center*, author Dallas Ducar, MSN, APRN, who is CEO of *Transhealth Northampton*, describes an innovative and one-of-a kind health-care organization for transgender and gender-diverse individuals across the lifespan from childhood to adulthood that provides gender-affirming care. The vision of *Transhealth Northampton* is, "… to transform the world so that trans and gender diverse adults, children and youth are empowered and celebrated as they work with an affirming team on own their healthcare journey." Ducar describes for the reader the historical context of the origins of this gender-affirming health-care organization and the discriminatory practices and gender-harming practices that created the need for *Transhealth Northampton*.

The background section of the chapter enlarges understanding of the challenges and barriers that the transgender and gender diverse population have encountered in accessing services that are responsive to their comprehensive needs for health services. Of particular interest for the reader, the author provides informed and insightful perspectives as one of the founders of *Transhealth Northampton* pertaining to the challenges and facilitators that were encountered with bringing this vision of gender-affirming care to fruition. As with any new endeavor, the service adjustments and visions for the future are reflective of the collective efforts of the dedicated leaders and team of *Transhealth Northampton*.

Dr. Barbara Speller-Brown details the health-care transition program for youth and young adults with Sickle Cell Disease (SCD) that was developed and implemented at Children's National Medical Center in Washington DC in the chapter entitled, *Transitioning from Pediatric to Adult Care in Sickle Cell Disease: An Innovative Nurse-Led Model*. As Dr. Speller-Brown notes, health-care transition service programs have become a necessity to ensure that youth and young adults with SCD transfer their care smoothly without interruption to adult health-care providers and transition to adulthood. In the 1970s, individuals with SCD were unlikely to survive into adulthood; today, the survival rates have changed dramatically as those with SCD are expected to survive into middle age.

As Dr. Speller-Brown describes, this program involves several components. The service model is based upon an interdisciplinary service model led by nursing as SCD affects many organ systems. The Sickle Cell Adolescent Team (SCAT) is composed of a Nurse Practitioner, who is the Program Director, Scheduler/RN Nurse Coordinator, and Social Worker. The roles and responsibilities of each of the SCAT are delineated providing the reader with an overview description of the activities in place to facilitate the youths and young adults transfer of care to adult providers. A notable feature is the ongoing survey follow-up using the Transition Health Care Transition Feedback Survey conducted to track outcomes of care quarterly during year 1, semiannually in year 2, and annually year 3 and beyond.

As presented in the chapter, *Evolution of a Complex and Home Care Program for Children with Chronic Diseases*, the author team, led by Lam Li Ying, describes the nurse-led home care program that was developed at KK Women's and Children's Hospital, the largest pediatric tertiary hospital in Singapore. This program, started over two decades ago, was established to address the complex medical needs of children who faced prolonged hospitalization, although medically stable as they were dependent on medical technology support. Children with medically complex needs served and who continue to be served in this program are those who require ongoing care and surveillance from three or more medical subspecialties and require one or more complex care supports that involve the assistance of oxygen therapy, mechanical ventilation, and tracheostomy care.

Other types of chronic care home support include children who require alternative nutritional support with tube feedings and those needing stoma care. Authors provide readers with the detailed planning that was undertaken that eventually resulted in the establishment of this program as a sustainable government service for children with complex medical needs. The service components of Children's Complex and Home Care Service (CCHS) as described in this chapter provide the reader with extensive detail.

Importantly, a vivid description is provided on the role of CCHS Home Care Nurse that involves transfer of care planning, ongoing patient assessment and monitoring conducted during home visits and tele-consultations, assistance with and management of medical equipment procurement and consumable supplies, patient and caregiving instruction. Other functions include care coordination with healthcare providers and consultation with medical equipment vendors. Authors offer insights as to the challenges and supports that were encountered with the development and implementation of this program as well as the service adjustments needed for sustainability. Their experience and expertise as described by these clinical experts provide important implications and application for clinical practice and research worldwide.

The authoring team led by Angela Kirk describes the development and implementation of a nurse-led extracorporeal membrane oxygenation program at KK Women's and Children's Hospital, the largest pediatric hospital in Singapore in the chapter, *Caring for Patient on Extracorporeal Membrane Oxygenation (ECMO) in the Pediatric Intensive Care Setting*. As recounted in this chapter, this program evolved over many years during which this program expanded from initially providing ECMO supportive care managed by perfusionists for a small group of eligible patients with severe cardiorespiratory failure. Now this nurse-led service model, although considered to serve a small volume of patients, has enlarged its service capacity.

As described in this chapter, the organizational efforts to develop the curricular components of the training program and its implementation involved many levels of organizational and interdisciplinary leadership. The complexity and intensity of training needed to implement this program are well documented in this chapter. This nurse-led service model involves a complex arrangement of nurse administrators and advanced practice nurses. These nursing roles include the ECMO nurse coordinator, who serves as the liaison between the ECMO oversight committee, clinicians, technical and ancillary support team, and families; the ECMO specialist nurse who coordinates and provides clinical oversight for the care for ECMO patients. Other members of the team are the bedside nurses, who are senior-level nurses who provide the direct care to ECMO patients, and the multidisciplinary team composed of the specialty physicians and interdisciplinary health-care professionals. As the authors convey, this highly specialized nurse-led service model is dynamic, comprehensive, and responsive to the critical care needs of the neonatal and pediatric patients served.

Leveraging a Professional Nursing Organization to Create an Antitrafficking Care Model authored by Dr. Jessica L. Peck presents the account of the development by the National Association of Pediatric Nurse Practitioners (NAPNAP) of a public-facing 501(c)3 organization called *NAPNAP Partners for Vulnerable Youth*. This NAPNAP organization was formed to create nurse-led public health initiatives that focused on specialized education and advocacy targeting the needs of vulnerable youth. The first programmatic effort of *NAPNAP Partners for Vulnerable Youth* is the establishment of the *Alliance for Children in Trafficking (ACT)*. Dr. Peck describes for the reader the formidable efforts that have been undertaken by *ACT* to address this public health crisis that is estimated to affect 40 million individuals worldwide of whom approximately 25% of those who are abused and exploited are children.

In this chapter, the historic background of the efforts undertaken to create *ACT* is described as this initiative was uniquely different and situated to create a trauma-informed, culturally responsive, patient-centered approach to address the needs of this vulnerable population of children from a public health prevention perspective unlike prevailing programmatic efforts that are focused on criminal justice. The author provides the reader with an overview of the establishment of *ACT* beginning with the survey of NAPNAP membership to determine their recognition and support for addressing this public health crisis to the development and implementation of educational programs, advocacy, and policymaking efforts to effect changes in practice to provide trauma-informed care for children who are victims of human trafficking. *ACT* reflects an innovative nurse-led approach undertaken by a prominent pediatric nursing professional organization to create the educational and policy-related infrastructure to improve nursing practice at the local level.

In the chapter entitled, *Nurse-Led Service Models: Lessons Learned Over 25 Years,* Dr. Cecily Betz shares with readers, the 25-year evolution and history of nurse-led model development pertaining to the provision of health-care transition services to adolescents and emerging adults with special health-care needs. As described in this chapter, model development and implementation does not evolve in a linear manner. Service model development undergoes refinement and alterations over a prolonged period of time as circumstances change, practice approaches evolve based upon empirical evidence that emerges and team composition, to name a few. The lessons learned and insights gathered over this period of service development and implementation are described.

Erin Brandon, RN, NP, and Tessa Diaczun, RN, NP, both pediatric nurse practitioners, provide an overview of the NP-led clinic based upon the Patient-Focused Process for Advanced Practice Nursing (PEPPA) Framework (Bryant-Lukosius and Dicenso 2004) for children with medical complexity (CMC) needs at the Holland Bloorview Kids Rehabilitation Hospital in the chapter, *Canadian Nurse Practitioner-Led Pediatric Rehabilitation Complex Care Program*. In this chapter, the authors provide background information on Canadian NP scope of practice and the clinical environment for readers from other international settings to better understand the context of this nurse-led initiative, NP-led complex care neuromotor program.

As the authors describe the services provided for this population of children with CMC, the reader acquires an understanding of the clinical challenges that these children and their families face with lifelong care needs. The central focus of this nurse-led service model is based upon nursing plan of care in collaboration with the interprofessional team and the partnership of physicians. The challenges and facilitators that were faced with the development and implementation of this unique nurse-led care model provide insights and understanding that had to be addressed as this model of the NP-led complex care neuromotor program evolved into practice. As the authors describe, it is difficult if not entirely possible to have foreseen the unfolding of issues that arose with the implementation of this nurse-led model of care.

Theory-Driven Approaches to Care

The chapter, *The Social-Ecological Theory of Child Development: A Framework For Nurse-Led Initiatives And Models of Care*, authored by Dr. Linda Eanes, provides the reader with theoretical perspective and discussion of the core concepts of the Uric Bronfenbrenner Social-Ecological Theory (SET) (Bronfenbrenner 1977) for clinical application of comprehensive nurse-led initiatives and interventions for the health and well-being for pediatric populations from at-risk and socially, economically, and culturally disadvantaged circumstances. In this chapter, Dr. Eanes forcefully advocates for more broadly defined frameworks of care as exemplified by the Bronfenbrenner Social-Ecological Model, moving targets of care from narrowly defined focus on medically related problems to those that are embedded in person-centered and family-centered approaches. Throughout the chapter, the author provides evidence of improved outcomes associated with more expansive biopsychosocial approaches to care. Readers will observe this chapter includes an assessment tool-the Social-Ecological Needs Assessment (SENA), which reflects this comprehensive perspective. The SENA addresses assessment of housing instability, child and parental/caregiver educational attainment, child and parental/

caregiver gender, food insecurity, safety, and income. As evidenced throughout this text, models of nurse-led services are demonstrated examples of varied comprehensive approaches to the provision of care for children, adolescents, and families.

In the chapter entitled, *Interactional Model of Caring for Families of Children with Chronic Conditions*, the author team led by Lucila Castanheira Nascimento, RN, PhD, provides the reader with a thorough description of the Interactional Family Care Model (IFCM) that is used in pediatric nursing practice in Brazil. The development of the IFCM was influenced by the theories of Symbolic Interactionism (Blumer 1969), Family Vulnerability (Pettengill and Angelo 2005) and the Family Resilience Model (Walsh 2015). In particular, the *IFCM* provides a theoretical framework for the care of children with chronic health conditions with emphasis on promoting familial empowerment for families who are seen in the nurse-led Expanded Family Clinic, which is a family space established on the premises of the Integrated School Clinic (ISC) of the Integrated Health Institute of the Federal University of Mato Grosso do Sul (INISA/UFMS) in Campo Grande, Brazil. By fostering provision of nursing care based on the *IFCM* for Brazilian families whose children have a chronic condition, they are assisted to cope more effectively in dealing with the adversities they encounter along the life course of the child's chronic health condition.

This chapter provides extensive detail about the application of *IFCM* for nursing practice. The *IFCM* theoretical underpinnings of the assessment process, intervention strategies, and evaluation of outcomes are presented. This chapter provides insights for readers on care issues unique to Brazilian families and the nurse-led IFCM of care developed and implemented to address families' needs for services to care for their children with chronic conditions.

Staff Initiative

Author Dr. Vicki Freedenberg, writes in the chapter, entitled From *Patient Studies to a Hospital-Wide Initiative: A Mindfulness Journey* about the evolution of a pilot program on mindfulness that eventually evolved into a hospital-wide program for the staff of Children's National Hospital in Washington, DC. Initially Dr. Freedenberg developed a mindfulness program for a small group of adolescents with pacemakers or implanted cardiac defibrillators (ICDs) to assist them in alleviating their stress with this lived experience. This adaptive program for this adolescent group was based upon Mindfulness-Based Stress Reduction model developed by Dr. Jon Kabat-Zinn (1990) at the University of Massachusetts Medical School. Subsequently, this program was tested using a randomized control trial model with a larger group of adolescents and findings revealed that this program was effective in reducing the distress of those who participated in the intervention (Freedenberg et al. 2015; Freedenberg et al. 2017). These precursor efforts led to the development of an institutional-wide initiative, *Mindful Mentors* for the staff of Children's National Hospital. Dr Freedenberg provides the reader with the description of efforts undertaken to implement this innovative program for hospital staff (Freedenberg et al.

2020). Of particular interest, are the adaptations that were needed to adjust for the challenges encountered with the Pandemic. This nurse-led program is demonstrative of programmatic opportunities available at an institutional level focused on needs of not only nurses but the composite hospital workforce. This nurse-led model also exemplifies the developmental process of piloting a service model and its evolution for application with an entirely different target group.

Conclusion

As has been presented in this introductory chapter, a myriad of nurse-led innovations representing seven countries worldwide have been summarized that are featured in this publication. This text is unlike others published in the field of pediatric/paediatric and child health nursing given its focus on nurse-led models of care. Most often, texts in pediatric/paediatric and child health nursing focus on topics pertaining to the needs of hospitalized infants, children, and youth based upon traditional models of healthcare. This text advances nursing models of practice that are representative of the innovations in nursing practice for infants, children, and youth. These innovations in pediatric/paediatric and child health nursing will continue to emerge and will likely accelerate as independent nurse practice becomes more widespread worldwide.

References

Blumer H. Symbolic interactionism: perspective and methods. Englewood Cliffs, NJ: Prentice Hall; 1969.

Bronfenbrenner U. Toward an experimental ecology of human development. Am Psychol. 1977;32:513–31.

Bryant-Lukosius D, Dicenso A. A framework for the introduction and evaluation of advanced practice nursing roles. J Adv Nurs. 2004;48(5):530–40. https://doi.org/10.1111/j.1365-2648.2004.03235.x. PMID: 15533091.

Freedenberg VA, Thomas SA, Friedmann E. A pilot study of a mindfulness based stress reduction program in adolescents with implantable cardioverter defibrillators or pacemakers. Pediatr Cardiol. 2015;36(4):786–95.

Freedenberg VA, Hinds PS, Friedmann E. Mindfulness-based stress reduction and group support decrease stress in adolescents with cardiac diagnoses: a randomized two-group study. Pediatr Cardiol. 2017;38(7):1415–25.

Freedenberg VA, Jiang J, Cheatham CA, Sibinga EM, Powell CA, Martin GR, Steinhorn DM, Kemper KJ. Mindful mentors: is a longitudinal mind–body skills training pilot program feasible for pediatric cardiology staff? Glob Adv Health Med. 2020;9:2164956120959272.

Kabat-Zinn J. Full catastrophe living: the program of the stress reduction clinic at the. Worcester, MA: University of Massachusetts Medical Center; 1990.

Pettengill MAM, Angelo M. Family vulnerability: concept development. Revista Latino-Americana De Enfermagem. 2005;13(6):982–8. https://doi.org/10.1590/S0104-11692005000600010. Accessed 15 Dec 2021.

Walsh F. Strengthening family resilience. New York, NY: Guilford; 2015.

The Social-Ecological Theory of Child Development: A Framework for Nurse-Led Initiatives and Models of Care

Linda Eanes

Social-Ecological Theory

The social-ecological theory (SET) first advanced by Urie Bronfenbrenner (1977) postulates that a child's growth and maturity extend beyond individual genetics and biological development and is affected by dynamic overlapping interactions among complex environmental systems including the immediate family, surrounding community, socioeconomic conditions, peers, school, and political climate as well as the broad cultural values, practices, and beliefs that are upheld (Bronfenbrenner 1977; Kilanowski 2017). Thus, from a social-ecological perspective when applied to nursing, there is a cause-and-effect interrelationship between a child and the environment in which the child is a part (McLeroy et al. 1988).

While Bronfenbrenner's theory was first advanced for understanding human development, his theory has been broadly applied to nursing and other health disciplines. When used in nursing, the SET of child development is aligned with the nursing philosophy of the holistic model of care in that children are comprised of mind, body, and spirit in ever-changing environments. Thus, the SET enables nurses to provide a more holistic approach that considers the child's environmental conditions and policy context, as well as the physical, social, spiritual needs that affect both development and overall health (Salis et al. 2008). Through nurse-led health models of care and innovative initiatives that take into account the complex environmental, social, and cultural systems underlying health disparities, nurses can lead the way toward building strong partnerships and interprofessional relationships directed toward eliminating inequalities in health care for disadvantaged pediatric

L. Eanes (✉)
University of Texas Rio Grande Valley, Edinburg, TX, USA

© The Author(s), under exclusive license to Springer Nature
Switzerland AG 2023
C. L. Betz (ed.), *Worldwide Successful Pediatric Nurse-Led Models of Care*,
https://doi.org/10.1007/978-3-031-22152-1_2

populations. Across the globe, nurses can be instrumental in promoting positive changes in communities, as well as public, clinical, and acute care health systems at multiple levels to help improve the quality of life for underprivileged children.

A Need for Change

For the past two decades, there has been a shift in attention from the traditional patient-centered acute care medical model concentrated primarily on the treatment of disease or curative care to a greater emphasis on population-based health promotion and disease prevention grounded in socioecological theory of care. Factors contributing to and driving the need for this transformation in the delivery of health care include evidence published demonstrating the problems associated with the limited framework of care that include fragmented care with suboptimal outcomes, unsustainable cost, and access disparities among low-income disadvantaged groups (Andermann 2016; Salmond and Echevarria 2017; Cheng et al. 2016). According to the World Bank and World Health Organization (2017), children and young people residing in low-income or developing countries, most notably in Sub-Saharan Africa and Southern Asia, face multiple challenges and inequitable access to quality health care.

While the focus on health promotion and disease prevention has helped bridge the gaps in health care, pediatric populations from low-income circumstances remain at high risk not only for developmental delays but for both acute and chronic diseases. According to Blair and Raver (2016), children living in impoverished conditions are at a significant risk for developing stress-related emotional, physical, and cognitive health deficits. To further narrow the gaps among disadvantaged children across the globe, more consideration should be given to social and cultural circumstances in which children are conceived, born, live, learn, play, grow, and develop that affect quality-of-life outcomes and health risks (Goutevitch 2019; WHO 2018). Hence, given a child's overall health and illnesses are determined by the interaction amid and between social, cultural, and environmental factors make viewing the health needs of children through a broader perspective essential.

Although worldwide, there has been a consequential reduction in child and youth morbidity and mortality over the past 20 years, considerable sociocultural inequities that can have direct and indirect effects on their health and well-being persist (Schellenberg and Berhanu 2020). Evidence shows that whether born in the world's poorest countries or in the most highly economically developed countries, children growing up in poor families fare worse than children growing up in more affluent families. Poverty has a significant influence on child morbidity and mortality, as well as affecting the growth and development of children from conception to birth, through childhood, to adolescence and into adulthood (Hansen and Paintsil 2016; Heaton et al. 2016; Spencer et al. 2019). Globally, children born into poverty are twice as likely to die before age 5 years compared to those of middle-income or wealthier families (WHO 2020).

There are many environmental conditions that may explain why children of poverty are at greater health risks compared to more children from affluent backgrounds. Children residing in low-income communities often lack access to a wide range of services and supports that are essential for promoting health such as full-service grocery stores, affordable fresh produce, and public transportation or safe recreational areas (Denney et al. 2020). Other community-based conditions that may increase a child's vulnerability to disease are immigration status of the child and parents especially noncitizen mothers, raised in a single-family structure, born to teenage mothers with a low educational level, lack of social cohesion among family or neighbors, and degraded home conditions with more exposure to environmental pollutants (Andermann 2016; Blair and Ford 2019; Denney et al. 2020; Eanes et al. 2021; Hansen and Paintsil 2016; Linton et al. 2019; Salmond and Echevarria 2017). Children living in adverse social and economic conditions are also more likely to be exposed to violence, parental incarceration, substance abuse, and discrimination (Halfon 2017). In other words, the socioeconomic conditions in which children are conceived and born can either promote or compromise healthy child development.

According to the United Nations Inter-Agency Group for Child Mortality Estimation (UN IGME; 2020), over seven million children and young people under age 25 years have died mostly from preventable causes. Evidence indicates that neonates born to impoverished immigrant mothers with low educational status (less than a high school education) are at a significantly greater risk for premature births, low birth weights (less than 2500 g), poor neurodevelopment, adult-onset diabetes, as well as increased risk of early death even in countries with universal healthcare (Marete et al. 2020; Martinson et al. 2016; Spencer et al. 2019; Stylianou-Riga et al. 2018; UNICEF 2019). Additionally, children who are foreign born, refugees, or raised in low-income immigrant families without legal status are also more likely to experience chronic conditions such as malnutrition, stunting (below median height-for-age), and obesity. Other various conditions associated with children of low-income immigrant families include hypertension, hyperlipidemia, arthritis, diabetes, and sleep apnea (Datar and Chun 2015; Eanes et al. 2017). Moreover, in addition to physical health problems, children from low-income refugee or immigrant families can experience extreme emotional stressors, such as political violence or family separation, that places them at increased risk of posttraumatic stress disorder, substance abuse disorders, and depression, as well as premature mortality (Datar and Chun 2015; Khan et al. 2020). Children born into poor resource settings are also at a significantly increased risk of acquiring serious communicable diseases. HIV/AIDS, tuberculosis, malaria, and pneumonia, commonly referred to as diseases of poverty, disproportionately affect children from the world's poorest regions and are considered major causes of death among children under 5 years (Hansen et al. 2020; Ngocho et al. 2019; Paintsil 2016; UNICEF 2020). Diarrhea, and acute protein malnutrition among children and adolescents from low-resource countries also remain notably high as leading causes of death (Reiner et al. 2019). Thus, nurses need to recognize that it is no longer sufficient to simply address an immediate medical problem with a short-term perspective (Michel et al. 2018).

Applying Social-Ecological Theory to Care

Nurse-led models of care and initiatives amplify the framework of nursing practice as presented in the American Nurses Association, Nursing: Scope and Standards of Practice, Third Edition (2015).

> Nursing is the protection, promotion, and optimization of health and abilities, prevention of illness and injury, facilitation of healing, alleviation of suffering through the diagnosis and treatment of human response, and advocacy in the care of individuals, families, groups, communities, and populations (American Nurses Association 2015, p. 11).

Through nurse-led models of care and nurse-led initiatives based upon nursing practice frameworks of care that are child-and family-centered, address healthcare needs comprehensively and that take into account social and cultural drivers of health. These socio-cultural determinants of health include the parental socioeconomic status, educational level, health literacy, and important cultural values, beliefs, and practices that influence the health and well-being of children. Given their comprehensive and inclusive framework of care, nurses are well-positioned to serve as vanguards in the promotion of health and in the care of children who develop poverty-related infectious and chronic diseases.

Bronfenbrenner's SET can be used at all levels of nursing to help guide policy and practice that recognizes the importance of preventing illness and promoting children's health and development. Whether at the individual, community, regional, national, or international level, nurses are capable and well within their scope of practice to evaluate the socioecological needs of children and their families and to serve as their advocates. At the individual level, nurses can take a leading role in developing and initiating protocols directed toward gaining an understanding of potential social and cultural barriers to achieving optimal health, that includes screening for behavioral and emotional problems in children and mental status of their parents (Francis et al. 2018). To reduce health risks and improve health outcomes of children from underserved families, whether in a hospital, clinic, or community setting, involves moving beyond traditional, paternalistic, curative care and educational models that are narrowly focused on lifestyle modification strategies and treatment regimens to improve health outcomes (Andermann 2016). Within this traditional model, patients are viewed as passive recipients of care and, little, if any attention is given to the challenges or barriers patients may face in meeting professional recommendations. For example, although counseling patients on lifestyle modifications to promote healthy eating is important, providing education alone may be an ineffective strategy for those residing in food-insecure households where fresh produce are unavailable or unaffordable (Cahill et al. 2020; Eanes et al. 2021).

While nurses are expected to incorporate patient education into all aspects of their practice, today's nurses need to acquire informed knowledge about population-based inequities and challenges that are explicit to underserved pediatric populations under their care. When assessing patients and families to determine specific social and cultural factors influencing their health decisions, nurses need to be skilled in communicating in a nonjudgmental manner that promotes trust and caring (Thomas-Henkel and Schuman 2017). Thus, utilizing Peplau's Interpersonal

Relation model as a frame where interactions between the nurse and the patient are based on mutual trust, nurses can advance the development of culturally sensitive therapeutic relationships (Arabaci and Tas 2019). It is through active listening and treating patients with respect that a nurse can begin to understand the challenges that pediatric patients and their families face, gain pertinent information, or deliver educational information (Hagerty et al. 2017). Self-management skills and improved health outcomes can be facilitated when educational information is tailored to account for the patient's and family's relevant cultural considerations. Comprehensive assessment of patient and family learning needs includes the patient's developmental status and family's educational level, preferred language, and health literacy, as well as socioeconomic factors influencing their health decisions, behaviors, and willingness or ability to be engaged with treatment instructions (Marcus 2014).

Integrated models of nursing care within health-care systems can be utilized to assist children and their families living in poverty. Nurses are in a unique position to improve treatment engagement and reduce treatment attrition by incorporating the SET into the nursing framework of care starting with assessment of health needs that include social determinants for all children particularly children from socioeconomically disadvantaged families (Hodgkinson et al. 2017; Pinto et al. 2019). A routine nursing social and ecological needs assessment for all patients, notwithstanding basic patient and family characteristics or current medical diagnosis is expanded that takes into account social disparities, such as housing instability, educational attainment, gender, food security, safety, and income. A comprehensive nursing assessment (Box 1) that includes a focus on social determinants of care can reduce provider biases and enhance identification of additional needs of support and expedite referrals to community services (Phillips et al. 2012).

Box 1 Social-Ecological Needs Assessment
- Housing Instability
  - Trouble in paying rent
  - Excessive amount of income paid for housing
  - Moves frequently
  - Reliant on extended family/relatives
  - Crowded living arrangements
  - Eviction
  - Homelessness
  - Staying at an emergency shelter
  - Living in a car/tent
  - Living in a hotel
  - Living in transitional housing
  - Living in unsheltered locations
  - Living in Permanent Supportive Housing
- Educational Attainment
  - Parental/caregiver level of education
  - Literacy

- Health Literacy
- Children's grade level
- Regular or special education student
- Child's access to health-related and/or academic accommodations
- Gender
  - Parent/caregiver
    Male
    Female
    Transgender
    Nonbinary
    Others
  - Child
    Male
    Female
    Transgender
    Nonbinary
    Others
- Food Insecurity
  - Lack of access to sufficient amounts of food
  - Duration of food insecurity
  - Lack of funds for food
  - Enrollment in food assistance programs (i.e., Women, Infants, and Children (WIC) program)
  - Parent/caregiver employment status
  - Limited neighborhood access to grocery stores
  - Lack of transportation to access food supplies ("food deserts")
  - Living in rural area
  - Living in neighborhood with low opportunities
  - Racial/Ethnic Disparities
- Community Safety
  - At-risk community
  - Domestic violence
- Income
  - Socioeconomic status
  - Enrollment/access in social service programs (i.e., income assistance programs)
  - Parental/caregiver employment status
  - Family composition

Orlando et al. (2020), United States Department of Housing and Urban Development, Office of Community Planning and Development (2021), United States Department of Health and Human Services, Office of Disease Prevention and Health Promotion (2020).

Application to Practice, Training, and Research

The state of a child's health or illness should be understood as product of distinct individual, social, cultural, and shared communal determinants and their relationship with each other. Nurses can be influential in screening, analyzing, and implementing plans that address the social and cultural needs and challenges of pediatric populations living in poverty. Nurses can also assist patients and families by providing them with resource material in the patient's preferred language using plain language guidelines, and in facilitating effective referral systems for local support services. Moreover, nurses can serve as a liaison or contact person for those seeking assistance, such as helping to coordinate care with social workers, community-based health centers, or government supplementation services.

Through an interprofessional collaborative model of care in diverse settings, nurses can best meet the complex health needs of underserved children and their families. Given that nursing is holistic and client-centered, nurses can take the lead in creating a cultural change in the delivery of healthcare, to one that is equitable for children living in poverty. To improve the quality and access to health-care services for these children, nurses can work together with other health professionals with different backgrounds and expertise to deliver a more holistic and effective care. For example, in Sweden, nurses and physicians worked well together in making regular team-based home visits targeting children and families to assess and address special needs of children and families (Nygren et al. 2021). To foster professional collaboration, enhance understanding of others' professions, and to identify a nurse's role within a multidisciplinary team, nursing faculty can play an integral part in developing and implementing models of interprofessional education that build a culture of cooperation among students from multiple disciplines (Bridges et al. 2011). Results from a study by Singh and colleagues (2019) examining the effects of poverty immersion simulation as a method of teaching and training interprofessional students on understanding barriers to health and healthcare showed an increased mindfulness of poverty and should be considered an essential educational tool.

At the community level, nurses can play an important role in creating and advocating for societal policy changes that lead to transformations in healthcare. It is through nursing models of care that take into account the importance of establishing long-term partnerships with the public sector that infectious and chronic diseases affecting children of poverty can be reduced or eliminated (Alsan et al. 2011). Nurses can be instrumental in appraising a population's health risks and needs, as well as in the planning and implementing initiatives directed toward ameliorating acute and chronic conditions that negatively affect children residing in underserved areas (Phillips et al. 2012). For example, in Sub-Saharan African areas where the prevalence of prenatal HIV and infant mortalities is high and human and financial resources are limited, nurse-led home-based models of care have shown to aid underserved children and families overcome some barriers to accessing healthcare, help personalize care, and improve both maternal and child health (Wood et al. 2018).

Given the importance of the social determinants of health to a child's well-being, nurse-led programs directed toward improving the health outcomes of children living in low resource areas are essential. Evidence shows nurses should take a broad population health perspective that is focused on addressing not only the individual health of a child but the multilayered and interacting social, cultural, and collective health challenges within the child's environment (Eriksson et al. 2018). While a systematic review by Wood et al. (2018) was directed toward adults, the results showed that nurse-led home-based interventions could help people diagnosed with HIV/AIDS in adherence to antiretroviral therapy and improve their mental health. Nurses could also partner with other professionals in the adoption of home-based interventions directly targeting the care of children with HIV to promote positive health outcomes (Multambo et al. 2019). Additionally, data from a study by Wynn et al. (2017) showed that a community-based nurse-led model of care that included pre- and postnatal home visits to mothers residing in low resource settings in South Africa could be a cost-effective way to improve health outcomes for mothers and their children.

Nurses can take a leading role in forming strategic partnerships with key community stakeholders in providing educational health promotion programs. For example, to fill the gaps in nutrition education for children residing in underserved communities where educational resources are limited, nurses can establish partnerships between university schools of nursing and key leaders of rural underserved communities to provide health education to disadvantaged children and adolescents attending local schools (Eanes et al. 2019). In an innovative nurse-led innovative interdisciplinary model of care, nurses can also play an integral role in assessing, planning, making referrals to interagency services, monitoring, and evaluating health outcomes and needs of disadvantaged children and adolescents (Betz et al. 2015) In university settings, nurses can lead in developing interprofessional simulation learning activities as an essential education tool directed toward preparing students from multiple health disciplines in identifying key socioecological factors that impact a child's health and well-being (Singh et al. 2019).

Conclusions

Nurses can be instrumental in eliminating health disparities and in bringing hope to underprivileged children across the globe. Nurses are uniquely positioned to take the lead in transforming healthcare as it relates to understanding and addressing social determinants of health identified as having significant effects on a child's health and well-being. Through nursing models of care and innovative strategies, a culture of health can be built and, enable strong leadership and community support that narrows the gaps between healthcare and social determinants affecting the health and well-being of children across the globe (Francis et al. 2018). But first, nurses need to recognize that poverty, as a major determinant of health, has been inextricably linked to adverse conditions affecting both immediate- and long-term health and development of children (Cheng et al. 2016; Denney et al. 2020). To attend to social-ecological determinants of health, provision of nursing services needs to move beyond focusing merely on curative care at an individual level, to recognizing the intertwined relationships that exist between children and their environments. This is accomplished by addressing the specific social, cultural, political, and health system environments affecting their health-related issues, such as nutrition, physical functioning, mental health, intellectual development, and social support (Gombachika et al. 2012; Reiner et al. 2019) Recognition of both acute and chronic diseases as well as developmental conditions shown to disproportionately increase morbidity and mortality risk among children from diverse poor and vulnerable populations will provide opportunities to create nurse-led services and initiatives to address these health challenges (Braveman and Gottlieb 2014).

References

Alsan MM, Westerhaus M, Herce M, Nakashima K, Herce M. Poverty, global health, and Infectious disease: lessons from Haiti and Rwanda. Infect Dis Clin N Am. 2011;25:611–22. https://doi.org/10.1016/jidc.2011.05.004.

American Nurses Association. Nursing scope and standards of practice. 3rd ed. Silver Spring, MD: American Nurses Association; 2015.

Andermann A. Taking action on the social determinants of health in clinical practice: a framework for health professions. Can Med Assoc J. 2016;188(18):E474. https://doi.org/10.1503/cmaj.16017.

Arabaci LB, Tas G. Effect of using Peplau's interpersonal relation nursing model in the care of a juvenile delinquent, Journal of Psychiatric. Nursing. 2019;103:218–26. https://doi.org/10.14744/phd.2019.54366.

Betz CL, Smith KA, Van Speybroeckm A, Hernandez FV, Jacobs RA. Movin' on up: an innovative nurse-led interdisciplinary health care transition program. J Pediatr Health Care. 2015;30(4):323–37. https://doi.org/10.1016/j.pedhc.2015.08.005.

Blair LM, Ford JL. Neighborhood context and the risk for developmental disabilities in early childhood. Matern Child Health J. 2019;23(9):1213–9. https://doi.org/10.1007/s10995-01902757-w.

Blair C, Raver C. Poverty, stress, and brain development: new directions for prevention and intervention. Acad Pediatr. 2016;16(3 Suppl):S306. https://doi.org/10.1016/j.acap.2016.01.010.

Braveman P, Gottlieb L. The social determinants of health: it's time to consider the causes of the causes. Publ Health Rep Reposit. 2014;129(Suppl 2):19–31. https://doi.org/10.1177/00333549141291S206.

Bridges D, Davidson RA, Odegard PS, Maki IV, Tomkowiak J. Interprofessional collaboration: three best practice models of interprofessional education. Med Educ Online. 2011;16:1. https://doi.org/10.3402/meo.v1610.6035.

Bronfenbrenner U. Toward an experimental ecology of human development. Am Psychol. 1977;32:513–31.

Cheng TL, Johnson SB, Goodman E. Breaking the intergenerational cycle of disadvantage: the three generation approach. Pediatrics. 2016;137(6):e20152467.

Datar A, Chun PJ. Changes in socioeconomic, racial/ethnic, and sex disparities in childhood obesity at school entry in the United States. J Am Med Assoc Pediatr. 2015;169(7):696–7.

Denney JT, Brewer M, Kimbro RT. Food insecurity in households with young children: a test of contextual congruence. Soc Sci Med. 2020;263:113275. https://doi.org/10.1016/j.socsimed.2020.113275.

Eanes L, Fuentes LA, Bautista B, Garza DD, Salazar D. Bridging the gaps: evaluating the teaching effectiveness of graduate nursing students in helping children in underserved schools learn about healthy eating. Journal of. Nurs Sci. 2017;3(6):50–6. ISSN: 2381-1056 (Print); ISSN: 2381-1064 (Online).

Eanes L, Fuentes L, Bautista B, Garcia D. Bridging the gaps through nurse-led nutrition education to underserved children. Hispanic Health Care Int. 2019;17:1–9. https://doi.org/10.1177/1540415319830762.

Eanes L, Huerta C, Fuentes LA, Bautista B. Nurse practitioner students' perceptions on delivering culturally congruent care to vulnerable Mexican immigrants: a qualitative study. Hispanic Health Care Int. 2021;20:1–10. https://doi.org/10.1177/15404153211020417.

Eriksson M, Ghazinour M, Hammarström A. Different uses of Bronfenbrenner's ecological theory in mental health research: what is their value for guiding public mental health policy and practice? Social Theory Health. 2018;16:41–433. https://doi.org/10.1057/s41285-018-0065-6.

Francis L, DePriest K, William M, Gross D. Child poverty, toxic stress, and social determinants of health: screening and coordination. J Issue Nurs. 2018;23(3):2.

Gombachika BC, Fjeld H, Chirwa E, Sundby J, Malata A, Maluwa A. A social ecological approach to exploring barriers to accessing sexual and reproductive health services among couples living with HIV in Southern Malawi International Scholarly Research Network. ISRN Publ Health. 2012;2012:825459, 13 p.

Goutevitch MN. Determinants of health: healthy people. J Am Med Assoc Netw Open. 2019;2(4):e192200. https://doi.org/10.1001/jamanetworkopen.2019.2200.

Hagerty TA, Samuels W, Norcini-Pala A, Gigliotti E. Peplau's theory of interpersonal relations: an alternate factor structure for patient experience data? Nurs Sci. 2017;30(2):160–7. https://doi.org/10.1177/089431841769326.

Hansen C, Paintsil E. Infectious diseases of poverty in children: a tale of two worlds. Pediatr Clin N Am. 2016;63(1):37–66. https://doi.org/10.1016/j.pcl.2015.08.002.

Heaton TB, Crookston B, Pierce H, Amoateng Y. Social inequality and children's Health in Africa: a cross sectional study. Int J Equity Health. 2016;15:92. https://doi.org/10.1186/s12939-016-0372-2.

Hodgkinson S, Godoy L, Beers S. Improving mental health access for low-income Children and families in the primary care setting. Pediatrics. 2017;139(1):e2011175.

Keleb A, Sisay T, Alemu K, Ademas A, Lingerew M, et al. Pneumonia remains a leading public health problem among under-five children in preurban areas of North-Eastern Ethiopia. PLoS One. 2020;15:e0235818. https://doi.org/10.1371/ournal.pone.02.35818.

Khan F, Eskander N, Limbama T, Salman Z, Siddiqui PA, Hussaini S. Refugee and Migrant children's mental healthcare: serving the voiceless, invisible, and the vulnerable Global citizens. Cureus. 2020;12:e9944. https://doi.org/10.7759/cureus.9944.

Kilanowski JF. Breadth of the socio-ecological model. J Agromed. 2017;22(4):295–7.

Linton JM, Green A, AAP Council of Community Pediatrics. Providing care for children of immigrant families. Pediatrics. 2019;144(5):e20192077.

Marcus C. Strategies for improving the quality of verbal patient and family education: a review of the literature and creation of the EDUCATE model. Health Psychol Behav Med. 2014;2(1):482–95. https://doi.org/10.1080/2164250.2014.900450.

Ngocho JS, de Jonge MI, Minja L, Olomi GA, et al. Modifiable risk factors for community-acquired pneumonia in children under 5 years of age in resource poor settings: a case-control study. Trop Med Int Health. 2019;24(4):484–92. https://doi.org/10.1111/tmi.13211.

Nygren US, Tindberg Y, Erikson L, Erikson H, Sandberg H, Nordgren L. Team-based visits within Swedish child healthcare services: a national cross-sectional study. J Interprofess Care. 2021:1–18. https://doi.org/10.1080/13561820.2021.1902960.

Orlando MS, Vable AM, Holt K, Wingo E, Newmann S, Shapiro BJ, Borne D, Drey EA, Seidman D. Homelessness, housing instability, and abortion outcomes at an urban abortion clinic in the United States. Am J Obstet Gynecol. 2020;223(6):892.e1–892.e12. https://doi.org/10.1016/j.ajog.2020.07.002. Epub 2020 Jul 5. PMID: 32640198.

Phillips JL, Rolley JX, Davidson PM. Developing targeted health service interventions using the PRECEDE-PROCEED model: two Australian case studies. Nurs Res Pract. 2012;2012:279431. https://doi.org/10.1155/2012/279431, 8 p.

Pinto AD, Bondy M, Rucchetto A, Ihnat J, Kaufman A. Screening for poverty and intervening in primary care settings: an acceptability and feasibility study. Fam Pract. 2019;36:634–8. https://doi.org/10.1093/fampra/cmy129.

Reiner R, Obsen H, Breda CT, Echko MM, Ballestreros ET. Diseases, injuries, and risk factors in child and adolescent health, 1990 to 2017. Findings from the Global Burden of Diseases, Injuries, and Risk Factors 2017 Study. J Am Med Assoc Pediatr. 2019;173(6):e190332. https://doi.org/10.1001/jamapediatrics.2019.0337.

Salis JF, Owen N, Fisher EB. Health behavior and health education. San Francisco, CA: Jossey-Bass; 2008. p. 1–5, Chapter 20. https://www.med.upenn.edu/hbhe4/part5-ch20.shtml.

Salmond S, Echevarria M. Healthcare transformation and changing roles for nursing. Orthop Nurs. 2017;36(1):12. https://doi.org/10.1097/NOR.0000000000000308.

Schellenberg J, Berhanu D. Major gaps in child survival by ethnic group. Lancet. 2020;8(3):E308–4.

Singh S, McKenzie N, Headley S-A, Mortland K, Woolford D. A teaching innovation on poverty for interprofessional students: cost of poverty experience simulation. Health Interprofess Pract Educ. 2019;3(4) https://doi.org/10.7710/2159.1253.1473.

Spencer N, Raman S, O'Hare B, Tamburlini G. Addressing inequities in child health and development: towards social justice. BMJ Paediatr Open. 2019;3:e000503. https://doi.org/10.1136/bmjpo-2019-000503.

Stylianou-Riga P, Kuis P, Kinni P, Rigas A, Papadouri T, et al. Maternal Socioeconomic factors and the risk of premature birth and low birth weight in Cyprus: a case-control study. Reprod Health. 2018;15:157. https://doi.org/10.1186/s12978-018-0603-7.

Thomas-Henkel C, Schuman M. Screening for social determinants of health in populations with complex needs: implementation considerations. Thomas, NJ: Center for Health Care Strategies; 2017.

UNICEF. Childhood diseases. New York, NY: UNICEF; 2019. https://www.unicef.org/health/childhood-diseases.

United Nations Inter-Agency Group for Child Mortality Estimation (UN IGME). Levels & trends in child mortality: report 2020, estimates developed by the United Nations Inter-Agency Group for Child Mortality Estimation. New York, NY: United Nations Children's Fund; 2020.

United States Department of Health and Human Services, Office of Disease Prevention and Health Promotion. Healthy people 2030. Food insecurity. Washington, DC: USDHHS; 2020. https://www.healthypeople.gov/2020/topics-objectives/topic/social-determinants-health/interventions-resources/food-insecurity. Accessed 27 Mar 2022.

United States Department of Housing and Urban Development, Office of Community Planning and Development. The 2020 Annual Homeless Assessment Report (AHAR) to Congress. Washington, DC: HUD; 2021. https://www.huduser.gov/portal/sites/default/files/pdf/2020-AHAR-Part-1.pdf. Accessed 27 Mar 2022.

Wood E, Zani B, Esterhuizen TM, Young T. Nurse led home-based care or people with HIV/AIDS. Health Serv Res. 2018;18:219. https://doi.org/10.1186/s12913-018-3002-4.

World Bank, WHO. Half the world lacks access to essential health services, 100 million still push into extreme poverty because of health expenses. Washington, DC: World Bank; 2017. https://www.worldbank.org/en/news/press-release/201/1213/orld-bank-who-half-world-lacks-access-to-essential-health-services-100-million-still-pu.

World Health Organization. About social determinants of health. Geneva: WHO; 2018. https://www.who.int/social.determinants/sdh.definition/.

World Health Organization (WHO). Children; Improving survival and well-being. Geneva: WHO; 2020. https://www.who.int/news-room/fact-sheets/detail/children-reducing-mortality.

Wynn A, Rotheram-Borus MJ, Leibowitz AA, Weichle T, Roux I, Tomlinson M. Mentor mothers program improved health outcomes at a relatively low cost in South Africa. Health Aff. 2017;36(11):1947–55. https://doi.org/10.1377/hithaff.017.0553.

Baby Steps: Improving the Transition from Hospital to Home for Neonatal Patients and Caregivers Through a Nurse-Led Telehealth Program

Danielle Altares Sarik and Yui Matsuda

Introduction

In the United States (US), close to one in every ten infants receives care in the neonatal intensive care unit (NICU) within the first month of life (Mahoney et al. 2020). Research has shown that the caregivers of infants hospitalized in the NICU experience high levels of stress (Green et al. 2021; Kuo et al. 2017; Yeh et al. 2021). At the point of discharge, many infants are likely to require ongoing specialized care at home (Kuo et al. 2017). The extent of care required depends on the acuity of their medical condition; some infants are technology dependent, have a gastric-tube or other feeding concerns (e.g., challenges with bottle feeding and/or breastfeeding), require oxygen at home, or need specialized care after surgical procedures.

In the NICU setting, infants receive around-the-clock care from trained nursing and medical staff. However, upon discharge, caregivers take primary responsibility to address medical needs and provide routine infant care (e.g., changing diapers, feeding). Caregivers of NICU graduates are already likely to experience elevated levels of stress and/or postpartum depressive symptoms, which could make the transition of roles overwhelming and potentially lead to increased risk of mental health concerns in the caregivers. The medically vulnerable state of recently discharged infants also places them at increased risk for readmission and unnecessary emergency department or urgent care use (Rubinos et al. 2021).

Although the transition of care period represents a critical time during which caregivers need support, there is often a disconnect between the hospital system and

D. A. Sarik (✉)
Nicklaus Children's Hospital, Miami, FL, USA
e-mail: Danielle.Sarik@Nicklaushealth.org

Y. Matsuda
University of Miami School of Nursing and Health Studies, Miami, FL, USA
e-mail: ymatsuda@miami.edu

© The Author(s), under exclusive license to Springer Nature
Switzerland AG 2023
C. L. Betz (ed.), *Worldwide Successful Pediatric Nurse-Led Models of Care*,
https://doi.org/10.1007/978-3-031-22152-1_3

25

the community or home setting. While the gap is known and costly, programs to address these critical moments of transition from hospital to home are lacking. Therefore, the *Baby Steps* program was conceptualized and created by an interprofessional team of researchers, clinicians, and telehealth experts and was funded by the Florida Blue Foundation. In this chapter, we provide background about our hospital and the *Baby Steps* program, as well as our service structure and the roles of team members. We then describe challenges and facilitating factors for implementing the program, as well as lessons learned throughout the first 2 years of implementation. Lastly, we illustrate the future directions of our Baby Steps program.

Background Information

The *Baby Steps* program was developed to provide assistance with transition of care, from hospital to home, for infants who received NICU services at Nicklaus Children's Hospital (Nicklaus), located in South Florida, United States. The NICU at Nicklaus has been designated as a Level 4 facility. Nicklaus is not a birth facility, which means that no babies are delivered in this setting; therefore, infants may be transferred from other hospitals in the region, the state, the nation, or even from international locations to receive care. The majority of international patients are transferred from locations in the Caribbean and South and Central America.

Additionally, due to the high level of care that is provided in this NICU, most infants who are admitted require some form of surgical intervention. The most common diagnoses seen and cared for in the NICU include congenital cardiac conditions, genetic anomalies, diaphragmatic hernia, respiratory distress, and other complex and often chronic health conditions. The high-acuity patient population at Nicklaus makes the care and discharge teaching needs for our patients unique.

Due to the hospital's location in South Florida, the hospital serves a predominantly Spanish-speaking population (~70% identify Spanish as the primary home language). Additionally, a majority of patients use public health insurance to access medical services (~75% Medicaid/public health insurance). Nicklaus also provides care to a large population of immigrant communities, including itinerant farm workers and seasonal hospitality workers. This cultural and language milieu adds to the complexity of our discharge teaching needs, as well as the importance of providing culturally appropriate and language-concordant care during the discharge process.

The *Baby Steps* study takes place within the Nicklaus NICU, which as previously mentioned is designated as a Level 4 facility. This rating indicates that this highly specialized and equipped unit is able to support/perform open heart surgery procedures, provide extracorporeal membrane oxygenation (ECMO), and care for micropreemies (fewer than 28 oz). Nicklaus is also the only stand-alone pediatric hospital in South Florida and is a Level 1 Trauma institution, which is the highest certification available. Additionally, the nursing care team at Nicklaus has received consistent recognition for the high-quality care provided to patients. One indicator of this care is the American Nurses Credentialing Center (ANCC) Magnet designation, a national certification awarded to institutions with a clear and exemplary dedication to patient safety, high-quality outcomes, and nurses' scope of practice (ANCC and ANA n.d.). Nicklaus is a four-time Magnet-designated facility, and is currently in the process of applying for its fifth certification. Additionally, Nicklaus is a Certified Safe Sleep Hospital, a recognition given to hospitals that promote infant safe sleep and prevent sudden infant death syndrome (Cribs for Kids n.d.). Given that Nicklaus is not a birth facility, patients and caregivers may need to travel a great distance to access care, and caregivers may be unable to remain physically present in the NICU during hospitalization. This geographic challenge adds another layer of complexity to the transition of care from hospital to home.

Why Develop *Baby Steps*?

The impetus for the development of the *Baby Steps* program stemmed from the identified need to provide additional support to families during the challenging transition period, from hospital to the home and community setting (Green et al. 2021). While this need is borne out in published literature, we also saw these needs and gaps in care first-hand. NICU admissions have been identified as emotionally and mentally difficult for caregivers, who experience high rates of anxiety and depression during NICU admissions (Alkozei et al. 2014). Compounding these mental and emotional health burdens, caregivers and families also have a difficult time in accessing needed pediatric or specialty services after discharge.

Due to the gap between in-patient care and access to specialist or pediatric support in the immediate postdischarge period, increased rates of emergency department (ED) and urgent care center (UCC) use were noted (Rubinos et al. 2021). Often, these visits addressed common health concerns or questions related to the NICU course of care. In many cases, these needs could be better met by a nurse or clinician who was involved in the NICU care trajectory.

Process to Develop the *Baby Steps* Service

In order to build *Baby Steps*, we first sought funding to support the needed services. Our team was awarded a Quality and Safety of Patient Care Grant from the Florida Blue Foundation, which fully funded the development and operation of the program for 3 years. This funding was key to the sustainability and feasibility of program development, and without it, the *Baby Steps* intervention would not have been possible. Such need for external funding is unfortunately common for many such programs and is a limiting factor when exploring new methods and models of care. In addition, this program represents a clinical-academic partnership between Nicklaus and the University of Miami School of Nursing and Health Studies (UM SONHS). The team leaders from each institution brought unique expertise needed for the *Baby Steps* program.

One of the first goals of the *Baby Steps* leadership was to develop an interprofessional team capable of providing the needed transition of care services. We recruited a telehealth lead and specialists, a NICU nurse lead and clinical specialist group, and academic and clinical nursing research experts. As the intervention was centered around the use of a telehealth framework, the expertise of our Nicklaus telehealth team was critical. Additionally, as this intervention began in the NICU setting and was embedded into the discharge process, the NICU nursing team included various nurse experts including registered nurses (RNs), advanced practice registered nurses (APRNs), Clinical Nurse Specialists, Managers, Directors, and a certified lactation consultant.

The lead NICU nurse for the *Baby Steps* program facilitated the day-to-day work of recruiting, enrolling, scheduling, and providing telehealth interventions, while also working to connect families to appropriate follow-up resources and to a higher level of care as needed. The nurse's role began in the NICU with daily rounding and patient monitoring to identify those infants and caregivers who would benefit from the *Baby Steps* program. Additionally, the nurse attended rounds with a team of physicians twice a week. After patients were identified as eligible (discharge to the home/community setting, residence within the state of Florida), the nurse would approach the bedside, explain the *Baby Steps* program, and assist the caregivers with enrollment. After the caregivers downloaded the platform onto their smart device, the nurse would teach them how to access the services and then facilitate a mock telehealth call in order to help the caregivers acclimate to the telehealth interface and feel comfortable using the services. Prior to discharge, the nurse would schedule a telehealth encounter for 24–48 h after the infant had been discharged to home. Additionally, the telehealth service was available at scheduled hours from Monday to Friday for on-demand patient questions.

Theoretical Framework: Theory of Transition (Meleis)

The *Baby Steps* program and intervention development was guided by Meleis's Theory of Transition. The Theory of Transition postulates that changes in health and illness of individuals create a process of transition, and that while in a state of transition, an individual may experience increased vulnerability and have unique needs (Meleis et al. 2000; Schumacher and Meleis 1994). At the time of discharge, caregivers may be experiencing multiple aspects of transition simultaneously, with situational (NICU to home or community setting), developmental (parenthood), and health-illness transitions (clinically complex infant) being among the most commonly experienced (Orr et al. 2020). Nurses are central in preparing individuals for health-related transitions, such as discharge from the NICU to the home setting in the *Baby Steps* study.

For our work, we conceptualized the discharge of an infant from the NICU setting to the home and community setting as a process of transition. In research examining the transition to motherhood for caregivers of infants with congenital health conditions, researchers describe the need for caregiver orientation in order to assist with transition and provision of optimal care (Korukcu et al. 2017). When Hua et al. studied inhibitors and facilitators of preterm infant discharge using Meleis's model, they identified several key themes that aligned with Meleis's Theory of Transition. Importantly, the knowledge and skills of caring for the infant were identified by both caregivers and health-care providers as a core need. Additionally, a common perspective among participants was that access to a provider was an important community condition to facilitate the discharge transition (Hua et al. 2021). Barimani et al. (2017) also explored factors that facilitated transition to parenthood using Meleis's model and found that, among the common themes noted, professional support and resources from the health-care team were needed (Barimani et al. 2017).

Taking into account the particular population of caregivers and infants the Nicklaus NICU serves, the *Baby Steps* program was built to support their unique situational, developmental, and health-illness needs. Elements of the transition of care model helped to guide program development, and provided a theoretical underpinning to the clinical care provided.

Description of Nurse-Led *Baby Steps* Model

In this section, elements of the nurse-led *Baby Steps* model are described. It begins with a description of the *Baby Steps* organizational components, followed by a description of the services provided, the roles, the responsibilities, and the position requirements of *Baby Steps* team members. Presentation of the *Baby Steps* model concludes with the methods of evaluation (Figs. 1, 2 and 3).

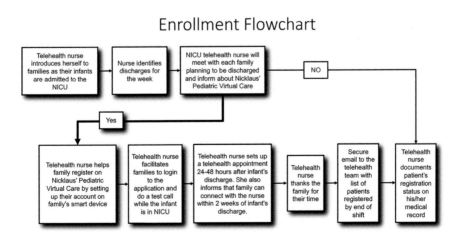

Enrollment Flowchart

Fig. 1 Flow chart of *Baby Steps* program

Figs. 2 and 3 Pictures of
Baby Steps in process.
(©Photographer name:
Photo acknowledgement:
Edgar Estrada, Nicklaus
Children's Hospital)

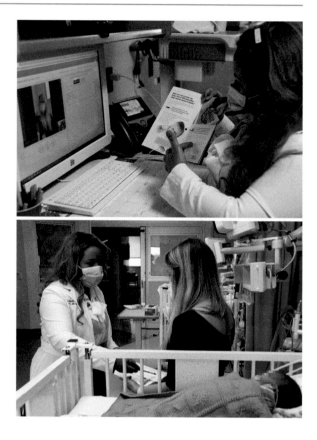

Organizational Components of *Baby Steps* Involve Several Interprofessional Teams

The main teams responsible for the build, operation, and evaluation of the *Baby Steps* program include the NICU team, the telehealth team, and the research team.

The NICU team is composed of a nurse lead, who is NICU-trained, as well a cadre of NICU RNs ($n = 8$) who have also been oriented to the program and received telehealth training and certification. This team of RNs is available to provide back-up services in case of illness or schedule conflict. Additionally, a team of NICU nurse leaders has been integrally involved in the development, implementation, and maintenance of the program, including a Clinical Nurse Specialist, NICU Nurse Manager, and NICU Nurse Director. These key stakeholders provide the needed clinical expertise to ensure the success of the program.

The telehealth team, comprised of the Director, Senior Telehealth Operations Specialist, and grants manager, is responsible for the training, education, certification, and day-to-day provision of telehealth services. These responsibilities include ensuring that patients are enrolled in the telehealth platform, calls/telehealth encounters are connected and working correctly, technological concerns are addressed, and the policies and procedures governing the use of telehealth are observed.

Additionally, at the end of each telehealth encounter, a brief survey is administered to caregivers to assess their experience, willingness to act on recommendations, and likelihood to use the service again or recommend it to their peers. This survey is maintained, and the results are tabulated, tracked, and presented by the telehealth team.

The last major team responsible for the development, implementation, and management of the *Baby Steps* program is the Research Team. This team, comprised of the Principal Investigator (Altares Sarik, Nicklaus) and Co-Principal Investigator (Matsuda, UM SONHS), represents a unique academic-clinical partnership. The research team collaborated on the writing of the original grant application that was submitted to the Florida Blue Foundation. The research team has also worked together to seek additional methods of funding and support for the program. Another major responsibility of this group is to provide leadership for the *Baby Steps* program. This is accomplished through regular group meetings (biweekly), transparent goals and project objectives, tracking and trending of data related to the program, and communication with the funder. This communication includes filing monthly progress reports, as well as more in-depth biannual reports on the project goals. The research team also leads the submission of manuscripts, poster and podium presentations, and internal and external communication of the grant including Podcasts, blogs, and institutional magazine articles.

Description of the Services Provided

The *Baby Steps* program is available to all infants and their adult caregivers who (1) receive care in the Nicklaus NICU; (2) are discharged to a home setting in the community; and (3) reside within the state of Florida. Prior to discharge, a trained *Baby Steps* nurse approaches a caregiver at the bedside to assess interest in program participation. If the caregiver expresses interest in receiving *Baby Steps* services and consents to participation, they are then led through the enrollment process. In order to access telehealth services, Nicklaus provides the Pediatric Virtual Care Telehealth Application free of charge to patients. To access this platform, a caregiver must first download the application to an internet-connected smart device, create an account, and be formally registered through Nicklaus. Once this process is completed, the lead *Baby Steps* nurse will engage the caregiver in a mock telehealth call to ensure familiarity with the application interface prior to discharge. While the majority of program enrollment occurs in the NICU setting, there are times when a discharge may occur before the nurse has had a chance to approach the caregivers directly. In these instances, the nurse will connect with caregivers via telephone after discharge and guide them through enrollment and registration remotely.

As an infant is nearing the time of discharge, the lead nurse will work with the caregivers to schedule a follow-up telehealth encounter, usually within 24–48 h after discharge from the NICU. This allows enough time for the family time to return to the community or home setting, and have a preliminary follow-up appointment with their pediatrician or a specialist, depending on patient needs. After the first postdischarge telehealth encounter, additional appointments can be made as needed to support the caregiver. On-demand calls to the NICU nurse can also be made for urgent issues that arise.

During the telehealth encounters, the NICU nurse has the ability to see the infant and the caregiver, and to visually assess the home environment. If the infant has been discharged with any technology needs, such as supplemental oxygen, feeding tubes, or other devices, the telehealth platform also facilitates visual inspection of these systems. If a caregiver expresses a concern, the NICU nurse is prepared to answer questions within her scope of practice, or to refer to a higher level of care if needed. For all patients, anticipatory guidance is reviewed in order to support evidence-based safety and health recommendations. Some of the standard information reviewed during these encounters includes feeding recommendations, human milk and lactation support, safe sleeping environments and reduction of risks associated with sudden infant death syndrome, and household safety (e.g., no smoking around baby, open flames around oxygen, pets in home). Additionally, if a caregiver is having difficulty connecting with a specialist or care provider, the NICU nurse will also assist with these efforts.

The telehealth encounters and nurse-led counseling all occur while the infant is in the home and community setting. At this time, the *Baby Steps* program is only available to infants who are discharged to a home setting, under the care of a designated adult caregiver who resides in the state of Florida. Due to restrictions associated with providing telehealth services across state lines, infants discharged to other states or who return to countries outside of the United States are not currently eligible for these services.

Role/Responsibilities of Team Members/Position Requirements of Those Involved with the Nurse-Led Model

Within our NICU specialist team, we have several key players: a lead NICU nurse, Clinical Nurse Specialist, Manager, and Director. The lead NICU nurse is a seasoned nursing professional, who has additional training in research and telehealth. From the moment the infant and caregiver are approached for enrollment into the *Baby Steps* program, the lead nurse is a part of the care process. Due to the multicultural nature of our facility, it is very important that the lead nurse is fluent in both English and Spanish and is comfortable interacting with caregivers and families from diverse backgrounds. The lead nurse enrolls the patient and caregiver in the *Baby Steps* program, ensures that the caregiver is comfortable with the Pediatric Virtual Care Telehealth Application, and schedules the follow-up telehealth encounter after discharge. The lead nurse facilitates the telehealth encounter, which includes providing care coordination, anticipatory guidance, assessment and teaching within the scope of nursing practice, and referral to a higher level of care as needed. It is important that this individual is a competent and confident nursing professional, is able to establish good rapport with families, and is self-directed in their work. In addition to the clinical responsibilities of this position, the lead NICU nurse also keeps detailed records of all encounters and helps with data management and review.

The NICU clinical nurse specialist is also a key team member who supports the lead nurse and the *Baby Steps* program. The clinical nurse specialist provides a unit-level understanding of the facilitators and barriers to care and is also able to provide expert clinical advice. This individual is a key member in creating program awareness, support for the initiative, and buy-in from stakeholders.

The NICU Manager and Director also participate in biweekly *Baby Steps* calls as needed and are instrumental in the success of the program through their support. The Manager works with the lead NICU nurse to ensure coverage for the role, working with the additional eight trained NICU nurses to cover for personal time off as needed. The Director provides oversight and executive approval for the program.

Nicklaus is fortunate to have a robust telehealth department. For the *Baby Steps* program, the Senior Telehealth Operations Specialist has been an indispensable team member since the conception of the program. In this role, the Operations Specialist creates a patient account within the telehealth application after registration and ensures that any technical difficulty is resolved. Additionally, this specialist is responsible for training all of our team members in telehealth and helping them to navigate the certification process. As part of the *Baby Steps* program, a survey is administered at the end of each telehealth encounter, and the Operations Specialist tracks and trends this data. The Director of the telehealth department is also highly involved in the program, participating in our biweekly meetings, academic presentations, and grant applications.

Uniquely, the grant and research coordination for the program is provided through an academic-clinical partnership between Nicklaus and UM SONHS. The Principal Investigator (Altares Sarik) is a pediatric nurse scientist responsible for directing nursing research and evidence-based practice (EBP) activities at Nicklaus. Her research training is in health services research and outcomes research, and her clinical training and practice is in pediatric primary care. Through her academic and research experience, she has gained project development and coordination skills. Her personal research interests are focused on improving the care provided to patients and caregivers, especially during the transition of care process.

The Co-Principal Investigator (Matsuda) is a nurse scientist specializing in public health nursing, whose research is focused on family-centered approaches to care. She is a faculty member at a research-intensive academic institution (UM SONHS). Specifically, she contributes to the *Baby Steps* program through her research expertise in addressing the needs of parents and caregivers who have children with chronic illnesses or special healthcare needs. Matsuda leads grant work aimed at preparing the future nursing workforce by exposing nursing students to telehealth nursing. To achieve this aim, Matsuda created the *Baby Steps Simulation*, a complementary program, which she continues to implement (please refer to Matsuda et al. 2022 for details). Through her research work, she has expertise in project development, management, and coordination.

Methods of Evaluation

While the *Baby Steps* program is clinical in nature, one of the major considerations in the development of the program was creating robust tracking mechanisms to ensure that outcomes of the work could be evaluated. The metrics identified and reviewed include demographic measures (sex, race/ethnicity, socioeconomic status, geographical distribution), total number of infants and families served, number of encounters (total, as well as telehealth versus telephone), 30-day readmission rates, emergency care use (ED and UCC), and caregiver experience measures (as collected by survey).

In the first 24 months of the program (April 2020 to April 2022), a total of 450 infants were enrolled in the *Baby Steps* program. Of these infants, 63% lived in Miami-Dade County, and the rest lived in other Florida counties. The majority of the infants enrolled were male (54%) and Hispanic (52%). While socioeconomic status is difficult to measure, 60% of our population uses public health insurance (Medicaid) to access medical care. We are in the process of exploring this data using geospatial coding to gain a more nuanced understanding of the environments in which our infants and families live.

During the first 24 months of the program 492 total visits were conducted (265 through the platform, 227 by phone), with the majority (59%) occurring via the Pediatric Virtual Care Telehealth Platform. Due to concerns about whether all caregivers would have access to a smart device, tablets were obtained through the grant to be used as needed. However, during the time reported, every caregiver and family in the program had access to their own smart device and internet or cellular service.

Of primary interest to the *Baby Steps* team was the impact of the service on the outcomes of emergency care use and 30-day readmission, as these outcomes are costly and emotionally burdensome to patients and caregivers (King et al. 2021). Of infants enrolled in the program 1.11% experienced a readmission within 30 days ($n = 5$). Compared to the baseline level of readmission for the group, this represents a 56% decrease. Additionally, during a time when we strived to keep infants out of the ED and UCCs due to the COVID-19 pandemic, we were happy to see that our rates of emergency care use sharply declined in the infants enrolled in the *Baby Steps* program. Within 30 days of discharge 14% of patients enrolled in the program sought care at an emergency care setting ($n = 63$), compared to 23% in patients not enrolled in the program during the same time frame.

In order to measure the experience of caregivers, a survey was presented electronically at the end of each telehealth encounter. The survey assessed perception of the program, likelihood to use again, likelihood to act on recommendations, and parental self-efficacy (selected questions from Barnes and Adamson-Macedo 2007). We found that 99.2% of caregivers would either highly recommend or recommend the *Baby Steps* service ($n = 141$), indicating high satisfaction with the service.

Challenges and Facilitators

Challenges

We faced several challenges as we started the *Baby Steps* program. The first challenge we addressed related to our team and the history behind the effort to provide transition of care services to caregivers and patients upon NICU discharge. While there have been several attempts to provide telehealth services to infants discharged from the NICU in the past, there was a lack of support and resources to make these attempts successful. In order to be sensitive to this shared history, the team was encouraged to have open dialogue about challenges encountered in the past, any unresolved concerns, and how best to move forward to ensure program success. These transparent discussions helped to unite the team and highlight the importance of each member.

As with any intervention that incorporates technology, there were some technological challenges encountered at the program onset, as well as a learning curve for all team members. Technical issues that interrupted telehealth encounters often required immediate intervention and were escalated to the telehealth team for their expertise.

An early challenge for the team also centered around the best way to communicate and work together. In order to facilitate coordination of the program, a biweekly meeting was established to check in on grant progress, identify concerns, and share wins. These meetings allowed the team to troubleshoot together, have a clear view of what each member was working on, and offer their unique experience and contributions. In these meetings, the team discussed the importance of the telehealth nurses regularly incorporating anticipatory guidance for the infants and their families. As an outcome of this discussion, the lead nurse spent more time addressing these topics with families during encounters. These examples illustrate that team communication has been critical in continuing to provide high-quality telehealth services.

An additional challenge was noted in regards to data collection and management. The nurse researchers considered the nature and context of the project to determine the amount of data to be collected: (1) The *Baby Steps* program focuses on providing services to infants and their families in the community setting (service-oriented versus research-oriented); and (2) caregivers are already burdened with caring for fragile infants. As a result, nurse researchers, with the help of the lead telehealth nurse, selected only five questions from the 20-item parenting self-efficacy scale to be added to the post-telehealth visit survey. Thus, the nurse researchers decided to seek quality improvement project approval given the scope of the work, instead of an institutional review board approval, which would be required for a research study.

Ensuring adequate professional staffing is another challenge we have faced with the *Baby Steps* program. We are thankful to have a lead telehealth nurse with NICU expertise direct the clinical encounters on a part-time basis (0.5 FTE). However, gaps in care due to the COVID-19 pandemic and associated time out of office for illness and exposure occur at times. One way that we have addressed these concerns is by training a cohort of additional NICU nurses who are able to step in to provide coverage as needed. With this approach, we have been able to offer telehealth coverage continuously since the start of the program, despite gaps in the availability of the lead NICU nurse.

Even though pediatric patients have not been as heavily affected by COVID-19 as adults, children's hospitals, like other hospitals, have experienced staff burnout, clinician strain, and interruptions to normal operations. These systemic issues contributed to challenges with program implementation. Our funding period started in November 2019, and we planned to launch the telehealth program in April 2020. Despite the World Health Organization declaring the COVID-19 pandemic on March 11, 2020, the team was able to launch the program as planned. However, due to changes in visitation policies, infection prevention practices, and general changes to hospital operations during the pandemic, we did need to adjust our program and approach.

Facilitators

While many challenges exist, several facilitators have made the program successful. One of our strengths is having a team of dedicated telehealth experts as active members of our project team. These telehealth experts maintain the telehealth infrastructure and telehealth-related data collection (e.g., post-visit survey). Their contributions have been critical in operating the program smoothly. The telehealth unit has been actively operating since before the pandemic; therefore, Nicklaus already had in place the necessary capacity and resources to manage and support telehealth care as the pandemic accelerated.

Additionally, we are thankful to have as cornerstones of the *Baby Steps* program a dedicated telehealth nurse with NICU expertise and expert nurse clinicians. These nurses are "insiders" to the NICU team given their experience in the NICU prior to their work on *Baby Steps*. Their familiarity with the unit, hospital, and community has been indispensable to our program's success. The lead telehealth nurse transitioned seamlessly into her new role as she was previously incorporated into the daily routines in the NICU and would introduce herself to caregivers as the infants were admitted to the unit. As a result, the lead telehealth nurse was able to establish rapport with the caregivers and build trust as a team member representing the program.

The COVID-19 pandemic served as an unexpected facilitator. Developed prior to the pandemic, the *Baby Steps* program was designed to be a telehealth intervention because it was determined to be the best way to connect with families of infants at home. With the COVID-19 pandemic, telehealth became more widely used and accepted, which we believe worked in our favor to increase participation in the *Baby Steps* program.

Financial Challenges and Opportunities

The *Baby Steps* program has been generously funded through the Florida Blue Foundation's Quality and Safety of Patient Care Grant Program ($300,000 for 3 years). This funding supports the majority of the program costs; however, some support comes from the personnel's in-kind contributions (e.g., part of the nurse researchers' time, NICU leadership team participation). The service cost is fully covered by the grant at this time; however, we are investigating additional methods for reimbursement or additional grant funding for further sustainability of the program.

During the pandemic, temporary changes in policies allowing the reimbursement of telehealth services have helped to facilitate expansion of these services (Curfman et al. 2021). It is fortunate that such policy changes have allowed the reimbursement of telehealth services provided not only by APRNs, but also by RNs (Sensmeier 2020). However, reimbursement policies differ by state, and federal policy concerning telehealth may change abruptly. Thus, incorporating the reimbursement of telehealth services as a viable mechanism to sustain the program will be explored.

Service Adjustments Made

The *Baby Steps* team has continuously adjusted program services in order to best support caregivers' needs. For example, the lead telehealth nurse's work environment emerged as a challenge at the start of the program. She had a desk in a room at the NICU that was shared with residents and other team members. To reduce noise and ensure privacy, the telehealth team set up a telehealth suite for use by the *Baby Steps* nurse. This provided a quiet environment to provide telehealth services as needed.

Moreover, at the beginning of the program, the NICU nurse was physically present in the hospital for enrollment and to provide telehealth services. However, we have since flexed to allow the lead NICU nurse to conduct telehealth visits from home as needed. This flexibility was important, and the team supported the ability to work from home. This change has allowed the telehealth nurse to tend to the families' requests in a more flexible manner.

In addition, there are times when families prefer to talk by telephone due to convenience and caregiver preference or owing to difficulty using the telehealth application. Difficulty using the telehealth application may be partly because of poor Internet services. In any of these instances, at the discretion of the lead NICU nurse, phone calls can be substituted for the telehealth encounter. This flexibility in the program has allowed the *Baby Steps* telehealth nurses to reach more families, potentially those who need the service most. Literature has demonstrated the importance of allowing both telephone calls and telehealth visits as ways to communicate with patients and caregivers, as lack of access to the Internet and data services may be barriers to utilizing telehealth services, particularly among those who are economically disadvantaged (Saeed and Masters 2021).

Lessons Learned

We learned many lessons during the development, planning, and implementation of the *Baby Steps* program. Of primary importance was the need to secure early stakeholder buy-in and transparency across the project group. Additionally, learning how to work with an interprofessional team with different communication style preferences helped set the program up for success. Finally, creating a forum in which clinical team members could voice concerns and challenges allowed our team to be flexible and to address barriers before they caused major delays or led to workarounds.

When the grant was first submitted, only a few of the team members were able to work on the application. While all teams (NICU, telehealth, and research) were represented, there were early leadership changes that led to some misunderstandings. As this gap in care from NICU to home had been evident for some time, previous teams had tried to launch a telehealth follow-up program for NICU patients in the past. However, as there was no dedicated leadership or individual clinician time to support this work, it was unsuccessful. This history was not clearly understood at the time that the grant was awarded, and as such it represented a potential barrier to team cohesion and function.

From this experience, we learned the importance of cultivating stakeholder buy-in early, as well as fully vetting the history and context of any large programmatic change. Due to the superb leadership of our NICU and telehealth teams, as well as their flexibility and willingness to give this effort another try, we were able to build the program in such a way that addressed past concerns and ensured future success.

In order to demonstrate the value of each team member's contribution and role, biweekly meetings are held to share information and address concerns as a group. In these calls, each team presents on their progress, identifies any barriers that have arisen, and shares thoughts and ideas with the group. The biweekly meetings allow for quick escalation of challenges to the team member who is best situated to resolve the concern, and feedback is given in a timely manner. We use a video platform for our calls, which has also given us an opportunity to learn more about each other and to develop trust in each other as colleagues despite not being present in the same physical location.

Baby Steps was funded for 3 years, and more funding will be needed to continue this service. Programs such as *Baby Steps* have the ability to greatly improve the transition of care from the hospital to home for neonates/infants and caregivers, but only if investments are made to create and sustain these efforts. It seems prudent to begin to look for more funding once an initial funding announcement is received to ensure smooth transition of funding sources.

Finally, the importance of having the right individual as a lead nurse cannot be overstated. The program has benefited greatly from having highly skilled, experienced, and caring nursing leads. Due to their work in the NICU, as well as their personal experiences, they are skilled at connecting with caregivers and providing needed support. Without these dedicated nurses, the work of *Baby Steps* would not be possible.

Future Implications for Clinical Practice and Research

The *Baby Steps* program has grown and evolved since its conception, but the central goal of the program remains the same: to provide expert nurse guidance and transition support to infants and their caregivers after discharge from the NICU. While the program has experienced broad support and exceptional uptake among this patient population, additional aspects could be incorporated into the program that would strengthen the model, help ensure its sustainability, and facilitate expansion of the service model to other organizations.

A 3-year investment by the Florida Blue Foundation made the *Baby Steps* program possible. As we begin to plan for the future, we will need additional foundation or institution funding to continue the program in its current form. The need for a sustained funding source, or a mechanism to pay for provision of these services, is currently one of the major foci of our work. As a research team, we have applied for several additional funding opportunities, and have successfully competed for two: a grant from the UM Citizens Board and a foundation grant from the Nicklaus Children's Young Ambassador organization. These investments will allow us to expand aspects of the program not directly related to clinical care, such as a study of *Baby Steps Simulation* to educate nursing students in conducting telehealth visits and qualitative exploration of the experience of caregivers who have used the *Baby Steps* service.

While we began the *Baby Steps* work in the neonatal/infant population, one possible future direction for research is to expand the program into the medical/surgical or step-down units for high-risk children and their families. For the population of children with developmental or chronic illness challenges, there may be value in having a supported transition of care program from hospital to home. Additionally, while the program is currently available during the week, it is part-time and staffed by a 0.5 FTE nurse. In order to provide more support for a larger number of infants and caregivers, expanding to a full-time role, or a team of transition specialists, would be key.

This pilot program focused on the needs of caregivers of infants discharged from the NICU but only extended as far as clinical care of the infant. During the course of our work, we have seen a need to identify and address the mental health needs of caregivers as well. A robust body of research has shown the intricate link between caregiver mental health and that of children (Matsuda et al. 2021a, b). As such, a natural extension of the transition of care work would be to provide screening for mental health concerns, and referrals and advice as appropriate. While most new mothers in the United States will receive a postpartum exam and screen for mental health concerns at the 6-week mark postdelivery, this may not be adequate for persons who have given birth to an infant requiring NICU care. Depending on diagnosis and clinical progress, many infants may still be in the NICU setting at 6 weeks, and these caregivers may experience unique stressors that could potentially contribute to mental health concerns after the discharge of their infant.

Yet another implication for clinical practice gleaned from this work is the importance of enculturation of a discharge service and a plan for real-time connection with families during the process of transition. Currently, in many organizations, there is no standardized transition of care follow-up; instead, this important piece of the care journey is often decided on a patient-to-patient or unit-to-unit basis. Using data from this program, we plan to advocate for standardized follow-up care and nurse-led telehealth services as a standard intervention for improving outcomes.

Conclusion

During its first 24 months, the *Baby Steps* program has demonstrated great success and feasibility. *Baby Steps* has garnered high satisfaction from caregivers, significant improvement on key patient outcome metrics (30-day readmission, emergency care utilization), and high levels of enrollment (81%). Additionally, this program has helped to create evidence for the capability of a nurse-led telehealth program to facilitate transition for the neonatal/infant population. As a result, we hope our findings will translate into opportunities to scale up and/or replicate our model. We plan to continue growing and expanding the program, and will seek additional funding in order to realize the continued success of *Baby Steps*.

Useful Resources

- Pediatric Virtual Connect Pamphlet

Appendix: *Baby Steps* Program Brochure

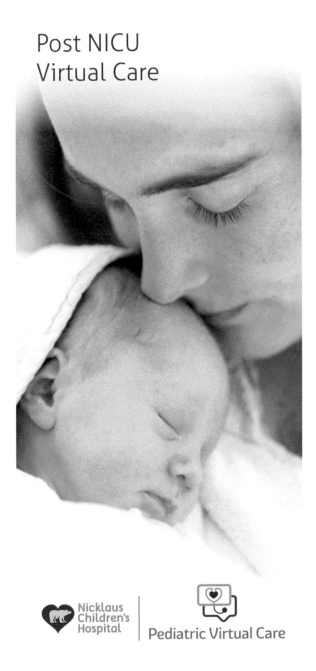

Connect with a Nicklaus Children's Expert from the Comfort of Home with Post NICU Virtual Care

Going home with an infant who has just spent weeks or even months in a neonatal intensive care unit (NICU) can be a daunting task for even the most experienced parent.

You may have questions about feeding, changing, bathing or how to use unfamiliar medical equipment and devices in the home, which can be overwhelming.

Now help is at hand with Baby Steps, post-NICU virtual care, a telehealth service from Nicklaus Children's Hospital that provides you direct access to your specialist healthcare team from the comfort of your own home.

Using a desktop computer, mobile phone or tablet with internet access, you can videoconference with one of our experienced NICU team members. They can provide guidance, advice and support for everything from basic newborn care to support of babies with tracheostomies, gastrostomies, central lines and other specialized medical equipment.

Download the Nicklaus Children's Virtual Care app and create your account, call in to the telehealth service during hours of operation to connect with a NICU team member and get instant peace of mind.

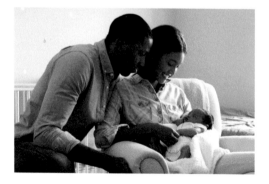

Expert Reassurance When You Need It

- Get expert pediatric guidance and advice for your baby
- No cost to families post discharge
- Accessible via computer, tablet or mobile app. Download the Nicklaus Children's Pediatric Virtual Care application on the Apple Store or Google Play Store.

Our experienced NICU team members can provide essential guidance and support for a range of infant care issues, including:

- Basic newborn care (bathing, skin care, umbilical stump care)
- Administering medication
- Back to sleep (newborn safety and SIDS prevention)
- Home ventilator/ aerosol/ suction equipment

- Pulse oximetry
- Oxygen therapy
- Central line care
- Gastrostomy care
- Tracheostomy care
- Ostomy care
- Wound care
- Pavlik harness

How to Connect

Nicklaus Children's Pediatric Virtual Care uses your video camera to connect. To set up a video-conference consultation with a NICU team member by phone/tablet:

Download the Nicklaus Children's Pediatric Virtual Care App from from the Apple Store or Google Play Store.

Or

Visit **app. nicklauschildrensvirtualcare.org** using Google Chrome from a computer or laptop with webcam.

Once registered, you can schedule a consult at your convenience.

Your Username

Your password

For more information, please contact the telehealth team by calling **305-662-8353** or **1-800-811-9350** (toll free) or email *Telehealth.office@nicklaushealth.org*

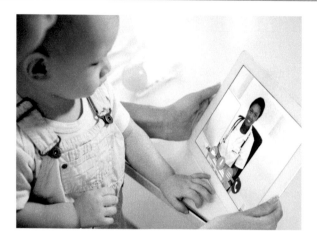

About Nicklaus Children's Pediatric Virtual Care

Nicklaus Children's Pediatric Virtual Care is the telehealth service of Nicklaus Children's Health System, parent organization of Nicklaus Children's Hospital, South Florida's only licensed specialty hospital exclusively for children. With more than 800 attending physicians and more than 475 pediatric specialists, the 309-bed nonprofit hospital - known as Miami Children's Hospital from 1983 through 2014 - is renowned for excellence in all aspects of pediatric medicine and routinely has many programs ranked among the nation's best by *U.S. News & World Report.*

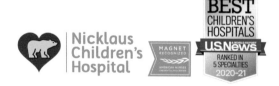

3100 SW 62 Avenue, Miami, FL 33155
305-666-6511
nicklauschildrens.org

11656MAMC-RDP072020

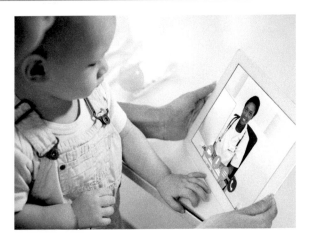

Horario

De lunes a viernes, de 9 a.m. a 1 p.m.

Acerca de Nicklaus Children's Pediatric Virtual Care

Nicklaus Children's Pediatric Virtual Care es el servicio de telesalud de Nicklaus Children's Health System, organización matriz de Nicklaus Children's Hospital, único hospital autorizado y especializado en el sur de la Florida, exclusivamente para niños. Con más de 800 médicos a cargo y más de 475 subespecialistas pediátricos, el hospital, de 309 camas y sin fines de lucro - conocido como Miami Children's Hospital desde 1983 hasta el 2014 - es reconocido por su excelencia en todos los aspectos de la medicina pediátrica y rutinariamente tiene muchos programas clasificados por *U.S.News & World Report* entre los mejores de la nación.

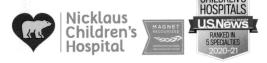

3100 SW 62 Avenue, Miami, FL 33155
305-666-6511
nicklauschildrens.org

Conéctese con un Experto de Nicklaus Children's desde la Comodidad de su Hogar a través de Cuidados Infantiles Nicklaus Children's Pediatric Virtual Care

El regresar a casa con un infante que acaba de pasar semanas o tal vez meses, en una unidad neonatal de cuidados intensivos (NICU por sus siglas en inglés) puede ser una tarea intimidante hasta para el padre más experimentado.

Quizás tenga preguntas acerca de alimentación, cambio de pañales, baños o acerca de cómo usar en casa, ciertos equipos médicos y aparatos poco familiares, lo cual puede ser abrumador.

Ahora existe ayuda a la mano con Cuidados Infantiles Nicklaus Children's Virtual Care, un servicio de telesalud de Nicklaus Children's Hospital que le brinda acceso directo a su equipo de especialistas en cuidados de salud desde la comodidad de su propio hogar.

Usando una computadora, teléfono celular o tableta con acceso a internet, usted podrá comunicarse mediante videoconferencia con un miembro experimentado del equipo de la Unidad de Cuidados Intensivos Neonatales (NICU). Nuestro personal puede brindar orientación, consejo y apoyo en todo, desde cuidados básicos para recién nacidos hasta apoyo a bebés con traqueotomías, gastrostomías, líneas centrales y otros equipos médicos especializados.

Descargue y cree su cuenta en Nicklaus Children's Pediatric Virtual Care, llame al servicio de telesalud durante las horas de operación para conectarse con un miembro del equipo de NICU y obtenga tranquilidad inmediata.

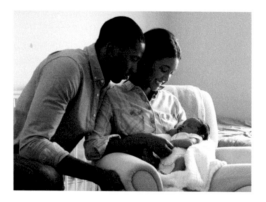

Seguridad y Confianza de los Expertos Cuando lo Necesite

- Obtenga orientación pediátrica y consejos de expertos para su bebé.
- No hay costo para las familias una vez dado de alta al paciente
- Accesible a través de una computadora, tableta o aplicación móvil. Descargue la aplicación Nicklaus Children's Pediatric Virtual Care la tienda virtual de aplicaciones de Apple o Google Play

Nuestro equipo experimentado de la unidad neonatal de cuidados intensivos (NICU por sus siglas en inglés) puede brindar orientación y apoyo esencial para diferentes áreas en el cuidado de infantes, incluyendo:

- Cuidado básico del recién nacidos (baño, cuidado de piel, cuidado del cordón umbilical)
- Administración de medicinas
- Programa "Back to Sleep" o "Volviendo a Dormir" (seguridad del recién nacido y prevención de síndrome de muerte súbita infantil – SIDS por sus siglas en inglés)
- Respirador artificial para el hogar/aerosol/equipo de succión
- Oximetría de pulso
- Terapia de oxígeno
- Cuidados de línea central
- Cuidados de gastrostomía
- Cuidados de traqueotomía
- Cuidados de ostomía
- Cuidados de heridas
- Arnés de Pavlik

Cómo Comunicarse

Nicklaus Children's Pediatric Virtual Care utiliza su cámara de video para comunicarse. Para establecer una consulta con un miembro del equipo de la unidad neonatal de cuidados intensivos (NICU) a través de su teléfono celular o tableta:

- Baje la aplicación Nicklaus Children's Pediatric Virtual Care de la tienda virtual de applicaciones de Apple o Google Play

- Visite **nicklauschildrensvirtualcare.org** usando el navegador Google Chrome desde su computadora o tableta con cámara web

Una vez registrada(o), puede programar una consulta de Cuidado Infantil a su conveniencia.

Su Nombre de Usuario

Su Contraseña

Para mayor información, por favor comuníquese

con el equipo de telesalud llamando al **305-662-8353** o al **1-800-811-9350** (sin costo), o envíe un correo electrónico a *Telehealth.office@nicklaushealth.org*

Cuidados Infantiles
de Telesalud

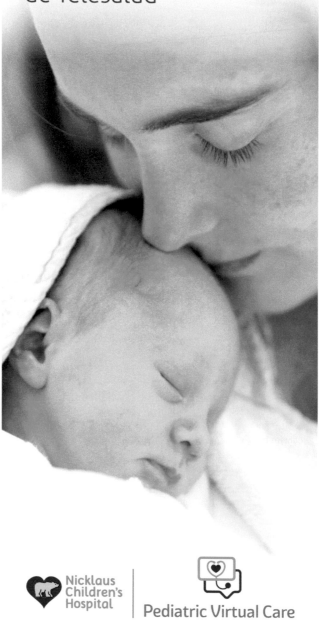

Nicklaus Children's Hospital | Pediatric Virtual Care

References

Alkozei A, McMahon E, Lahav A. Stress levels and depressive symptoms in NICU mothers in the early postpartum period. J Matern-Fetal Neonatal Med. 2014;27(17):1738–43.

ANCC, ANA. Magnet Recognition Program. Silver Spring, MD: ANCC. ANA; n.d.. https://www.nursingworld.org/organizational-programs/magnet/. Accessed 31 Jan 2022.

Barimani M, Vikström A, Rosander M, Forslund Frykedal K, Berlin A. Facilitating and inhibiting factors in transition to parenthood - ways in which health professionals can support parents. Scand J Caring Sci. 2017;31(3):537–46.

Barnes C, Adamson-Macedo EN. Perceived maternal parenting self-efficacy (PMP S-E) tool: development and validation with mothers of hospitalized preterm neonates. J Adv Nurs. 2007;60(5):550–60.

Cribs for Kids. Hospital certification. Pittsburgh, PA: Cribs for Kids; n.d.. https://cribsforkids.org/hospitalcertification/. Accessed 28 Feb 2022.

Curfman A, McSwain SD, Chuo J, Yeager-McSwain B, Schinasi DA, Marcin J, Herendeen N, Chung SL, Rheuban K, Olson CA. Pediatric telehealth in the COVID-19 pandemic era and beyond. Pediatrics. 2021;148(3):e2020047795.

Green J, Fowler C, Petty J, Whiting L. The transition home of extremely premature babies: an integrative review. J Neonatal Nurs. 2021;27(1):26–32.

Hua W, Wang L, Li C, Simoni JM, Yuwen W, Jiang L. Understanding preparation for preterm infant discharge from parents' and healthcare providers' perspectives: challenges and opportunities. J Adv Nurs. 2021;77(3):1379–90.

King BC, Mowitz ME, Zupancic JAF. The financial burden on families of infants requiring neonatal intensive care. Semin Perinatol. 2021;45(3):151394.

Korukcu O, Deliktaş A, Kukulu K. Transition to motherhood in women with an infant with special care needs. Int Nurs Rev. 2017;64(4):593–601.

Kuo DZ, Lyle RE, Casey PH, Stille CJ. Care system redesign for preterm children after discharge from the NICU. Pediatrics. 2017;139(4):e20162969.

Mahoney AD, White RD, Velasquez A, Barrett TS, Clark RH, Ahmad KA. Impact of restrictions on parental presence in neonatal intensive care units related to coronavirus disease 2019. J Perinatol. 2020;40(Suppl 1):36–46.

Matsuda Y, McCabe BE, Behar-Zusman V. Mothering in the context of mental disorder: effect of caregiving load on maternal health in a predominantly Hispanic sample. J Am Psychiatr Nurses Assoc. 2021a;27(5):373–82.

Matsuda Y, Schwartz TA, Chang Y, Beeber LS. A refined model of stress–diathesis relationships in mothers with significant depressive symptom severity. J Am Psychiatr Nurses Assoc. 2021b;27(3):240–50.

Matsuda Y, Valdes B, Salani D, Foronda C, Roman Laporte R, Gamez D, et al. Baby Steps Program: telehealth nursing simulation for undergraduate public health nursing students. Clin Simul Nurs. 2022;65:1–10.

Meleis AI, Sawyer LM, Im EO, Hilfinger Messias DK, Schumacher K. Experiencing transitions: an emerging middle-range theory. ANS Adv Nurs Sci. 2000;23(1):12–28.

Orr E, Ballantyne M, Gonzalez A, Jack SM. The complexity of the NICU-to-home experience for adolescent mothers: Meleis' Transitions Theory applied. ANS Adv Nurs Sci. 2020;43(4):349–59.

Rubinos LH, Foster CC, Machut KZ, Snyder A, Simpser E, Hall M, et al. Risk factors for hospital readmission among infants with prolonged neonatal intensive care stays. J Perinatol. 2021;42:624–30.

Saeed SA, Masters RM. Disparities in health care and the digital divide. Curr Psychiatr Rep. 2021;23(9):61.

Schumacher KL, Meleis AI. Transitions: a central concept in nursing. Image J Nurs Sch. 1994;26(2):119–27.

Sensmeier J. Enhancing the patient and provider experience through telehealth. Nurs Manag. 2020;51(11):8–15.

Yeh AM, Song AY, Vanderbilt DL, Gong C, Friedlich PS, Williams R, et al. The association of care transitions measure-15 score and outcomes after discharge from the NICU. BMC Pediatr. 2021;21(1):7.

Canadian Nurse Practitioner-Led Pediatric Rehabilitation Complex Care Program

Erin Brandon and Tessa Diaczun

Introduction

A significant portion of pediatric health care costs in Canada can be linked to children with medical complexity (CMC) despite the fact that the population represents a relatively low percentage of the pediatric population. As a result, publicly funded health-care organizations face increasing demands to implement solutions to respond to the unique needs of this population. There is need for extensive care coordination including interprofessional collaboration within health and community sectors as well as targeted caregiver support for this population, making implementation considerations even more challenging. The integration of a Nurse Practitioner (NP)-led clinic at a children's rehabilitation hospital, specifically for medically complex patients, demonstrated positive results including decreased wait-times and a high degree of collaboration as well as caregiver and interprofessional team satisfaction. A description of the implementation approach following the Patient-Focused Process for Advanced Practice Nursing (PEPPA) Framework is presented here, along with challenges and facilitators to the model of care,

E. Brandon
Holland Bloorview Kids Rehabilitation Hospital, Toronto, ON, Canada

University of Toronto, Toronto, ON, Canada

The Hospital for Sick Children, Toronto, ON, Canada
e-mail: erin.brandon@sickkids.ca

T. Diaczun (✉)
British Columbia Children's Hospital, Vancouver, BC, Canada

University of British Columbia, Vancouver, BC, Canada
e-mail: tessa.diaczun@cw.bc.ca

© The Author(s), under exclusive license to Springer Nature
Switzerland AG 2023
C. L. Betz (ed.), *Worldwide Successful Pediatric Nurse-Led Models of Care*,
https://doi.org/10.1007/978-3-031-22152-1_4

required clinical adjustments and future clinical and research considerations to support the improvement and access to high-quality healthcare for CMC in an NP-led clinic.

Background

NP Scope of Practice in Ontario

Nurse Practitioners have been part of the Canadian health-care landscape since the 1960s when their roles were primarily in northern, remote regions. Since the 1970s, interest in the NP role increased and educational programs became available. In 1997, NPs became regulated as a profession (Canadian Nurses Association 2020). Opportunities vary across Canada for NPs, as provinces implement the role with varying priorities and focus. In 2020, Ontario had employed over 50% of NPs in Canada (Canadian Nurses Association 2020).

NPs are registered nurses with additional, graduate level education and clinical experience, which enables them to practice with an expanded scope of practice. In Canada, NPs autonomously diagnose and treat illness, order and interpret diagnostic tests, prescribe medications, perform medical procedures, admit and discharge from hospitals, and initiate referrals. They provide comprehensive, coordinated care with a whole person approach, collaborating with other health-care providers thereby reducing pressure on the health-care system (Canadian Nurses Association 2017). NPs work in many settings across Canada including community care, long-term care, hospitals and NP-led clinics. Extensive research has consistently shown that the NP role improves timely access to high-quality, cost-effective care in a variety of settings. Canadians overwhelmingly report high satisfaction with NP care, with 93% of Canadians reporting their confidence that NPs meet their day-to-day health needs (Canadian Nurses Association 2020).

The Children's Rehabilitation Hospital

Holland Bloorview Kids Rehabilitation Hospital (HBKRH) is Canada's largest children's rehabilitation hospital. As an academic teaching center affiliated with the University of Toronto, HBKRH is a provincial resource for children with cerebral palsy and other developmental disabilities. In 2010, HBKRH set a number of strategic goals to improve access to care for outpatient clients with neuromotor concerns. The goals of the program were generated from a needs assessment of wait times, utilization statistics, and results from semistructured key informant interviews, which highlighted a number of unmet health-care needs for clients with complex neuromotor problems (Cox and DiCenso 2009).

Population Description (Children with Medical Complexity)

CMC represent a small but distinct group who have extraordinary needs and require services and supports from across acute, rehabilitation, and primary healthcare as well as education and community sectors. This population is characterized by the presence of chronic, severe health conditions, major functional limitations, substantial family-identified service needs, and high health-care use (Cohen et al. 2011). For example, Fatima is a child with medical complexity who is 4-years old. She and her mother are refugees. They live in social housing in a large urban center. She has global developmental delay, severe spastic quadriplegic cerebral palsy, and intractable seizures. She uses a wheelchair for mobility, requires feeding via gastrojejunostomy tube, takes multiple medications, requires frequent suction and repositioning to manage secretions, and requires full care. Children like Fatima account for one-third of all provincial child health spending despite representing only 0.67% of all children in the province (Cohen et al. 2012a; Shannon and French 2005). Studies from the USA show similar results of health-care utilization among CMC (Berry et al. 2014; Cohen et al. 2012a; Kuo et al. 2011).

In addition to the enormous fiscal impact on the health-care system, families of CMC struggle under the emotional, financial, and caregiving burden of meeting their child's needs (Altman et al. 2018; Arauz Boudreau et al. 2012; Kuo et al. 2011; Sacchetti et al. 2000; Slonim et al. 2013). For example, Fatima has exceptionally high care demands, requiring close observation day and night given her frequent seizures, need for respiratory support and repositioning. Her single mother is unable to work, because Fatima has one to three appointments per week and it takes up to two hours to travel to some of the appointments given their reliance on public transit. Her mother coordinates appointments endlessly and many of the providers at those appointments do not communicate with one another, leaving her navigating recommendations from multiple providers within a siloed system of care. Fatima's mother speaks and reads English; however, low literacy, cultural differences, language, and financial barriers are some factors leading to psychosocial complexity (Altman et al. 2018), adding further complexity to the situation families face. Not surprisingly, caregivers face increased unemployment and underemployment, significant financial burden and out-of-pocket expenses, increased physical and mental health concerns, and children have unmet medical needs despite multiple medical appointments per year (Arauz Boudreau et al. 2012; Dewan and Cohen 2013; Kuo et al. 2011).

Community primary care providers also face challenges caring for CMC. The health system lacks mechanisms to ensure good communication between hospital and community health-care providers leaving care fragmented and community providers "out of the loop." CMC are at greater risk of medical errors in part due to this poor communication (Burke and Alverson 2010; Burns et al. 2010; Dewan and Cohen 2013). Additionally, primary care providers in the community have limited time and resources to provide care coordination and often lack the experience to manage the multiple medical issues present for CMC (Altman et al. 2018; Canadian Association of Pediatric Health Centres 2018).

Nurse Practitioner-Led Model

Model Development

The Participatory, Evidence-Based, Patient-Focused Process for Advanced Practice Nursing (PEPPA) framework was chosen to guide the development and implementation of the NP-led clinic for children and youth with medical complexity at HBKRH in 2010. The nine-step framework addresses the unique implementation issues specific to advanced practice nursing roles and reinforces the value of conducting a comprehensive needs assessment to determine the capacity and readiness to integrate an NP into an existing system (Bryant-Lukosius and DiCenso 2004) (see Fig. 1).

HBKRH senior leaders and key stakeholders formed a steering committee to explore how an NP role, based on the PEPPA framework, might address the needs and gaps within the neuromotor program, an outpatient program providing assessment, diagnosis, and follow-up to children and youth with cerebral palsy and other developmental delays. The framework facilitated the steering committee members in thinking about a new model of care and the suitability and potential of the NP role (Cox and DiCenso 2009). Guiding questions facilitated a shift in thinking from focusing on health problems (e.g., cerebral palsy) to health needs (e.g., care coordination). Several months into this process, a Nurse Practitioner was hired and the PEPPA framework continued to guide model of care development. The NP engaged in a 5-month orientation, which provided an opportunity for the NP to become familiar with the program, work with and build trust with the interprofessional team, and see first-hand the challenges and gaps in care for children, youth, and their families. The NP's clinical experience as well as mentorship and collaboration with NPs in the near-by acute care hospital complex care program further guided development of the model of care.

Gaps and Challenges with the Pre-existing Model of Care

The model of care prior to the initiation of the NP-led complex care neuromotor program consisted of developmental pediatricians leading assessments for all new and follow-up clients. The wait time for new clients exceeded 1 year, contributing to caregiver stress and delays in addressing health concerns. Families and the healthcare team identified further challenges including infrequent follow-up visits, lack of community medical follow-up, and inadequate care-coordination. A subset of children within the neuromotor program are those with medical complexity. It was evident that caregivers of CMC need access to a health-care provider who can address the child's or youth's complex health problems as issues arise while also coordinating care among members of the interprofessional team (Berry et al. 2013). In addition to medical care, these families require a model that addresses mental and social needs of children/youth, caregivers, and family members, and provides support through transitions (Dewan and Cohen 2013).

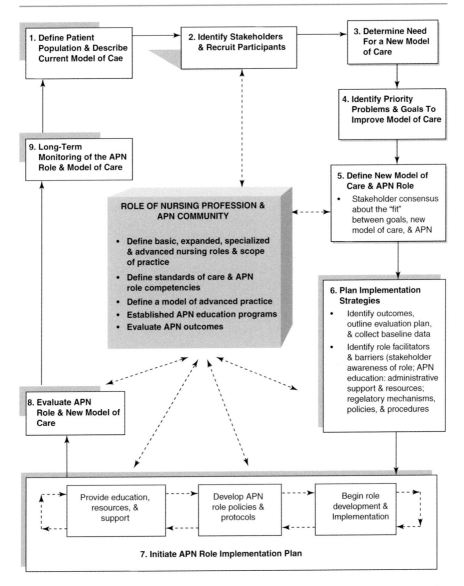

Fig. 1 The PEPPA framework: a participatory, evidence-based, patient-focused process for advanced practice nursing (APN) role development, implementation, and evaluation. (Reprinted with permission from Bryant-Lukosius and DiCenso 2004)

Through use of the PEPPA framework, the steering committee identified CMC within the neuromotor program as having unique needs that could be addressed by an NP. The goals of the new model of care were to increase access to care for children waiting to be seen in the neuromotor program, increase care coordination and follow-up for children with cerebral palsy (CP) and medical complexity, and ensure family satisfaction with the new model of care.

Description of the New Model of Care

The literature as well as local knowledge and experience was drawn upon to inform the NP-led complex care neuromotor program. In order to avoid duplication across acute care, rehabilitation, and community services, it was important to work with the near-by acute care hospital complex care program. The NP maintained open communication with the acute care complex care team about any children who were shared or transitioning between programs.

Referral criteria developed using the definition of CMC (Cohen et al. 2011) have evolved over time as the program became established. Most of the children/youth followed in the clinic at the outset had a diagnosis of cerebral palsy, were technology dependent (e.g., enteral feeding tube), and required assistance with mobility and communication. There was emphasis placed on acceptance of children and youth receiving a significant number of services and supports at HBKRH, in the community and at school. The local acute care complex care program followed those children who required more acute care admissions. Referrals were generated from the developmental pediatrician within the HBKRH outpatient neuromotor program after an initial assessment and diagnosis, so that the focus of the Complex Care Neuromotor NP clinic could be on follow-up and coordination of care. External referrals are not accepted.

There is flexibility in the timing and place of care delivery. Clients are seen every 6–12 months or with increased frequency based on clinical presentation and need. Appointments occur in the clinic, at home, virtually or in the community (e.g., school, respite agency) and are often coordinated with other members of the circle of care. The NP is also available by telephone, e-mail, and, since the COVID19 pandemic, virtually.

Significant attention is paid to what Feudtner and Hogan (2021) refer to as judgment, uncertainty, and shared control work. This work is described as working with families and providers within the circle of care to create a common understanding of the situation, an appreciation for goals of care, and an agreed-upon care plan. This work is done in the context of uncertainty given their child's complexity and fragility. Families and caregivers are faced with trade-offs as they try to make the best decision for their child and family in the face of this uncertainty.

In alignment with recommendations from the literature, a care plan is created by the NP, in collaboration with each client and family. This document summarizes the child's medical issues and care needs and is intended to enhance communication between care providers involved in the client's care and prevent errors across transitions through multiple settings (Adams et al. 2013). The care plan is also a tool to define who on the team is responsible for what and ensure shared understanding, which may be a critical ingredient in complex care programs (Feudtner and Hogan 2021).

Collaboration with Physician Partners

The NP who leads the program for children and youth with medical complexity practices autonomously, providing specialized medical and developmental follow-up care with consultation and/or referral to physicians internal and external to HBKRH when needed. Prior to changes in provincial legislation, hospital leadership facilitated adjustments to referral criteria for physician-led programs at HBKRH so that NP referrals would be accepted. Emphasis is placed on collaboration, communication, and coordination between the NP and these physicians. The NP also works closely with the child/youth's pediatrician who provides primary care in the community. The NP supports access to primary care and aims to keep the pediatrician "in the loop" with care being provided at the acute care and rehabilitation hospitals. As a result, reciprocal relationships have developed between the NP and many pediatricians/primary care providers where consultations occur both ways and expertise is shared between clinicians to provide comprehensive care of joint clients, appreciated by both parties.

Collaboration with the Interprofessional Team

The NP collaborates with the child/youth's interprofessional circle of care while acting as the "key worker" for families/caregivers. The literature describes a key worker as a single point of contact for a family with the ability to work collaboratively and help bridge the gap between and across services and sectors (Canadian Association of Pediatric Health Centres 2018; Drennan et al. 2015). Use of key workers has resulted in high levels of satisfaction of families and health-care providers (Rahi et al. 2004). The NP in the NP-led complex care neuromotor program is well positioned to support families given their scope of practice and specialized knowledge. Feudtner and Hogan (2021) describe the importance of specialized knowledge that providers in a complex care program must have, which includes knowledge and skills with various supportive technology, medications, and nutrition that these children and youth often require. Additionally, that knowledge needs to be customized to the unique child or youth, given their specific condition, history, and knowledge of what has worked and not worked in the past in any particular clinical situation. Through acting as a key worker for a child/youth and family, the NP in the HBKRH program has an opportunity to develop that customized knowledge.

The circle of care for CMC is vast and includes therapists (occupational therapy, physiotherapy, speech and language therapy), home care nurses, respite providers, school staff, dietitians, social workers, and others. The circle of care extends between sectors (health, education, child, and family services) and is often fragmented with poor communication between providers. The NP in the NP-led complex care neuro-motor program attends school team meetings, subspecialist appointments, and therapy appointments in an attempt to coordinate care. She also provides orders for home and respite staff, partners with families to ensure goals of care are heard during team meetings, and provides access to necessary services and supports in the community. The NP has developed a close working relationship with the social worker, therapists, and specialized therapist-led programs (i.e., specialized seating, augmentative communication) in the neuromotor program at HBKRH. This allows for sharing of expertise and effective communication between providers. This type of logistical case management work, as well as communication work is considered an important ingredient in complex care programs (Feudtner and Hogan 2021).

Provincial Framework Complex Care for Kids Ontario (CCKO)

After the implementation of the NP-led complex care neuromotor program at Holland Bloorview, a provincial strategy through the Provincial Council of Maternal and Child Health (PCMCH) was formed called Complex Care for Kids Ontario (CCKO). This provincial strategy was implemented with the intent to design models of care, which support integration and coordination of care for CMC in the province of Ontario and improve linkages between tertiary and community providers (Provincial Council of Maternal and Child Health 2017). The CCKO framework model of care is an NP-led outpatient clinic in a tertiary hospital setting, which is team-based, supporting collaboration between a pediatrician, social worker, dietitian, community service provider, and therapy supports. This model provides a one-stop shop model of care in Ontario (Provincial Council of Maternal and Child Health 2017). The CCKO complex care strategy has facilitated development of standards of care for complex care programs; care plans; and mechanisms to operationalize and standardize the values of the complex care approach to care delivery for CMC in the province. The standards of care have become essential resources for clinic development and support a systematic, consistent approach to care for CMC across the province and have been highly valuable to the NP-led complex care neuromotor program at HBKRH. This one-stop shop model, established through CCKO, is resource intensive and may have higher associated organizational costs than a single provider model like the HBKRH model. The CCKO model has not yet been compared to other models of care for CMC.

Evaluation

The NP-led complex care neuromotor program was evaluated over an 8-month period, 2 years after the NP role was implemented. Access and efficiency of care, caregiver satisfaction, and interprofessional collaboration were considered important outcomes in the context of the organizational strategic plan. Workload data and statistics including wait times, frequency of clinic visits and minutes of telephone contact points with families on a weekly basis were collected. Findings revealed improvements in wait times and access to care (Gresley-Jones et al. 2015). Data were gathered to compare no-show service rates of the NP-let complex care neuro-motor program (11%) with that of the previous developmental pediatrician-led model (30%). The differences of no-show rates were attributed to the frequency of NP support which include telephone contacts and the use of care plans.

Service satisfaction measures were administered to caregivers with the support of a research assistant. Measurements of interprofessional collaboration and satisfaction were obtained from providers. Tools utilized had reliable and valid psychometric properties. The Client Satisfaction Questionnaire (CSQ-8) was chosen as a global measure of client satisfaction that is widely used within the health-care system (Larsen et al. 1979; Please provide Bibliographic details n.d.). The Family Professional Partnership Scale was used to measure satisfaction, specifically satisfaction with family-professional partnerships. Scores and free text responses obtained from both of these measures revealed overall positive satisfaction with NP services. Interprofessional team collaboration and satisfaction was measured using the Provider Collaboration Survey (PCS) (Way and Jones 2001). The PCS was emailed to 52 interprofessional team members (internal and external to HBKRH) who worked with the NP on a regular basis. Findings revealed that interprofessional respondents viewed communication and collaboration with high rates of satisfaction.

This evaluation provided important feedback on the provision of NP services. As the data indicated, the services provided in the NP-led complex care neuromotor program were in alignment with organizational goals and priorities. Future evaluation plans include repeat satisfaction and collaboration measures as well as a cost analysis comparing models of care. For additional information on the findings of this programmatic evaluation, the reader is referred to a previously published article that provides details of the evaluation plan and findings (Gresley-Jones et al. 2015).

Challenges and Facilitators

Challenges

Adult transition from the pediatric health system has contributed to moral distress for the NP and significant stress for families and caregivers. Advancements in medical care, and specialized medical service models have led to a growing population of children with medical complexity and childhood onset disabilities reaching adulthood (Tennet et al. 2010). The transition to adulthood has been associated with lower levels of satisfaction for family/caregivers and transition aged youth, leaving them feeling abandoned in a geriatric focused, fragmented medical system (Shannon and French 2005). In Ontario, young adults and their families are left with a single provider model of care, limited care coordination, and a multisite model, which spans over a large geographic area. This is in stark contrast to the one-site pediatric counterpart with comprehensive supports to which they have become accustomed

(Brandon et al. 2019). Families and youth are then left to act as service navigator, medical historian, and care coordinator in an unfamiliar and more complicated system.

The challenge of transition to adulthood remains significant for families and the provider in the NP-led complex care neuromotor program. Specifically, it has been difficult to identify adult subspecialty and primary care providers to accept patients with complex medical needs. As a result, transition to adult care is left dis-jointed, unresolved, with multiple gaps to service and no available providers to take over the holistic care approach. Existing transition programs have been unable to address this gap for the unique and growing population of youth with complex medical needs. Most transition programs in Ontario that do exist were developed on a model of self-advocacy and independence which is not relevant to many youth with complex medical needs. Subsequently, families are left to access subspecialty care and primary care services through urgent care and emergency services.

Caseload Limits are required to provide adequate clinical support and care coordination for CMC. The size of the NP's caseload must be considered carefully. Analysis of other NP roles caring for CMC has shown that families appreciate timely connection to a clinician for support and a short turnaround for medical forms, prescriptions, and support letters (Looman et al. 2013). An increased caseload can directly impact the NP's availability to clients and families to provide these necessary and valued supports. Ideally, an NP would have a caseload of 80–85 CMC. This ratio is consistent with other complex care programs in Canada and the United States (Kingsnorth et al. 2013). However, this ratio exists in the context of the most responsible provider (NP or physician) having access to a multidisciplinary team. With increasing costs of healthcare, resource shortages, and increased accountability for health-care expenditures, there are increased pressures for health-care efficiencies and cost-saving measures (Shannon and French 2005). Caseload challenges exist in the context of these pressures for the NP-led complex care neuromotor program with a current caseload for one NP being well above the recommended provincial standard. This leaves the NP at risk for burnout and families with decreased access to the NP's support.

Administrative/Allied Supports remains a limitation for the NP-led complex care neuromotor program, specifically clerical, administrative, and dietitian supports. This places increased demands on the NP, further decreasing time available to support CMC and families. Through ongoing advocacy and support from leadership, a resource has been provided to support scheduling, coordination of appointments, and tasks such as sending referrals, prescriptions, and medical documentation. This is critical, since heavy caseloads in combination with lack of clerical/administrative supports have been found to directly impact NP's ability to take on more leadership roles (committee representation, program expansion, and management positions) (Elliott et al. 2016). CMC require an individual approach and advanced clinical expertise in nutrition to optimize provision of their nutritional requirements (Mazzeo and Mascarenhas 2021). Most CMC in the NP-led complex care neuromotor program are fed via feeding technology (gastrostomy or gastrojejunostomy tube). Many have gastrointestinal comorbidities, which contribute to challenges with feeding. Lack of dietitian support in the clinic places increased demands on the NP to have advanced knowledge and skills or spend time accessing consultative dietitian services.

After-hours coverage on evenings and weekends is not available for children or families followed by the NP-led complex care neuromotor program. Instead, families must access urgent care and emergency services during these hours. There continues to be challenges with securing medical coverage for vacation/sick time for the NP and vacation coverage is informally supported by other NPs within the organization for urgent issues only (prescription refills, medical support/triage). This is not unlike other single provider NP-led models of care where formalized coverage is lacking.

Facilitators

The PEPPA framework guided the implementation process for the NP-led complex care neuromotor program. Use of the 9-step framework identified specific actionable items, guided processes and assisted in the integration and evaluation of this NP role at HBKRH. Involving key stakeholders was critical to the implementation of this role, and ongoing success of the clinic. The use of the framework to identify gaps and program needs and establishing a comprehensive orientation assisted with addressing issues around role clarity, boundaries, acceptance, and identification of potential barriers and facilitators for the role implementation (Bryant-Lukosius and DiCenso 2004). The collaborative and inter-disciplinary orientation facilitated the development of trusting relationships with team members, enhanced other individuals' understanding of the NP role and scope of practice and allowed the NP to gain necessary expertise in daily clinical functioning to expand their autonomy and expertise. Guidance from the steering committee and the key findings of the initial key informant interviews, identified priority gaps in service and priorities of care for CMC's at HBKRH. This framework supported the development of a defined new model for care and establishment of a specific referral criterion for the clinic. Frequent check-in meetings and stakeholder involvement encourage the removal of barriers, facilitated change, and expanded the NP's role and scope of practice throughout the implementation period. The evaluation process characterized a model of care that provided support, access, and care to an underserviced population at HBKRH through an NP-led role.

Support from organizational leadership as key stakeholders was essential from the onset. Consistent with the literature, the use of the PEPPA framework facilitated the development and implementation of the NP role and promoted engagement of key stakeholders without power imbalance by valuing their contributions and collectively addressing problems (Bryant-Lukosius and DiCenso 2004). The NP met regularly with leadership to address role clarity, role acceptance, barriers, and strategies to ensure success of the program. Operational and senior leadership support assisted in the removal of barriers, facilitating change in scheduling, developing information systems templates to reflect care provision, adapting the referral processes/criteria and electronic documentation practices to accommodate NP scope of practice. Physician and other health-care providers' willingness to collaborate with the NP was due, in part, to the development of a trusting, collaborative partnership between the NP and the interprofessional team, which started during orientation and developed over time. Leadership supported this 5-month orientation, which was valuable both clinically, but also in terms of relationship building. Strong partnerships with operational management have been essential to the stability of this role, autonomy of the NP, and value perception at an organizational level for the program's contributions.

Community partnerships with primary care physicians were paramount for ongoing collaboration and continuity of care. Primary care providers have increased demands to see high patient volumes, limited time to provide comprehensive care to CMC's, and low reimbursement for complex medical assessments (Agrawal et al. 2013; Cohen et al. 2012b; Petitgout et al. 2013). There is recognition in the benefits for this population having a health home, which is a hub where clients and families receive timely provision and access to coordinated care (American Academy of Paediatrics 2013; College of Family Physicians of Canada 2011). Identifying the challenges faced by primary care providers, the NP-led complex care program was designed to provide a nontraditional medical home with comprehensive, coordinated care for children with medical complexity and their families, in partnership with their primary care providers. The NP provides specialized medical and developmental follow-up care and acts as the "key worker" for families, while the primary care provider continues involvement by supporting primary care responsibilities such as immunizations and sick visits. Partnerships between the two services, though not formalized, have been essential for improving continuity in care, communication between health-care providers and strengthening access to care for this population in the community.

Clinician autonomy for NPs increased with the expansion of the role in the province of Ontario. In 2009, the Government of Ontario passed Bill 179 (the Regulated Health Professions Statue Law Amendment Act), which supported the expansion of the scope of practice for NPs in the province for the purpose of improving timely access to healthcare for the public (Ministry of Health and Long Term Care 2009). 'This and subsequent expansions to the role have enabled NPs to practice autonomously across the province and has allowed for timely access to assessments, investigations, treatment, and specialty consultation for the clients followed in the NP-led complex care neuromotor program.

Positive impact on client/family therapeutic relationship was critically important in the development of this NP-led program. The NP provides a holistic approach to care acting as a "key worker" for families and caregivers of CMC. Additionally, a nursing and family-centered care model is central to care delivery, which is known to support goals that are most important to the child/family/caregiver, improve overall health outcomes, decrease acute care service requirements, and improve quality of life outcomes (Bonner et al. 2020). The clinic provides families/caregivers with access to care via e-mail, phone, and virtual platform, removing the requirement for families to take time off work and/or travel to yet another medical appointment.

Service Adjustments

Improvements for Access to Care

CMC require ongoing support for their complex and chronic health conditions from multiple subspecialists, requiring multiple appointments. There are a multitude of barriers and conflicting priorities, which contribute to challenges attending these appointments. Missed appointments can then be inefficient, costly, and strain clinician resources (Ballantyne and Rosenbaum 2017). Barriers for appointment keeping include challenges with transportation, competing priorities for the child/family and scheduling impacting their ability to attend (Ballantyne et al. 2019). Adding flexibility in scheduling to improve access to care was identified as a priority for the NP-led complex care neuromotor program. Opening appointment availability of the clinician, coordinating joint appointments with other service providers, providing service where the family is (including home/virtual appointments), and offering telephone support in between appointments have been key service adjustments to improve access to care for this population.

Appointment scheduling was adjusted in the NP-led program to support increased scheduling availability of the clinician. One week appointment times are available on Monday, Wednesday, or Friday and the alternating week appointments are available on Tuesday or Thursday and continue to alternate week by week. This provides flexibility in available appointment dates to correspond with parent/caregiver schedules. Additionally, later appointment time slots of 1600–1800 were added to accommodate for school attendance and parent/caregiver employment. Flexibility in appointment scheduling supports access to services provision (Cameron et al. 2014).

Coordinated Care is of significant value for CMC and their families and has the potential to decrease parental stress (Berry et al. 2013). At HBKRH, coordinated appointments are routinely arranged between providers to improve access to services and strengthen communication between providers centered on goals of care. Families in the NP-led complex care neuromotor program have identified that coordinated and collaborative visits with feeding therapy, hypertonia management, clinical seating, and orthotics services are most valued. Coordination of these joint appointments has also reduced frequency of appointments for families, strengthened clinical practice among providers and provides support during therapy sessions for medical issues that otherwise would have gone unaddressed.

Phone/E-mail Communication especially since the COVID 19 pandemic, has been highly valued by families. Unfortunately, organizational privacy and confidentiality policies, which require written consent, are a barrier to efficient and effective communication (Adams et al. 2021). Still, email and other forms of electronic communication (e.g., virtual platform, video conferencing, or telemedicine) have been essential to supporting families in the NP-led complex care neuromotor program between appointments. The ability for families to receive support at home in a timely way is key to preventing unnecessary hospitalizations and emergency visits. The clinic navigates organizational policies by routinely requesting consent for the NP to support families with the type of communication they prefer.

Home/virtual consultation provides access and connection to the child and family in their home environment. In this context, the NP is more able to understand and acknowledge social determinants of health, which contribute to the child's or youth's medical complexity (Heale et al. 2018). Home visits allow for earlier identification of supports required in the home and adaptation of clinical recommendations to suit the space, child, and family. In many cases, these support needs would have gone unrecognized in a traditional clinic visit, when family dynamics, living arrangements, and barriers might be hidden from clinician view. Home visits also eliminate the need for families to travel and allow for a more family-centered approach rather than a clinician-centered approach. Though there have been barriers to home visits during the COVID19 pandemic, the expansion of virtual health platforms for clinical care has maintained many of the benefits of home visits. Incorporating virtual, email, telephone, and in person options supports a holistic approach to care and can provide an improved understanding of the lived experience of the family in their home environment.

Lessons Learned

Building Relationships

Primary care providers often feel ill-equipped, strapped for time, and poorly compensated to participate actively in the care of CMC (Agrawal et al. 2013; Cohen et al. 2012b; Petitgout et al. 2013). It can take significant time and effort to build relationships with primary care providers and that engagement of primary care is critical in improving care moving forward (Kingsnorth et al. 2013). Networking, collaboration, and communication with primary care providers are essential for the care of CMC. Partnership building, though time consuming, ultimately improves care for the child and builds capacity in the provider.

The tools utilized to measure caregiver satisfaction for the evaluation of the NP-led program uncovered the benefits of the therapeutic relationship that develops between the NP and families over time. Results are consistent with the literature, suggesting NPs are well positioned to act as key workers for clients and families, given their clinical knowledge and scope of practice, their commitment to health education and health promotion, as well as their ability to act as care coordinators for CMC (Kingsnorth et al. 2013). Children with medical complexity represent an important group of patients who have multiple complex needs, which can be overwhelming for parent or caregiver. Having a "key worker" can support families to not feel like they are on an island by themselves, it can bridge trust and support a therapeutic relationship that is family centered.

Approach to Care of CMC

Utilization of the International Classification of Functioning, Disability and Health (ICF) framework when approaching clinical care of CMC can be helpful to support personalized pathways for care provision. The ICF framework developed by the World Health Organization (WHO) supports clinicians with a way to think about the health and well-being of clients in terms of health condition, body function, activities, participation, and environmental factors (World Health Organization 2001). This framework provides a neutral way for thinking about health, disability, and well-being that can support clinicians with joint goal setting and personalized medical management. Recent reframing of the ICF by Rosenbaum and Gorter (2011) into the "F-words" for childhood disability has further incorporated the ICF framework into a specific approach for childhood disability. The approach recognizes that personalized management plans should incorporate Function, Family, Fitness, Fun, Friends and Future in order to meet children's individual overall needs for care management (Rosenbaum and Gorter 2011).

Future Implications for Clinical Practice and Research

NP as Most Responsible Provider (MRP)

In Canada, MRP generally refers to a physician who assumes the overall responsibility for the care of an individual patient. NPs in Ontario are increasingly identified as MRP across health-care settings. Research has shown that the NP's role positively impacts client care, particularly when it comes to client satisfaction, interprofessional team collaboration, and coordination of care (Ontario Nurses Association 2017). NPs as MRP in acute care settings for complex aging seniors has highlighted that not only are NPs able to function in full capacity as MRP on an acute care medicine ward but additionally, they yielded high patient, family and staff satisfaction, and improved quality of care (Acorn 2015). The NP-led complex care neuromotor program already functions with the NP practicing autonomously, with consultation to internal and external physicians and interprofessional team members for clinical support. Although the NP provides care autonomously, it has been recommended that the NP be identified as the MRP within the electronic medical record and health system. This would support a streamlined referral process directly to the NP clinic rather than the currently required internal physician referral where the internal physician remains listed as the MRP.

Transition to Adulthood for Complex Care Population

Lack of access to coordinated care in adulthood increases risks for caregiver burn-out, medical errors, and a decompensation/decline in the young adult's overall health outcomes during the initial years of transition for CMC (Peter et al. 2009). Improvement in overall transition strategies, research, and system resolution for this population are essential to improve health outcomes during a transition period when they are at high risk for medical decompensation. Considerations for early transition planning (prior to the age of 16), access and partnership with adult primary care providers, and connection with transition/adult rehabilitation or physiatry programs requires further study and evaluation to support the transition process and aid in the elimination of gaps in service provision for this at-risk population with complex medical needs.

Evaluation of Long-Term Impact

The initial evaluation of the NP-led complex care neuromotor program was developed and carried out as a quality improvement project to measure access to care, efficiency, and caregiver and interprofessional team satisfaction, all of which were important initial outcomes in the context of the organizational strategic plan. Both a qualitative and quantitative approach was used to measure the efficiency and effectiveness of the NP-led clinic. The current economic climate in health-care forces administrators and clinicians to ensure that high-quality, safe care is provided in the context of an efficient and effective care delivery model. Further program evaluation is required to assess cost analysis and safety outcomes that were not previously evaluated during the early phase of the program. Though several studies in the United States and Canada have assessed health-care cost and utilization for CMC before and after enrollment in a complex care program, these are based on physician-led models of care. These studies provide promising evidence that programs designed to provide accessible, comprehensive, and coordinated care save health-care dollars (Berry et al. 2013). It is postulated that this NP-led complex care program likely will result in those same outcomes.

Conclusion

NPs require strong leadership and quality improvement skills as they lead the development and introduction of new clinical models of care for the population of CMC. The PEPPA framework is a useful guide to support the implementation of new NP roles, guiding the user through critical components of NP role planning, implementation, and evaluation. Program evaluation, which considers the impact of the NP role on clinical outcomes, care provision, coordination of service, and patient/family satisfaction, is essential to the success of such programs in the future. NPs are well positioned to act as key workers for clients and families, given their clinical knowledge, scope of practice, commitment to health education, and health promotion, as well as their ability to act as care coordinators for CMC (Kingsnorth et al. 2013). CMC represent an important group of patients who have multiple complex needs, which can be overwhelming for primary care providers to manage and treat in the community on their own. Significant work has been done to understand the cost and health-care utilization of this population and further development of best practices and ideal models of care to address their significant needs in ongoing. The lessons learned from the integration of the NP role and this new model of care may support other NPs and administrators successfully develop similar NP-led programs in their organization for CMC.

Useful Resources

1. Complex Care Kids Ontario (CCKO)—https://www.pcmch.on.ca/health-care-providers/paediatric-care/complex-care-kids-ontario/
2. AACPDM—https://www.aacpdm.org
3. Children's Healthcare Canada, CYMC Guidelines
4. Canadian Foundation for Healthcare Improvement. Programs: https://www.cfhi-fcass.ca/sf-docs/default-source/on-call/a-snapshot-of-transition-programs.pdf.
5. CanChild—https://www.canchild.ca/en/research-in-practice/f-words-in-childhood-disability

References

Acorn M. Nurse practitioners as most responsible provider: impact on care for seniors admitted to an Ontario Hospital. Int Nurse Clin Pract. 2015;2:126.

Adams S, Cohen E, Mahant S, Friedman S, Macculloch R, Nicholas D. Exploring the usefulness of comprehensive care plans for children with medical complexity (CMC): a qualitative study. BMC Pediatr. 2013;13:10.

Adams S, Beatty M, Moore C, Desai A, Barlett L, Culbert E, Cohen E, Stinson J, Orkin J. Perspectives on team communication challenges in caring for children with medical complexity. BMC Health Serv Res. 2021;21:300.

Agrawal R, Shah P, Zebracki K, Sanabria K, Kohrman C, Kohrman A. The capacity of primary care pediatricians to care for children with special health care needs. Clin Pediatr. 2013;52(4):310–4.

Altman YZ, Breen C, Hoffmann T, Woolfenden S. A qualitative study of health care providers' perceptions and experiences of working together to care for children with medical complexity. BMC Health Serv Res. 2018;18:70.

American Academy of Paediatrics. National center for medical home implementation: how to implement – getting started. Itasca, IL: American Academy of Paediatrics; 2013. http://www.medicalhomeinfo.org/.

Arauz Boudreau AD, Van Cleave JM, Gnanasekaran SK, Kurowski DS, Kuhlthau KA. A medical home: relationships with family functioning for children with and without special health care needs. Acad Pediatr. 2012;12(5):391–8.

Ballantyne M, Rosenbaum PL. Missed appointments: more complicated than we think. Paediatr Child Health. 2017;22:164–5. https://doi.org/10.1093/pch/pxx039.

Ballantyne M, Liscumb L, Brandon E, Jaffar J, Macdonald A, Beaune L. Mothers' perceived barriers to and recommendations for health care appointment keeping for children who have cerebral palsy. Glob Qualitat Nurs Res. 2019;6:1–13.

Berry JG, Agrawal RK, Cohen E, Kuo DZ. The landscape of medical care for children with medical complexity. Alexandria, VA; Overland Park, KS: Children's Hospital Association; 2013.

Berry JG, Hall M, Neff J, Goodman D, Cohen E, Agrawal R. Children with medical complexity and Medicaid: spending and cost savings. Health Aff. 2014;33:2199–206.

Bonner A, Havas K, Stone C, Abel J, Barnes M, Tam V, Douglas C. A multimorbidity nurse practitioner-led clinic: evaluation of health outcomes. Collegian. 2020;27:430–6.

Brandon E, Ballantyne M, Penner M, Lauzon A, McCarvill E. Accessing primary health care services for transition-ages young adults with cerebral palsy; perspectives of young adults, parents and physicians'. J Transit Med. 2019;1:20190004.

Bryant-Lukosius D, DiCenso A. A framework for the introduction and evaluation of advanced practice nursing roles. J Adv Nurs. 2004;48(5):530–40.

Burke RT, Alverson A. Impact of children with medically complex conditions. Pediatrics. 2010;126(4):789–90.

Burns KH, Casey PH, Lyle RE, Bird TM, Fussell JJ, Robbins JM. Increasing prevalence of medically complex children in US hospitals'. Pediatrics. 2010;126(4):638–46.

Cameron E, Heath G, Redwood S, Greenfield S, Cummins C, Kelly D, Pattison H. Health care professionals' views of paediatric outpatient non-attendance: implications for general practice. Fam Pract. 2014;31:111–7. https://doi.org/10.1093/fampra/cmt063.

Canadian Association of Pediatric Health Centres. CAPHC guideline for the management of medically complex children and youth through the continuum of care. CAPHC complex care community of practice. Ottawa, ON: CAPHC; 2018.

Canadian Nurses Association. The nurse practitioner [Position statement]. Ottawa, ON: Canadian Nurses Association; 2017. https://cna-aiic.ca/~/media/cna/page-content/pdf-en/the-nurse-practitioner-position-statement_2016.pdf?la=en.

Canadian Nurses Association. Nurse practitioners – untapped resource. Infographic. Ottawa, ON: Canadian Nurses Association; 2020. https://hl-prod-ca-oc-download.s3-ca-central-1.amazonaws.com/CNA/2f975e7e-4a40-45ca-863c-5ebf0a138d5e/UploadedImages/documents/Infographic_nurse-practitioners-untapped-resource.pdf.

Cohen E, Kuo D, Agrawal R, Berry J, Bhagat S, Simon T, Srivastava R. Children with medical complexity: an emerging population for clinical and research initiatives. Pediatrics. 2011;127(3):529–38.

Cohen E, Berry JG, Camacho X, Anderson G, Wodchis W, Guttmann A. Patterns and costs of health care use of children with medical complexity. Pediatrics. 2012a;130:e1463–70.

Cohen E, Lacombe-Duncan A, Spalding K, MacInnis J, Nicholas D, Narayanan UG, Gordon M, Margolis I, Friedman JN. Integrated complex care coordination for children with medical complexity: a mixed-methods evaluation of tertiary care-community collaboration. BMC Health Serv Res. 2012b;12:366. https://doi.org/10.1186/1472-6963-12-366.

College of Family Physicians of Canada. A vision for Canada: family practice - the patient's medical home. Mississauga, ON: The College of Family Physicians of Canada; 2011. http://www.cfpc.ca/A_Vision_for_Canada/.

Cox S, DiCenso A. Setting the stage: using an evidence-informed approach to address implementation of nurse practitioners within a pediatric rehabilitation and complex continuing care hospital. Ontario Training Centre in Health Services and Policy Research. (Unpublished fellowship dissertation). 2009.

Dewan T, Cohen E. Children with medical complexity in Canada. Paediatr Child Health. 2013;18(10):518–22.

Drennan A, Wagner T, Rosenbaum P. The 'key worker' model of service delivery. Keeping Current. 2015. https://www.canchild.ca/en/resources/85-the-key-worker-model-of-service-delivery.

Elliott N, Begley C, Sheaf G, Higgins A. Barriers and enablers to advanced practitioners' ability to enact their leadership role: a scoping review. Int J Nurs Stud. 2016;60:24–45.

Feudtner C, Hogan AK. Identifying and improving the active ingredients in pediatric complex care. JAMA. 2021;175:1.

Gresley-Jones T, Green P, Wade S, Gillespie R. Inspiring change: how a nurse practitioner-led model of care can improve access and quality of care for children with medical complexity. J Pediatr Health Care. 2015;29:478–83.

Heale R, James S, Wenghoder E, Garceau M. Nurse practitioner's perceptions of the impact of the nurse practitioner-led clinic model on the quality of care of complex patients. Prim Health Care Res Dev. 2018;19:553–60.

Kingsnorth S, Lacombe-Duncan A, Keilty K, Bruce-Barrett C, Cohen E. Inter-organizational partnership for children with medical complexity: the integrated complex care model. Child Care Health Dev. 2013;41(1):57–66.

Kuo DZ, Cohen E, Agrawal R, Berry JG, Casey PH. A national profile of caregiver challenges among more medically complex children with special health care needs. Arch Pediatr Adolesc Med. 2011;165:1020–6.

Larsen DL, Attkisson CC, Hargreaves WA, Nguyen TD. Assessment of client/patient satisfaction: development of a general scale. Eval Progr Plan. 1979;2(3):197–207.

Looman W, Presler E, Erickson M, Garwick A, Cady R, Kelly A, Finkelstein S. Care coordination for children with complex special health care needs; the value of the advanced practice nurse's enhanced scope of knowledge and practice. J Pediatr Health Care. 2013;27(4):293–303.

Mazzeo P, Mascarenhas M. Feeding and nutrition in children with medical complexity. Curr Probl Pediatr Adolesc Health Care. 2021;51(9):101071.

Ministry of Health and Long Term Care. Regulated health professions statue law amendment act. Toronto, ON: Ministry of Health and Long Term Care; 2009. https://www.health.gov.on.ca/en/common/legislation/bill179/default.aspx.

Ontario Nurses Association. Nurse practitioners: improving access to quality care for Ontarians. Toronto, ON: Ontario Nurses Association; 2017. https://www.ona.org/wp-content/uploads/ona_npsimprovingaccesstoqualitycareforontarians_201710.pd.

Peter NG, Forke CM, Ginsburg KR, Schwarz DF. Transition from pediatric to adult care: internists' perspectives. Pediatrics. 2009;123:417–23.

Petitgout JM, Pelzer DE, McConkey SA, Hanrahan K. Development of a hospital-based care coordination program for children with special health care needs. J Pediatr Health Care. 2013;27(6):419–25.

Please provide Bibliographic details. n.d.

Provincial Council of Maternal and Child Health. CCKO functions of a complex care clinic and program standard. Toronto, ON: Provincial Council of Maternal and Child Health; 2017. https://www.pcmch.on.ca/wp-content/uploads/2017/10/CCKO-Functions-of-a-Complex-Care-Clinic-and-Program-Standard-.pdf.

Rahi JS, Manaras I, Tuomainen H, Hundt GL. Meeting the needs of parents around the time of diagnosis of disability among their children: evaluation of a novel program for information, support, and liaison by key workers. Pediatrics. 2004;114:477–82.

Rosenbaum P, Gorter J. The 'F-words' in childhood disability: I swear this is how we should think!'. Child Care Health Dev. 2011;38(4):457–63.

Sacchetti A, Sacchetti C, Carraccio C. The potential for errors in children with special health care needs. Acad Emerg Med. 2000;7:1330–3.

Shannon V, French S. The impact of the re-engineered world of health-care in Canada on nursing and patient outcomes. Nurs Inq. 2005;12:231–9.

Slonim A, Lafleur B, Ahmed W. Hospital reported medical errors in children. Pediatrics. 2013;111:617–21.

Tennet P, Pearce M, Bythell M, Rankin J. 20-year survival of children born with congenital anomalies: a population-based study. Lancet. 2010;375(9715):649–56.

Way D, Jones L. Improving the effectiveness of primary health care through nurse practitioner/family physician structured collaborative practice. Health Canada's Health Transitions Fund. Ottawa, ON: University of Ottawa Department of Family Medicine and School of Nursing; 2001.

World Health Organization. The international classification of functioning, disability and health (ICF). Geneva: WHO; 2001. https://www.who.int/classifications/international-classification-of-functioning-disability-and-health.

Leveraging a Professional Nursing Organization to Create an Antitrafficking Care Model

Jessica L. Peck

Introduction

The Alliance for Children in Trafficking (ACT) is a nurse-led model of care established by the National Association of Nurse Practitioners (NAPNAP) Partners for Vulnerable Youth (NNPVY) (Peck 2021). As the first professional society for nurse practitioners established in 1973, NAPNAP remains the only organization in the world dedicated to supporting the advanced practice nursing role to optimize access to high-quality care for children. NAPNAP leveraged its relational, reputational, and resource capital to launch NNPVY and ACT, which represented a cohesive organizational response from the nursing profession to help reframe the criminal justice paradigm of trafficking response to one centered on public health (Peck 2021).

More than 40 million people are exploited and abused through trafficking worldwide, according to estimates by the International Labour Organization (ILO). One in four are children (ILO 2022). Contrary to widespread misconception, human trafficking is not confined to only sex trafficking. Globally, trafficking occurs primarily through forced labor, but also encompasses debt bondage, involuntary domestic servitude, child sexual abuse material production, commercial sexual exploitation of children, sex trafficking, organ trafficking, baby trafficking, child marriage, and child soldiering (United Nations Office on Drugs and Crime [UNDOC] 2020). In the United States (US), trafficking occurs mainly through forced labor and sexual exploitation and abuse (U.S. Department of State 2021). A formalized US federal definition of trafficking was first codified in the Trafficking Victims Protection Act in 2000, setting the stage to create a criminal justice-centered response framework. Law enforcement entities employed a

J. L. Peck (✉)
Louise Herrington School of Nursing, Baylor University, Dallas, TX, USA
e-mail: Jessica_Peck@Baylor.edu

© The Author(s), under exclusive license to Springer Nature
Switzerland AG 2023
C. L. Betz (ed.), *Worldwide Successful Pediatric Nurse-Led Models of Care*,
https://doi.org/10.1007/978-3-031-22152-1_5

downstream approach steeped in tertiary prevention for persons already victimized with significant and long-lasting traumatic effects on holistic health (United States Department of Justice 2022).

Studies estimate 60–87% of trafficked persons encounter a health-care professional at some point during exploitation without being identified (Chisolm-Straker et al. 2016; Goldberg et al. 2017; Lederer and Wetzel 2014). However, human trafficking did not begin to emerge in health sciences literature until around 2015, catalyzed largely by the widely cited study by legal scholars Lederer and Wetzel published in 2014 as well as federal statute establishing the Office of Trafficking in Persons as a division of US Health and Human Services. At this time, some continuing education courses emerged, but very few were designed for health professionals in clinical settings. Courses often were provided by well-meaning but ill-informed advocacy organizations or law enforcement professionals who received little guidance in adapting messaging for an audience of clinicians. With a dearth of professional clinical literature, practice guidelines, professional health-care organization guidance, curricular standards, and no other organizational standards for health systems accreditation, awareness remained low (Peck 2021).

The ACT nurse-led model has three main working components: standard setting, replication, and dissemination (Fig. 1). With more than 23 diverse and interprofessional organization partners, ACT's success spurred a train-the-trainer program to amplify the ability to reach more health professionals, training more than 10,000 clinicians in its first 3 years (Peck 2021). ACT also coauthored federal guidelines from the US Department of Health and Human Services, establishing core competencies for response to trafficking by individual clinicians, health systems, and academic institutions (National Human Trafficking Training and Technical Assistance Center [NHTTAC] 2021).

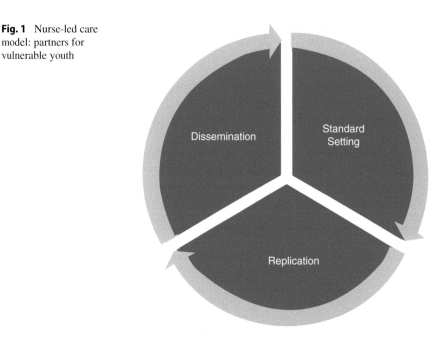

Fig. 1 Nurse-led care model: partners for vulnerable youth

Background

Human Trafficking: A Public Health Threat

While the concept of slavery is a tale as old as time, modern modalities through human trafficking are occurring unrecognized and in epidemic proportions. Of the 21 million people trafficked globally each year, experts estimate eight million are children with 5.7 million exploited through labor and 1.8 million for sex (ILO 2022). Prevalence and incidence are widely debated with contributory challenges including lack of common nomenclature, absence of reporting standards, and the illicit nature of a criminal enterprise (Peck et al. 2020). However, the National Trafficking Hotline in the United States receives thousands of calls each year reporting potential victimization, and many of those at-risk persons reported are accessing health-care environments (Peck 2019). Table 1 reviews possible trafficking modalities and environments.

The United States government first authorized the Trafficking Victims Protection Act in 2000, creating the first legal pathway for human trafficking cases. Despite this, more than 15 years passed before the first emergence of organized health-care response in this well-established criminal justice response framework. In 2016, the Association of Women's Health, Obstetric, and Neonatal Nurses (AWHONN) became the first professional nursing organization to issue policy directives to equip nursing response to human trafficking. The federal SOAR (Stop, Observe, Ask Respond) to Health and Wellness Act, which provides resources to engage health-care providers through establishment of the Office of Trafficking in Persons, was not signed into law until December 2018. However, since then only eight of 110 nursing organizations have policy directives or advocacy resources for members to effectively respond to trafficking risk despite a well-documented knowledge gap in the presence of widely rising acknowledgement by nurses that trafficking is a very real and present health threat (Peck and Doiron 2022).

Table 1 Modalities and environments where human trafficking risk occurs

Sex trafficking	Labor trafficking
Forced prostitution	Work camps
Modeling	Agricultural environments (farms, fishing)
Stripping or exotic dancing	Construction (quarries, building, mines)
Massage parlors	Domestic servitude
Child sexual abuse material production	Hospitality industry (restaurants, hotels)
Escort services	Door-to-door magazine sales
Sex tourism	Forced peddling or street begging
Survival sex	Day laborers
Forced marriage	Massage parlors/spa or beauty industries

Target Setting: Professional Nursing Organizations

Although human trafficking is a relatively new concept in the collective public conscious, nursing response to public health threats is not new. In the early history of nursing as an organized profession, leaders such as Florence Nightingale, Jane Addams, and Lillian Wald achieved a significant historical presence influencing policy development, especially in the spheres of women's, children's, and environmental health (Peck 2022). In modern nursing practice, however, individual nurses possess limited political self-efficacy, effectively restraining activism to voting and correspondence with legislative representatives. Although nurses are highly trained with professional assessment skills, seldom are these skills used in the context of evidence-informed health policy (O'Rourke et al. 2017). Training and education specific to health-related policy matters yields more effective nursing immersion and engagement to positively impact public health. There is critical opportunity for professional nursing organizations to leverage collectively advanced knowledge and professional skillsets to catalyze nurses to promote a unified policy agenda uniquely supported with operational resources and professional networks (O'Rourke et al. 2017; Peck 2022). Professional nursing organizations have voice, connection, and resources to influence innovative responses to complex health threats. Nurses have the professional skillset to navigate complex and often antagonistic or controversial environments with quickly changing contexts. Specific relevant strategies include establishing a policy agenda, employing effective decision-making frameworks and engagement pathways, and creating collaborative advocacy alliances (Chiu et al. 2020). A relevant current example of leveraging influence using the principles outlined above is the American Nurses Association (ANA), which succeeded in advocacy efforts to procure $100 billion in federal funding for needs surrounding personal protective equipment during the SARS-CoV-2 pandemic. ANA President Ernest Grant provided Congressional testimony and accepted an invitation with other nursing leaders to have an audience with the President of the United States along with other high-level policy stakeholders (ANA 2020).

Continued member engagement augments nursing impact in policy arenas. Prioritizing and cogently marketing direct impacts of organizational policy action strengthens nursing engagement in continued innovative initiatives to engage in advocacy or action responding to public health threats (Taylor 2016). NNPVY is a showcase of the aggregate power professional nursing organizations can harness to create a compelling policy initiative. ACT is an exemplar of engaging and equipping nurses to identify and respond to human trafficking in the clinical setting. This nursing model of organizational response created greater potential for successful impact than was possible through the actions of individual nurse leaders (Peck 2022).

Impetus for Model Development

Nursing is the largest and most trusted health-care profession in the world and plays an important role in recognizing and responding to risk and victimization with therapeutic communication skills guiding evidence-based, trauma-informed, culturally responsive care modalities (NHTTAC 2021). Nurses are on the front lines to identify at-risk and trafficked persons and connect them to holistic health services. Nurses are strong coordinators of care for social, mental, health, and housing services. However, awareness in the health professions remains exceptionally low. Many nurses lack knowledge and skills to identify persons victimized through trafficking, because it is not taught in academic health programs and is rarely prioritized in continuing education. When the NAPNAP Executive Board became aware of child trafficking as an emerging public health threat, a membership survey was employed to evaluate knowledge, beliefs, and attitudes of pediatric-focused advanced practice registered nurses (APRNs) (n = 799).

Survey findings dramatically demonstrated that pediatric-focused APRNs felt trafficking was a critical health threat and they were likely to encounter it in clinical practice, but less than one-quarter of those surveyed felt adequately prepared to respond. There were no comprehensive resources, policy supports, or curricular or certification standards guiding evidence-informed response. Leaders were justifiably concerned raising awareness without creating pathways for nurse response would create moral distress in the profession. This prompted NAPNAP to plan a comprehensive response using an innovative nurse-led model (Peck and Meadows-Oliver 2019).

Theoretical and Conceptual Frameworks

Recognizing a need to transition from a criminal justice framework to a public health prevention framework was critical in the foundational stages of theoretical and conceptual frameworks. The process of adopting a programmatic model that served to guide the development of National Association of Nurse Practitioners (NAPNAP) Partners for Vulnerable Youth (NNPVY) involved a process that ultimately incorporated several theoretical and conceptual frameworks. These were the Social Ecological Model (Bronfenbrenner 1979), Policy Circle Model (Yoder-Wise 2020; Peck 2022) and Public Health Intervention Wheel (Schaffer et al. 2022). An overview of the model integration for the NNPVY is provided below.

The first step undertaken to develop this framework was to conduct an integrative review. The Social Ecological Model (Bronfenbrenner 1979) was used to guide an integrative review of the literature and categorize risk factors for trafficking. The outcomes of this review resulted in the identification of four categories of risk factors: societal, community, relationship, and individual. The societal risk factors included sociocultural norms, social inequality, and determinants of health. Community risk factors consisted of connection to financial resources, housing opportunities, organizational policy and legislation developments, and multidisciplinary partnerships. The relationship category of risk factors involved team-based prevention and mentoring programs, peer-to-peer education, and community training. For further information, the reader is referred to Peck et al. (2020) publication that can be found in the reference list.

The Policy Circle Model is a conceptual framework to foster change with effective application for comprehensive interventions planned and implemented to address child trafficking in a professional nursing organization setting (Yoder-Wise 2020; Peck 2022). This framework guided the planned policy change that was the envisioned with the implementation of NNPVY. The Policy Circle Model elements provided a step-wide process for policy implementation for (Peck 2022).

Finally, the Public Health Intervention Wheel is a reputable population-centered care model used in public health practice that spans community, systems, and individual or family levels with 17 targeted public health interventions (Schaffer et al. 2022). It was used to direct specific interventions for nurses responding to trafficking and trafficking risks in school settings (Peck and Doiron 2022).

The Alliance for Children in Trafficking

Standard Setting for Education and Policy

NNPVY was designed as an umbrella organization to house multiple initiatives addressing at-risk populations with the goal of improving physical and mental health through early intervention and prevention efforts. The first of these initiatives launched was ACT, under the initial leadership of a steering committee with transition to an executive board of directors. Twenty-two nursing and interprofessional partner organizations joined NPVY with a statement of support. Program goals were established to improve nursing awareness, engage and equip health professionals with evidence-informed tools and resources, and collaborate with interprofessional health disciplines and systems. In addition, plans were made to deploy a robust advocacy strategy to support legislative and regulatory frameworks, which create and sustain a health framework focused on prevention and patient-centered services (Peck 2021). After analysis of the needs assessment survey, ACT moved forward with engaging in standard setting related to human trafficking (Peck et al. 2020). Examples of these efforts are listed in Table 2. After robust development of continuing education materials, resources, and supports, ACT's current Chair accepted an invitation to co-author interprofessional core competencies from the National Human Trafficking Training and Technical Assistance Center (NHTTAC), a division of the Office of Trafficking in Persons at the United States Department of Health and Human Services.

Replication Through the ACT Advocates Program

Shortly after launching standard setting education, it quickly became apparent that demand would exceed supply. NPVY could not effectively meet the needs requested for additional education. At the national conference for the Emergency Nurses Association in 2019, the fire marshal had to be called to turn people away after

Table 2 Standard setting by the alliance for children in trafficking (ACT)

Education standards	• Established 22 partner stakeholders for expert consultation and interprofessional collaborative efforts
	• Consulted a nationally recognized survivor advocate as keynote speaker for 2018 keynote speaker at 2018 annual conference
	• Conducted an organizational needs-assessment to direct education efforts and create standard clinical practice guidelines
	• Partnered with the McCain Institute and National Student Nurses' Association for nationwide distribution of Student Alliance Against Trafficking Toolkit
	• Supported a 2-h intensive workshop taught by a national nurse expert in collaboration with Shared Hope International, an advocacy organization for members to attend to enhance knowledge
	• Participated in standard setting for continuing education on trafficking as published by Health, Education, Advocacy, Linkage (HEAL) Trafficking
	• Developed a 1-h continuing education in collaboration with the American Academy of Pediatrics, including expert interprofessional stakeholders and survivor leaders; dual accreditation for physicians and nursing professionals
	• Developed an intensive 3-PARRT comprehensive, on-demand training for a more advanced level of competency for interprofessional clinicians
	• Joined in partnership as the nursing representative with the National Human Trafficking Training and Technical Assistance Center to create interprofessional Core Competencies
Policy standards	• Successfully suggested an amendment to SOAR to Health and Wellness to include professional organizations in funding opportunities for programmatic resources
	• Delivered professional consultation to Congressional forums concerning the FOSTA
	• Partnered with attorney and film producer Mary Mazzio to provide screening of documentary I Am Jane Doe to launch a call-in effort for successful passage of the FOSTA
	• Contributed to bill language, securing bipartisan cosponsorship, testimony, advocacy, and successful passage of House Bill 2059 in Texas (now referred to as The Texas Model) requiring evidence-based standards for health professional training on human trafficking, now being replicated in other states
	• ACT Advocates serve as expert consultants and resources in implementing organizational and institutional policies and protocols in congruence with best practices
	• Conducted a media tour for policy advocacy public awareness campaign with a reach of 4.3 million listeners

hundreds overflowed the educational session. At that point, a train-the-trainer program called ACT Advocates was developed wherein health-care providers complete a curated, evidence-based training curriculum aimed at expanding training capacity for health-care providers. ACT Advocates serve as community grassroots experts to conduct education sessions for their peers in health-care and community settings. They serve as policy advocates at the national and state level as well as media experts and thought leaders representing the antitrafficking movement. To date, more than 50 ACT Advocates in 25 U.S. states have trained more than 15,000 providers around the world (Peck 2021).

Dissemination Through Contributions to Scientific Literature

ACT made a concentrated effort to leverage interprofessional partners and experts to monitor and synthesize trafficking research literature and generate professional clinical literature issuing evidence-based education, practice guidelines, and policy directives. These are strategically aimed from a narrow to a broader audience using the Social Ecological Model (Bronfenbrenner 1977) for categorization: (1) Individual (written for individual pediatric nursing professionals to enhance education and skills), (2) relationship (focused on team-based prevention, mentoring, peer-to-peer education), (3) community (organizational, legal, regulatory, and ethical implications for interprofessional partnerships), and (4) societal (exploring sociocultural influencers and social determinants of health). The most significant work is the Core Competencies (Fig. 2) with the credibility of federal support, widespread professional endorsement, and dissemination to clinical audiences.

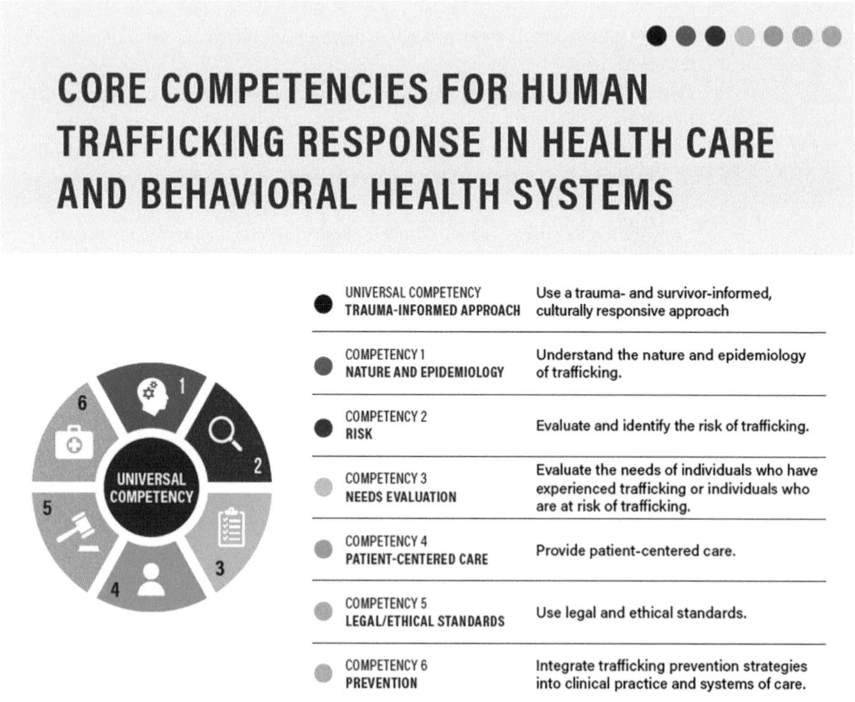

CORE COMPETENCIES FOR HUMAN TRAFFICKING RESPONSE IN HEALTH CARE AND BEHAVIORAL HEALTH SYSTEMS

UNIVERSAL COMPETENCY TRAUMA-INFORMED APPROACH	Use a trauma- and survivor-informed, culturally responsive approach
COMPETENCY 1 NATURE AND EPIDEMIOLOGY	Understand the nature and epidemiology of trafficking.
COMPETENCY 2 RISK	Evaluate and identify the risk of trafficking.
COMPETENCY 3 NEEDS EVALUATION	Evaluate the needs of individuals who have experienced trafficking or individuals who are at risk of trafficking.
COMPETENCY 4 PATIENT-CENTERED CARE	Provide patient-centered care.
COMPETENCY 5 LEGAL/ETHICAL STANDARDS	Use legal and ethical standards.
COMPETENCY 6 PREVENTION	Integrate trafficking prevention strategies into clinical practice and systems of care.

Fig. 2 Core competencies for human trafficking response in health-care and behavioral health systems

Batley et al. (2021). Core Competencies for Human Trafficking Response in Health Care and Behavioral Health Systems, Washington, DC: National Human Trafficking Training and Technical Assistance Center, Office on Trafficking in Persons, Administration for Children and Families, U.S. Department of Health and Human Services.

It is estimated only one-third of all professional human trafficking publications are in health journals, with prevailing reports in journals of law or social work. Only 10% of health literature on trafficking pertains to children. Nursing and healthcare continue to be largely excluded in dissemination of trafficking resources and guidelines. A recent literature review found only ten resources including federal and state government ($n = 7$), academic medical centers ($n = 1$), and nonprofit agencies ($n = 2$) to equip school policy makers and leaders to respond to trafficking. Only two of the ten addressed the role of the school nurse in leading, planning, and implementing effective response (Peck and Doiron 2022). A list of ACT publications can be reviewed in Table 3.

Table 3 Publication dissemination through ACT

Publication	Purpose	Audience
Peck, J.L. (2018). How nurse practitioners can help end modern-day slavery. *Journal of the American Association of Nurse Practitioners, 30*(11) 597–599. https://doi.org/10.1097/JXX.0000000000000152.	Call to awareness for nurse practitioners as requested by the Journal of the American Association of Nurse Practitioners	Relationship
Peck, J.L., & Meadows-Oliver, M. (2019). Human trafficking of children: Nurse practitioner knowledge, beliefs, and experience supporting the development of a practice guideline: Part One. *Journal of Pediatric Health Care, 33*(5) 603–611. https://doi.org/10.1016/j.pedhc.2019.05.006	Organizational member survey, needs assessment to direct educational interventions to the membership	Individual
Peck, J.L. (2020). Human trafficking of children: Nurse practitioner knowledge, beliefs, and experience supporting the development of a practice guideline: Part two. *Journal of Pediatric Health Care, 34*(2), 177–190. https://doi.org/10.1016/j.pedhc.2019.11.005	Integrative literature review, grading evidence using American Association of Critical Care guidelines and issuing the first clinical practice guidelines for trafficking	Individual
Peck, J.L. (2020). Human trafficking in the clinical setting: Critical competencies for family nurse practitioners. *Advances in Family Practice, 2,* 169–186. https://doi.org/10.1016/j.yfpn.2020.01.011	Invited submission to address educational needs of family nurse practitioners encountering situations of trafficking in primary care	Relationship

(continued)

Table 3 (continued)

Publication	Purpose	Audience
Peck, J.L., Meadows-Oliver, M., Hays, S., & Garzon-Maaks, D. (2020). White paper: Recognizing human trafficking as a critical emerging health threat. *Journal of Pediatric Health Care,* 35(3), 260–269. https://doi.org/10.1016/j. pedhc.2020.01.005	NAPNAP's first official White Paper, issuing a call to action in the profession for response from individual clinicians, health systems, and academic institutions	Relationship
Peck, J.L. (2020). Child trafficking victims in pediatric surgical environments: Implications for nursing care and advocacy. *Journal of Pediatric Surgical Nursing, 9*(4) 116–124. https://doi. org/10.1097/JPS.0000000000000266.	Invited manuscript following a conference presentation to raise awareness of sex and labor trafficking in pediatric surgical settings. This article was selected as the Article of the Year by the Journal of Pediatric Surgical Nurses and was a Hall of Fame Entry as selected by the International Academy of Nurse Editors	Relationship
Doiron, M., & Peck, J.L. (2021). The role of nursing in the school setting to lead efforts to impact child trafficking: An integrative review. *Journal of School Nursing,* online advance access. https://doi.org/10.1177/1059840520987533	Application of the Public Health Intervention Wheel to issue specific practice guidelines for nurses in the school setting	Relationship
Peck, J.L. (2021). A train-the-trainer programme to deliver high quality education for healthcare providers. *Anti-Trafficking Review 17(2021), 140–147.* https://doi.org/10.14197/atr.201221179.	Chronicling the history of the ACT Advocate program analyzing specific impacts and lessons learned	Community/ societal
Peck, J.L., Greenbaum, J., & Stoklosa, H. (2021). Mandated continuing education requirements for health care professional state licensure: The Texas model. Journal of Human Trafficking. Advance online publication. https://doi.org/10.1080/233227 05.2021.1981708	A policy analysis of House Bill 2059 in Texas and successful passage of mandated continuing education. This publication was funded by NAPNAP and HEAL Trafficking to be open access to be more accessible to legislators and was subsequently used to guide the Illinois state legislature	Community
Peck, J.L. (2021). Letter to the Editor. *Journal of Professional Nursing,* (38)1. https://doi. org/10.1016/j.profnurs.2021.10.009	Response to a trafficking study conducted by nursing with advisement for care in language and raising awareness of the Core Competencies	Relationship

Table 3 (continued)

Publication	Purpose	Audience
Peck, J.L. (2022). Partners for vulnerable youth and the alliance for children in trafficking: Using the policy circle model as a framework for change. *Journal of Pediatric Health Care*, advance online publication. https://doi.org/10.1016/j.pedhc.2020.10.001	Policy analysis chronicling the framework to develop and implement NPVY	Community
National Human Trafficking Training and Technical Assistance Center [NHTTAC]. (February 2021). *Core competencies for human trafficking response in health care and behavioral health systems.* U.S. Department of Health and Human Services, Administration for Children and Families [ACF], Office of Trafficking in Persons [OTIP], National Human Trafficking Technical Assistance and Training Center [NHTTAC]. Primary authors: Batley, C., Chon, K. (HHS OTIP), Garrett, A. (NHTTAC), Greenbaum, J. (International Centre for Missing and Exploited Children [ICMEC]), Hopper, E. (Justice Resource Institute), Murphy, L. (Sheffield Hallam University), Peck, J. (National Association of Pediatric Nurse Practitioners [NAPNAP]), Pfenning, E. (HHS OTIP), Robitz, R. (Department of Psychiatry and Behavioral Sciences, University of California Davis), Stoklosa, H. (HEAL Trafficking, Harvard Medical School). https://nhttac.acf.hhs.gov/resource/report-core-competencies-human-trafficking-response-health-care-and-behavioral-health	Critical first-of-its-kind resource issued from the United States Department of Health and Human Services.	Community/ societal
Peck, J.L., & Doiron, M. (2022). Human trafficking policies of professional nursing organizations: Opportunity for innovative and influential policy voice. Nursing Forum. In press.	This review mimicked a thorough review of medical organizations, which intentionally excluded nursing in the search criteria (Fang et al. 2019). This review systematically examined professional nursing organizations for trafficking policies and resources	Relationship
Peck, J.L., Kline-Tilford, A., Koppolu, R., & Sonney, J. (2022). NAPNAP partners position statement on implementation of the human trafficking core competencies. NAPNAP Partners for Vulnerable Youth. Journal of Pediatric Health Care. In press.	This is the first position statement released by NPVY endorsing universal health-care adoption of the Core Competencies and is endorsed by organizational partners.	Community

Dissemination also occurred through ACT Advocate presentations as previously described. After an initial organizational survey and needs assessment, an integrative literature review was completed to analyze the education-practice gap, resulting in clinical practice guidelines for human trafficking response in pediatric settings (Peck and Meadows-Oliver 2019) Dissemination was effective through partner organizations as well, who received and continue to receive a newsletter and invitations to share NPVY resources and news with their respective memberships. The American Association of Nurse Practitioners hosted a no-cost train-the-trainer session at an annual conference, partnered with ACT to provide a continuing education initiative to its membership, and featured the work of ACT on their internationally acclaimed podcast. The Emergency Nurses Association invited training for every member of their executive board to become an ACT Advocate, leading the way by example while also inviting a train-the-trainer program at their national conference.

Evaluation

Evaluation occurs primarily through ACT Advocate quantitative metrics including number of persons successfully completing evidence-based training, number of trainings held, number of ACT Advocates, and number of organizational partner endorsements of support. In addition, each ACT Advocate is given a QR code to direct participants to an evaluation of the education provided. Leaders review evaluation data and make revisions and recommendations accordingly. Because this program was launched prepandemic, it required standards for transition to adoption of virtual platforms, which were developed using evaluation data as a guide. Currently, a psychometrician is professionally engaged to establish reliability and validity of NPVY's original organization survey instrument, with a follow-up study to re-evaluate pediatric knowledge, beliefs, and attitudes concerning human trafficking. More planning is ongoing for possibilities to measure indirect impacts on patient outcomes including a standard measure/instrument to ensure comparison of outcomes across settings.

Challenges and Facilitators

Challenges

Challenges were multifaceted and complex, requiring innovation and resilience. Inclusion of nursing as a profession in national forums was scarce. Leaders who submitted abstracts were repeatedly rejected as presenters and had to start by simply attending and working to influence leadership to include health perspectives. Funding opportunities, particularly federal grant funding, primarily prioritizes criminal justice approaches. Highly accomplished scholars and awarded researchers experienced repeated rejections and denials. This is an ongoing challenge requiring innovation through crowd-sourced funding and seeking private donors. There is continued resistance within health professions to accept human trafficking as a legitimate threat. Stigma and bias endure, with common misconceptions that trafficking is rare, primarily occurs through sexual exploitation of White women, and that victims only present in emergency settings (NHTTAC 2021). The rise of misinformation and the hostage of the public narrative on trafficking through widely reported conspiracy theories severely damages and detracts from legitimate efforts to provide responsible, evidence-based, trauma-informed, and patient-centered solutions (Benton and Peterka-Benton 2021; Health, Education, Advocacy, and Linkages (HEAL) Trafficking 2021). Advocacy organizations popular with the public sometimes divert critically needed funds with little financial transparency as the opportunity for predation by preying on public sympathy is ripe. Funding and other infrastructure resource needs have been sparse, and success has relied almost entirely upon the labor-intensive efforts of volunteer leaders.

Facilitators

Most significantly, the sustained and enduring public trust in the nursing profession lends itself well to raise community awareness of an emerging health threat. That trust translated favorably to willingness of interprofessional organizational partners to support NPVY given the positive nature of press coverage partnering with nurses to respond to human trafficking. Favorability of the political climate to have a recorded collaborative success in a hyperpartisan, emotionally charged electorate opened doors widely that would not previously have been receptive to issues related to health policy. Conversely, overeagerness for political capital leads to haste in policy decisions with little regard for evidence, efficacy, or unintended harms. These are important elements to seek balance in future efforts, with an emphasis on the need to generate scholarly research and evaluation to support evidence-informed decision-making. In summary, organizational facilitators leveraged public trust in the nursing profession, created a partnership network to influence creation of education and policy standards, and established a credible international platform for dissemination.

Financial Support and Sustaining Strategies

NAPNAP contributed $50,000 in seed money and in-kind services to fund start-up and initial strategies. When grant funding efforts were unproductive, budget reliance on peer-to-peer fundraising and crowdsourcing funds brought a moderate degree of success, enough to continue to fund operations and promote growth alongside volunteer sweat equity. In 2020, initiation of a formal development committee to propose and direct long-term sustaining strategies was created. After being set back by the COVID-19 pandemic and related financial and resource competitors and stressors, the development committee is back on track working on a comprehensive plan for sustainable funding.

Service Adjustments

National Workgroup Development

Three national volunteer workgroups were created and sustained over a 1-year time frame to establish the major education standards to prepare for replication and dissemination. The first was continuing education authorship and delivery. This group developed a taskforce to seek a diverse and inclusive group of authors to create enduring education materials. This led to online, asynchronous on-demand modules (the first nationally available) as well as other materials including podcasts, professional journal manuscripts, and expert forums. The second group developed policies and procedures for the ACT Advocates program. This required legal counsel to ensure appropriate guidelines for representing the organization, and development of a robust policies and procedures manual to support the training guidelines and standards trainees must complete before being accepted into the program. This group had to create standards concerning scholarship dissemination to assure proper author credit and submission of materials to journals and conferences. The third group focused on critical evaluation of resources to create a resource intensive, evidence-based toolkit for all health-care providers. Staff assisted the executive board in developing a policies and procedures manual to govern NAPNAP NPVY, including by-laws, operating procedures, and lines of authority. It is the goal of NAPNAP NPVY to be self-sustaining with staff dedicated to this single organization, but currently, NAPNAP staff are allocated designated time for NPVY efforts.

Lessons Learned

Health Equity

NPVY values child health equity and endeavors to put actions behind values and goals. Although all children are at risk for trafficking, there is increased risk for children with complex vulnerabilities. These include but are not limited to child abuse and neglect; children in foster care and the juvenile justice system; youth who run away or experience homeless; individuals who identify as LGBTQIA+; undocumented persons; and children of color (Albright et al. 2020; Franchino-Olsen 2019; Peck et al. 2020). NAPNAP Partners' ACT initiative teaches nurses to identify at-risk populations of children and provide timely interventions to optimize their health while minimizing risk. Preventive and early intervention efforts decrease adverse childhood events, which have tremendously negative impacts on long-term health. As experts in pediatrics and advocates for children, NPVY is committed to equipping health-care providers with education and resources to advocate for child health equity. Every child deserves fairness, justice, and equitable opportunities for optimal health outcomes. NPVY is committed to advocating delivery of high-quality, accessible, affordable, evidence-based healthcare to all children regardless of their socioeconomic background, race, citizenship status, or sexual orientation.

Global Health Perspective

Trafficking is not unique to children in the U.S., and ACT has helped lead efforts in Indonesia, Malaysia, India, Australia, England, Ukraine, and other countries to mobilize and train health-care providers to respond to trafficking. Equitable collaboration with international partners is critical to overcome cultural barriers which view exploitation resulting from trafficking as shameful or taboo. Publications have been disseminated in international health journals, raising awareness of the need for global collaboration (Peck 2021; Peck et al. 2021).

Importance of Partnerships

Having national partners is a critical element of success in both building credibility as an expert and amplifying voice through dissemination. NNPVY's organizational partners have strengthened the work of ACT and widened the reach. Partnering with professional survivor advocates is an often overlooked but critical element of directing effective patient-centered interventions. Significant success is found in convening community collaborative efforts with partners including survivors, health-care sector representatives, elected officials, governmental resource entities, law enforcement, and community organizations providing advocacy and services.

Calls to Action

Nothing is impossible. There may be obstacles, which seem extraordinarily difficult, but with tenacity, innovation, and resilience, goals can still be accomplished. Professional organizations should be challenged leverage their resources to enact incremental change with specific, measurable, achievable, realistic, and timely (SMART) goals that equip their members to provide optimal patient care.

Future Implications for Clinical Practice and Research

Suicide Prevention and Foster Care

ACT's demonstrated success in successfully establishing a strategic and innovative pathway to expand an upstream preventive approach, leveraging the trusted power of nursing to reach two new populations. In 2021, the Alliance for Children in Foster Care and the Alliance for Children at Risk for Suicide were launched by NAPNAP Partners. Both populations experience a critical health intersection for trafficking risk. Both initiatives were modeled after ACT, using the same frameworks. A call for leaders was sent to the general membership with a careful vetting process to select a chair and cochair with remaining Alliance members named as "Champions." More work is needed in the area of primary prevention, funding procurement, and outcomes measurement.

Conclusion

The Role of Professional Nursing Organizations

The COVID-19 pandemic has led to increased prevalence of social isolation, depression, and anxiety among teens, contributing to increased vulnerability. Racial and social injustices, health inequities, and poverty are rapidly accelerating risk of exploitation, abuse, and mental health crises. NPVY successfully created a new and innovative nursing model of care to address the public health threat of human trafficking with new horizons including children in foster care and at risk for suicide. NPVY is emerging as an extraordinary national and international leader and advocate by engaging nurses to change the paradigm of trafficking response to an upstream public health approach. They are on a mission to shape public discourse surrounding human trafficking, to challenge the status quo of current reactive approaches, and to inspire nurses around the world to take action to promote child health equity, reducing risk for exploitation and victimization. NPVY works to decrease barriers to care access by engaging and equipping nurses (the nation's largest health-care workforce) with standardized education to skillfully employ trauma-informed health services with a patient-centered, culturally responsive approach for at-risk and victimized persons. This effort has been amplified by replication and dissemination. NPVY is a trailblazer in leading a way forward to engage nurses in a collective response, envisioning a world in which at-risk children are safe from abuse and exploitation.

Useful Resources

NAPNAP Partners	3-PARRT Training	www.napnappartners.org
	ACT Advocate Training	
	Provider Resource Page	
Missouri Department of Mental Health	Missouri Model for Trauma-Informed Care	https://dmh.mo.gov/media/pdf/missouri-model-developmental-framework-trauma-informed-approaches
Stanford Social Innovation Review	A Trauma Lens for Systems Change (the Missouri Model)	https://ssir.org/articles/entry/a_trauma-lens_for_systems_change
U.S. Department of Homeland Security	Blue Campaign—a national public awareness campaign to educate the public, law enforcement, and other industry partners to recognize and respond to human trafficking	https://www.dhs.gov/blue-campaign

U.S. Department of Health and Human Services; National Human Trafficking Training and Technical Assistance Center; Administration for Children and Families; Office on Trafficking in Persons; Office on Women's Health	SOAR to Health and Wellness Training	www.acd.hhs.gov/otip/training/soar-to-health-and-wellness-training/soar-onlineUs
	Core Competencies (with coauthors HEAL Trafficking, NAPNAP, and ICMEC)	
HEAL Trafficking	List-Serv	www.healtrafficking.org
	Protocol Toolkit for Developing a Response to Victims of Human Trafficking	
	Recent Publications and Reports	
	Webinars	
Dignity Health	Shared Learnings Manual	www.dignityhealth.org/hello-humankindness/human-trafficking
	PEARR Tool (A Trauma-Informed Approach to Victim Assistance in Healthcare Settings)	
Shared Hope International	State Report Cards	www.sharedhope.org/what-we-do/bringjustice/reportcards/2021-reportcards/
Polaris	National Human Trafficking Hotline	www.polaris.org
	Annual Statistics	www.humantraffickinghotline.org
U.S. Department of Homeland Security	Blue Campaign—public awareness campaign	www.dhs.gove/blue-campaign
Jones Day Human Trafficking and Health Care Provider Resource	Legal Requirements for Reporting and Education	https://www.jonesday.com/en/insights/2021/09/human-trafficking-and-health-care-providers

References

Albright K, Greenbaum J, Edwards SA, Tsai C. Systematic review of facilitators of, barriers to, and recommendations for healthcare services for child survivors of human trafficking globally. Child Abuse Negl. 2020;100:104289. https://doi.org/10.1016/j.chiabu.2019.104289.

American Nurses Association (ANA). Legislative and regulatory advocacy. Spring, MD: American Nurses Association; 2020. https://www.nursingworld.org/practice-policy/work-environment/health-safety/disaster-preparedness/coronavirus/what-you-need-to-know/legislative-and-regulatory-advocacy/.

Batley C, Chon K, Garrett A, Greenbaum J, Blank S, Hopper E, Murphy L, Peck J, Pfenning E, Robitz R, Stoklosa H. Core competencies for human trafficking response in health care and behavioral health systems. Washington, DC: National Human Trafficking Training and Technical Assistance Center, Office on Trafficking in Persons, Administration for Children and Families, U.S. Department of Health and Human Services; 2021.

Benton B, Peterka-Benton D. Truth as a victim: the challenge of anti-trafficking education. Anti-Traff Rev. 2021;17:113–31. https://doi.org/10.14197/atr.201221177.

Bronfenbrenner U. Toward an experimental ecology of human development. Am Psychol. 1977;32(7):513–31. https://doi.org/10.1037/0003-066X.32.7.513, https://psycnet.apa.org/record/1978-06857-001.

Bronfenbrenner U. The ecology of human development: experiments by nature and design. Cambridge, MA: Harvard University Press; 1979.

Chisolm-Straker M, Baldwin S, Bertille GT, Ndukwe N, Johnson PN, Richardson LD. Health care and human trafficking: we are seeing the unseen. J Healthc Poor Underserv. 2016;27(3):1220–33. https://doi.org/10.1353/hpu.2016.1031.

Chiu P, Duncan S, Whyte N. Charting a research agenda for the advancement of nursing organizations' influence on health systems and policy. Can J Nurs Res. 2020;52:185–93. https://doi.org/10.1177/0844532120928794.

Fang S, Nguyen P, Coverdale J, Gordon M. What are the human trafficking policies of professional medical organizations? J Hum Traff. 2019;7:137–44. https://doi.org/10.1080/23332705.2019.1698895.

Franchino-Olsen H. Vulnerabilities relevant for commercial sexual exploitation of children/domestic minor sex trafficking: a systematic review of risk factors. Trauma Violence Abuse. 2019;22(1):99–111. https://doi.org/10.1177/1524838018821956.

Goldberg AP, Moore JL, Houck C, Kaplan DM, Barron CE. Domestic minor sex trafficking patients: a retrospective analysis of medical presentation. J Pediatr Adolesc Gynecol. 2017;30(1):109–15. https://doi.org/10.1016/j.jpag.2016.08.010.

Health, Education, Advocacy, and Linkages (HEAL) Trafficking. Combating disinformation. Long Beach, CA: HEAL Trafficking; 2021. https://healtrafficking.org/combating-disinformation/.

International Labour Organization (ILO). Forced labour, modern slavery, and human trafficking. Geneva: ILO; 2022. https://www.ilo.org/global/topics/forced-labour/lang_en/index.htm.

Lederer LJ, Wetzel CA. The health consequences of sex trafficking and their implications for identifying victims in healthcare facilities. Annal Health Law. 2014;23(1):61–91. https://lawecommons.luc.edu/annals/vol23/iss1/5/.

National Human Trafficking Training and Technical Assistance Center [NHTTAC]. Core competencies for human trafficking response in health care and behavioral health systems. U.S. Department of Health and Human Services, Administration for Children and Families [ACF], Office of Trafficking in Persons [OTIP], National Human Trafficking Technical Assistance and Training Center [NHTTAC]. Primary authors: Batley, C., Chon, K. (HHS OTIP), Garrett, A. (NHTTAC), Greenbaum, J. (International Centre for Missing and Exploited Children [ICMEC], Hopper, E. (Justice Resource Institute), Murphy, L. (Sheffield Hallam University), Peck, J. (National Association of Pediatric Nurse Practitioners [NAPNAP], Pfenning, E. (HHS OTIP), Robitz, R. (Department of Psychiatry and Behavioral Sciences, University of California Davis), Stoklosa, H. (HEAL Trafficking, Harvard Medical School). 2021. https://nhttac.acf.hhs.gov/resource/report-core-competencies-human-trafficking-response-health-care-and-behavioral-health.

O'Rourke N, Crawford S, Morris N, Pulcini J. Political efficacy and participation of nurse practitioners. Pol Pol Nurs Pract. 2017;18(3):135–48. https://doi.org/10.1177/1527154417728514.

Peck J. Human trafficking of children: nurse practitioner knowledge, beliefs, and experience supporting the development of a practice guideline: Part two. J Pediatr Health Care. 2019;34(2):246–55.

Peck JL. A Train-the-trainer programme to deliver high quality education for healthcare providers. Anti-Traff Rev. 2021;17:140–7. https://doi.org/10.14197/atr.201221179.

Peck JL. Partners for vulnerable youth and the alliance for children in trafficking: using the policy circle model as a framework for change. J Pediatr Health Care. 2022;36(2):144–53. https://doi.org/10.1016/j.pedhc.2020.10.001.

Peck JL, Doiron M. The role of nursing in the school setting to lead efforts to impact child trafficking: an integrative review. J Sch Nurs. 2022;38(1):15–20. https://doi.org/10.1177/1059840520987533.

Peck J, Meadows-Oliver M. Human trafficking of children: nurse practitioner knowledge, beliefs, and experience supporting the development of a practice guideline: Part one. J Pediatr Health Care. 2019;35(3):603–11. https://doi.org/10.1016/j.pedhc.2019.11.005.

Peck JL, Meadows-Oliver M, Hays SM, Maaks DG. White paper: recognizing child trafficking as a critical emerging health threat. J Pediatr Health Care. 2020;35(3):260–9. https://doi.org/10.1016/j.pedhc.2020.01.005.

Peck JL, Greenbaum J, Stoklosa H. Mandated continuing education requirements for health care professional state licensure: the Texas model. J Hum Traff. 2021; https://doi.org/10.1080/23322705.2021.1981708.

Schaffer MA, Strohschein S, Glavin K. Twenty years with the public health intervention wheel: evidence for practice. Public Health Nurs. 2022;39(1):195–201. https://doi.org/10.1111/phn.12941.

Taylor MRS. Impact of advocacy initiatives on nurses' motivation to sustain momentum in public policy advocacy. J Prof Nurs. 2016;32(3):235–45. https://doi.org/10.1016/j.profnurs.2015.10.010.

The United Nations Office on Drugs and Crime (UNODC). Global report on trafficking in persons 2020. Vienna: UNODC; 2020. https://www.unodc.org/documents/data-and-analysis/tip/2021/GLOTiP_2020_15jan_web.pdf.

United States Department of Justice (DOJ). Key legislation. Washington, DC: DOJ; 2022. https://www.justice.gov/humantrafficking/key-legislation.

United States Department of State. Understanding human trafficking: fact sheet. Washington, DC: Office to Monitor and Combat Trafficking in Persons; 2021. https://www.state.gov/what-is-trafficking-in-persons/.

Yoder-Wise P. A framework for planned policy change. Nurs Forum. 2020;55:45–53. https://doi.org/10.1111/nuf.12381.

Evolution of a Complex and Home Care Program for Children with Chronic Diseases

Clara Li Ying Lam, Yanyin Zeng, Bettina Li Hoon Tan, Cristelle Chu-Tian Chow, and Yoke Hwee Chan

Introduction

Children with medical complexity (CMC) are a well-recognized population with high health-care needs globally and continue to be a growing phenomenon (Brenner et al. 2018). They represent about 3% of the pediatric population in the United States (Barnert et al. 2019) and approximately 0.7% in Canada (Orkin et al. 2019). In Japan, 9403 CMC were reported in 2005, increasing to 17,078 in 2015 (Matsuzawa et al. 2020).

CMC refer to children and youth with chronic conditions related to medical fragility, presence of functional limitations, increased health and other service needs, and escalated health-care expenditures (Cohen et al. 2018). They are often dependent on medical technology such as home ventilation, oxygen therapy, tracheostomy care, and gastrostomy or tube feeding to allow a reasonable quality of life. Conventional health-care systems are unable to address the holistic care required for CMC, which requires significant coordination between tertiary hospital and

C. L. Y. Lam (✉) · Y. Zeng · B. L. H. Tan
Nursing Clinical Services, Division of Nursing, KK Women's and Children's Hospital, Singapore, Singapore
e-mail: Lam.Li.Ying@kkh.com.sg

C. C.-T. Chow
Division of Medicine, KK Women's and Children's Hospital, Singapore, Singapore

Y. H. Chan
Division of Medicine, KK Women's and Children's Hospital, Singapore, Singapore

Yong Loo Lin School of Medicine, National University of Singapore, Singapore, Singapore

Duke-NUS Medical School, Singapore, Singapore

© The Author(s), under exclusive license to Springer Nature Switzerland AG 2023
C. L. Betz (ed.), *Worldwide Successful Pediatric Nurse-Led Models of Care*,
https://doi.org/10.1007/978-3-031-22152-1_6

91

community resources (Berry et al. 2013; Cohen et al. 2012). With increasing evidence that the optimal environment for a developing child is in a caring home setting (Davies et al. 2014; Namachivayam et al. 2012) rather than in hospital, a nurse-led home care model of care was designed in our institution to improve the provision of community nursing care for CMC. Since 2001, this nurse-led program was developed allowing home care nurses to exercise autonomy in caring for children with complex health needs in Singapore. It focuses on coordination and planning for discharge of children from hospital and provides continual support to them after discharge. This innovative program shifted the emphasis from physician-led, hospital-based care to a nurse-led, community-based model, providing nurses with the opportunity to participate actively in program leadership and development.

This chapter provides an overview of a multidisciplinary nurse-led CMC program for CMC in Singapore. It includes the background on how the program has transformed over the past two decades, using a theoretical framework as a guide for service development, detailed description of the nurse-led role in the service, the challenges and facilitators faced in the development and implementation of the model, the lessons learned, and the future plans for the service.

Background

Medical advances have resulted in improved survival of children with critical care illness and chronic medical conditions, leading to a growing number of CMC (Burns et al. 2010; Cohen and Patel 2014). These children need significantly more healthcare services than their peers and are often dependent on medical technology (Berry et al. 2013; Glader et al. 2016). The "medical home" also known as a "health home" concept involves a patient-centered (Medicaid 2021), multidisciplinary model of care that is coordinated and holistic (Kingsnorth et al. 2015; Kuo 2019; Avritscher et al. 2019). This chapter chronicles the evolution of a Children's Complex and Home Care Program over a 20-year period, with highlights on the challenges faced and service adjustment over the years.

In 2000, a group of critical care nurses and physicians at the KK Women's and Children's Hospital (KKH), the largest pediatric tertiary hospital in Singapore, brought to attention an increased number of children dependent on medical technology who had prolonged intensive care unit (ICU) and hospital length of stay. If they are discharged, they inevitably required multiple hospital readmissions. This stemmed from the lack of community facilities to cater to the complex care needs of these children and the lack of a structured program to provide care coordination for home discharge. This sparked discussion among the team of health-care professionals consisting of ICU nurses, doctors, and allied health professionals (medical social workers (MSW), respiratory therapists, and physiotherapists) who were involved in the care of these children. This multidisciplinary team proposed a Pediatric Home Care Service (PHCS) as a pilot to enable the transition of children who are medically stable but require medical technology support, from hospital to home, in a safe and of holistic care manner, which is centered on the child and the family unit (Fig. 1).

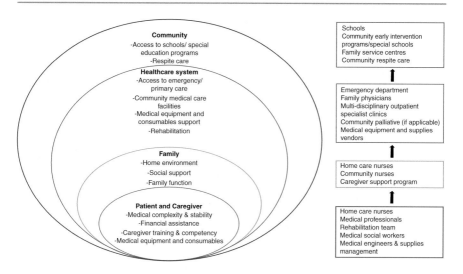

Fig. 1 Pediatric home care service (PHCS) model of care

Over the next 20 years, the service expanded in both scale and scope beyond children who require medical technology into the Children's Complex and Home Care Service (CCHS) to include CMC who require three or more pediatric subspecialties for care. It also transitioned from philanthropic to a more sustainable mainstream government-funded program.

This chapter chronicles the evolution of the PHCS to the CCHS over two decades.

Target Population and Setting

KKH is a women's and children's hospital that provides the majority of the tertiary care for obstetrics, neonatal and pediatric patients in Singapore. The PHCS was established in 2001 to facilitate safe and seamless home discharge for the group of children who required long-term support on medical technology including mechanical ventilation, oxygen therapy, tracheostomy care, gastrostomy or tube feeding, and stoma care. Children with acute illnesses who had stabilized and those with chronic conditions who require long-term support with medical technology were referred to the PHCS nurses for coordination of care and discharge planning. The service evolved into the CCHS in April 2017 with pediatricians providing care oversight, and expansion of service goals to deliver coordinated, cost-effective, and patient-and family-centered care to CMC and their families in addition to the existing nursing support provided to technology-dependent children without medical complexity. The referral criteria for CMC included children with (1) chronic illness requiring three or more subspecialty care services, (2) medical fragility, and (3) a need for care coordination.

Since 2001, more than 2300 technology-dependent children have successfully transited from hospital into the community. To date, 146 CMC have received care coordination from CCHS. As the CMC population grows, a transitional model of care from hospital to home was established to foster positive outcomes through understanding the needs and experiences of caregivers during transitions from hospital to home (Ronan et al. 2020).

Process Undertaken to Implement This Model

The PHCS was first set up in 2001 with the main objective to allow children who require long-term medical technology to be discharged home once they are medically stable. This program was based on the premise that there were suitable caregiver(s) and family support, and on the assumption that the child's recovery and development is best optimized in the home and community setting. The team aimed to build a model of care that was family- and patient-centered, where healthcare, community, and education services were built on this framework of care (Fig. 1). The development of the service involved several planning steps: (1) projection of service workload, (2) budget projection on operating, manpower, and capital equipment expenditure, (3) medical equipment and consumable acquisition and inventory management, (4) caregiver training modules, (5) care plans based on idealized patient journey and patient care, and (6) postdischarge follow-up.

Workload Projection

The team undertook a review of the workload of children who required long-term technology support from various medical specialties across pediatric surgical, medical, and neonatal departments in the hospital. It was estimated that the main support needed was nasogastric or gastrostomy feeding (60%), followed by naso/oropharyngeal suctioning (18%), oxygen therapy (13%), and tracheostomy care (9%). Majority (>70%) required only one type of technology support. Approximately 1 in 10 children would require home ventilation support, either invasive via tracheostomy or noninvasive via external interfaces, and these children were more likely to require more than two types of support at home. The team also projected a 20% year-on-year increase in workload in the initial years as majority of the children were likely to require support for more than a year.

Budget Planning

Based on the workload projection, a budget projection was planned out for manpower, capital equipment and consumables, and other operating expenditures. While Singapore residents were entitled to government subsidies for inpatient and outpatient bills based on financial means testing, no funding existed for portable medical equipment and consumables nor home visits by nurses for technology-dependent children at home. Additional resources for manpower, such as home care nurses, medical engineers, operations support for inventory management, were needed. Starting as a proof-of-concept model, the team secured philanthropic funding.

Home Medical Equipment and Consumables

The market for medical equipment and consumables for children was small, especially with the small national population of approximately 4.1 million in 2001 and the absence of a home model of care for technology-dependent children and adults. The team worked with the hospital medical engineering and procurement team to raise formal invitation to bid for a term service contract, as well as to engage equipment vendors to trial and identify suitable home medical equipment to cater for the different home care needs. Service agreements were also drawn up for round-the-clock equipment support, preventive maintenance, and inventory management.

Caregiver Training

The team felt that caregiver competency and comfort in caring for a chronic sick child with medical technology was a key element to the success of the service. The home care nurses devised clear instructions with pictorial guides and competency checklists for each medical technology. For safety and to prevent caregiver burnout, it was decided that there should at least be two trained and competent caregivers for each patient.

Care Plans

As each child had unique medical conditions and the service would cater for a heterogeneous group of patients, the team decided that a customized care manual that included the case summary, types of medical support, subspecialty care providers, medications, and emergency hotlines would be provided to each child before discharge. This would be planned by the CCHS home care nurse who would be the key worker and main liaison person, and revised based on the changing needs of the child.

Postdischarge Care

The care after discharge was comprised of two components: (1) home visits performed by the home care nurses and (2) outpatient specialist visits. Besides performing medical checks on the child with long-term conditions, the purpose of the home visits was also to assess the home environment, perform caregiver competency checks, and to check on the medical equipment. A home visit checklist was drafted to facilitate documentation.

In 2016, PHCS was renamed as Children's Complex and Home Care Services (CCHS) as CMC were identified to be growing in numbers. Subsequently, in 2018, a CCHS home care nurse was granted the Health Manpower Development Program (HMDP) award to Montreal Children's Hospital and Hospital for Sick Children in Canada to cognize how respective complex care services collaborate across their multidisciplinary team. By 2019, the nursing manpower of CCHS has expanded to seven registered nurses.

Theoretical Framework

It is essential to provide holistic care for every CMC to ensure that an effective, safety, and competent health-care delivery system is in place, so as to promote improved health-care quality with enhanced care coordination (Peterson et al. 2019). The theoretical framework for CCHS (initially named PHCS) transitional model of care from hospital to home is similar to the conceptual model of the Integrated Complex Care Model (ICCM) (Cohen et al. 2011a), delivering family- and child-centered care to every CMC. A pediatrician serves as both the clinical and system key worker, ensuring that both clinical and system needs are met. The focus of clinical needs is child-centered and includes overseeing of the medical/long-term care treatment, providing care coordination, and following through the care plan created for each CMC. System-related care needs refer to the provision of family-centered care. The main caregiver provides information about the child's condition to the CCHS home care nurses when required, allowing proper allocation of community resources for CMC's health needs. A CCHS home care nurse works as a system key worker performing various simultaneous tasks including the following: being a consistent source of contact through, providing nursing advice including caregiver training, troubleshooting and procuring medical equipment for home use, and assisting with the change of appointments and prescriptions.

The ICCM comprises of four main components and are classified into shared care, team-based care, joint accountability, and electronic care plans (Cohen et al. 2011a). These components emphasize that services are based on multidisciplinary collaboration and integrated care for every CMC.

Shared Care

The ICCM *shared care* component acknowledges that an individual organization cannot fulfill the lifelong care and comprehensive care requirements of a CMC, especially when the child reaches the transitional age of 16 and beyond. CMC will require ongoing community services including education and rehabilitation, respite care, home care, and at times palliative care across their lifespan (Cohen et al. 2012).

Additionally, transition of care to the adult setting requires a collaboration with adult hospital and providers and community services, home care support, and rehabilitation services. To scale up community resources for long-term and respite care for CMCs, the team lobbied and collaborated with community hospitals, nursing homes, and palliative care to provide the necessary training and medical support.

Team-Based Care

A multidisciplinary team ensures the delivery of high-value care to individual CMC. Team-based care is an approach to prevent miscommunication and medical errors that can lead to frustration of patients and caregivers, poor health outcomes, and inefficient and unnecessary expenditure of health resources (Cohen et al. 2011a). The CCHS team consists of pediatricians, home care nurses, physiotherapists, occupational therapists, speech and language therapists, dieticians, pharmacists, MSWs, care coordinators, administrative managers, biomedical engineers (BME), and materials and management department (MMD) staff (Table 1). The role of each team member is clearly defined while ensuring regular multidisciplinary team meetings for case discussions and consistency of care.

Table 1 Roles and responsibilities of team members

CCHS home care nurses
• Develops, implements, and evaluates the nursing care for the following group of patients requiring home care with
• Tracheostomies, invasive and noninvasive ventilators, oxygen devices, naso-gastric and naso-jejunal tube feeding, clean-intermittent catheterization, stoma care, home total parenteral nutrition, other specialized medical equipment and care that require home care services
• Performs caregiver training and assessment, equipment acquisition, and devise individualized care plans before discharge
• Performs home environment assessment
• Performs home visits
• Coordinates multidisciplinary clinics
• Coordinates multidisciplinary discussions
• Provides phone consults for caregivers
• Serves as a liaison person for clinical problem solving and professional issues for CCHS patients with Director of CCHS service, primary physician, other allied health-care professionals, medical equipment providers, BME staff, and voluntary support groups
• Understands and troubleshoot the technical aspects of the supportive equipment used by patients
Physicians
• Performs medical assessment and works with CCHS home care nurses on care planning

(continued)

Table 1 (continued)

Medical social worker
• Performs psychosocial assessment and if needed, counseling
• Performs financial assessment and if needed, financial assistance
• Assist patients with Early Intervention school application
• Collaboration with family service centers
• Collaboration with Ministry of Social and Family Development (MSF)

Care coordinator
• Assists CCHS home care nurses on care coordination, e.g., multidisciplinary clinics, home visits

Administrative manager
• Maintains home care database and equipment inventory
• Works with finance department on financial reporting and claims from funding agent (e.g., philanthropy and government sources)

Physiotherapist
• Assess gross motor skills
• Assess hip/swash braces and splints
• Assess and recommend suitable equipment

Occupational therapist
• Provision of equipment
• Assess patient's buggy to ensure good fitting
• Performs home visit for home modifications
• Assess on seating and positioning

Pharmacist
• Works with CCHS home care nurses and physicians on providing recommendations on medications
• Follow-up with outpatients to understand on their medical conditions and recommendation to physician on drug dosages
• Facilitation of consumables requisites for home care patients purchase

Biomedical engineer
• Works with home care nurses/physicians/respiratory therapists on trial of new equipment and assessment for suitability for home care
• Works on specifications home care equipment, raises call for tender, and closes contract with vendor
• Maintains preventive maintenance contract
• Monitors maintenance and repairs of home medical equipment

Materials and management department staff
• Sources for suitable home medical consumables and equipment

Joint Accountability

Integrated care is made possible when care providers are agreeable to uphold the care responsibilities of CMC. Collaboration with various community partners where CMC can be taken care at when they are stable to be discharged from acute hospital care settings. Star PALS (Paediatric Advanced Life Support) provides palliative care for CMC at home, while St. Andrew Community Hospital (SACH) and

Singapore Christian Home (SCH) provide both short-term and long-term care according to respective CMC's needs. As for respite care, Assisi Hospice provides it on a short-term basis and follow-up on care needs such as wound dressing during the stay.

Electronic Care Plans

Effective communication with multiple care providers is essential. The team leverages electronic care plans through electronic medical records to ensure care continuity with different health-care providers. Health-care professionals within the health-care system can access up-to-date information on CMC's clinical assessments, prescriptions, social background, investigations and appointments. As some external organizations do not have access to National Electronic Health Records (NEHR), communication with these partners takes the form electronic correspondence and teleconferences with proper documentation into the health records.

Organizational Component

The organizational components of the nurse-led home care model are illustrated in Fig. 2. The CCHS director oversees the operation of entire program. A team of CCHS pediatricians provide oversight on the overall care required for each CMC, mainly focusing on clinical aspects.

CCHS home care nurses play a pivotal role in care coordination and collaboration with external community partners to facilitate smooth transition from hospital to home. The position scope of practice is categorized into two aspects—clinical and administrative, which are further sub-categorized (Fig. 2). During hospitalizations, CCHS home care nurses equip caregivers of CMC with the appropriate knowledge and skills in managing the required medical technology at home. In addition, postdischarge follow-up is performed to monitor the progress of CMC through outpatient multidisciplinary clinic visits and regular home visitations. Caregivers also have access to on-demand assistance from CCHS home care nurses when required through a phone hotline, such as troubleshooting of medical equipment alarms, advice on tracheostomy as well as gastrostomy care, rescheduling of medical appointments, and requesting for medication prescriptions.

Apart from patient care, CCHS home care nurses perform administrative work such as evaluation, procurement, and maintenance of new and existing equipment, as well as preparation of consumable lists customized to each individual child's needs. This requires coordination with the medical team, MSW for financial assistance, external equipment and consumable vendors, BME, MMD, and pharmacy. CCHS home care nurses are also heavily involved in nursing education through in-service and skills trainings of nurses based in inpatient units and the community setting, such as community hospitals and nursing homes. Regular review of risk

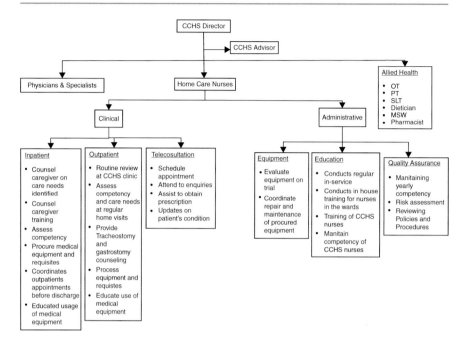

Fig. 2 Organizational components

assessment and policies are done to ensure patient safety such as assuring nursing practices and caregiver training modules are up to date, correct use of current and new medical equipment, as well as performing regular home visitations to caregivers are consistent in their care for CMC.

Service Components of CCHS

The involvement of CCHS home care nurses starts at the point of a referral from the primary clinical team. Firstly, a clinical interview is performed to ascertain caregiver understanding on patient's diagnosis, prognosis, and treatment plans. A detailed assessment of the social background is also determined, including identification of the primary caregiver and potential psychosocial stressors affecting the child and family. Specific caregiver concerns provide insight into the readiness for discharge. The common caregiver concerns are as follows:

1. Uncertainty of care ability: Caregivers often have self-doubt and lack confidence in caring for their children on medical technology, especially as laypersons without nursing experience.
2. Lack of appropriate caregiver support: Most families have a single parent as the sole caregiver of their technology-dependent child, while the other parent attempts to sustain employment to support the family financially. This results in

significant caregiver burden for the sole caregiver and strains on family relationships.
3. Lack of conducive environment: A conducive environment to care for CMC may not be available for some families due to challenging socioeconomic circumstances. Discharge planning can be delayed if the home environment is deemed unsuitable for the care of CMC.
4. Financial constraints: Expenses in supporting the care needs of CMC can be high, causing significant financial strain especially for low- to middle-income households.

As caregiver readiness contributes greatly to the success of transition from hospital to home, individualized plans based on caregiver concerns will be needed to establish caregiver readiness in preparation for home. A physical examination is done to determine a baseline on CMC's physical findings. This will help CCHS home care nurses to differentiate any abnormalities or new physical findings during postdischarge home visit.

Caregiver Training and Assessment

After identification of the primary caregiver(s), assessment of caregiver(s) learning needs, and the required home care procedures to be conducted are identified, a caregiver training (CGT) schedule is planned out. Depending on complexity of the patient's care needs, the average duration for completion of CGT ranges from 3 days to 1 month.

The procedures taught under CGT include (1) enteral feeding and care, (2) nasogastric tube insertion, (3) tracheostomy tube insertion and care, (4) invasive and noninvasive ventilation, (5) naso-oropharyngeal suctioning, and (6) oxygen therapy. The CCHS home care nurse provides a demonstration of the procedure and caregivers are required to perform at least three return demonstrations on the patient to be deemed competent. Caregivers are also taught infant or child cardiopulmonary resuscitation (CPR) skills just prior to discharge date.

Medical, Psychosocial and Financial Assessment

During the CMC's hospitalization, pediatricians conduct regular clinical assessments to ascertain medical fitness for discharge. An assigned MSW collaborates with CCHS home care nurses in performing psychosocial assessments to identify caregivers experiencing high levels of stress when providing psychosocial counseling and emotional support. Caregivers at high risk of clinical depression or anxiety are referred to psychiatrists or psychologists for further mental wellness interventions. The MSW conducts a financial assessment to determine eligibility for government or hospital financial assistance programs. This process facilitates the processing of medical equipment and consumables for discharge preparation.

Home Environment Assessment

There is significant variation in the level of care needs required by CMC, which can range from enteral feeding alone to invasive ventilation support via a tracheostomy. This correlates with the amount of medical equipment needed, which is operated at home. Additionally, most CMC have mobility limitations requiring mobility aids and devices such as wheelchairs and customized wheelchairs. A home environment assessment is therefore essential to ensure the suitability and safety of the home setting in catering to the CMC's specific care needs. This individualized home assessment is especially needed to prevent overloading of electrical points with multiple medical equipment, which may result in fire hazards (Samantha 2018). Appropriate recommendations are also provided on placement of medical equipment, medical consumables and patient's bed. Referrals to occupational therapists are made to facilitate the installation of ramps and handlebars to enhance the CMC's safety and accessibility at home.

Equipment and Consumables Assessment and Procurement

Selection of appropriate medical equipment and associated consumables required for CMC is performed by CCHS home care nurses. The decision-making process is influenced by various factors including clinical needs, equipment models and specifications, with consideration of cost effectiveness and logistical limitations.

CCHS home care nurses initiate the procurement process of medical equipment through submission of an electronic purchase request. This is processed via a materials and management department's (MMD) representative to a purchase order to the respective vendor(s) before the medical equipment is brought to BME department. BME engineers facilitate the commissioning of the medical equipment before it is certified safe for patient use. Subsequent to that, the medical equipment for home use is used by the patient with inpatient monitoring for a minimum of 24 h prior to hospital discharge.

Care Planning and Coordination

Care planning starts upon initiation of CGT. A training schedule is created with the goal of establishing caregiver competency in caring for CMC at home. Simultaneously, allied health professionals such as the physiotherapist, occupational therapist, speech and language therapist conduct CGT with a focus on the therapy procedures that should be performed at home. Upon confirmation of discharge date, the pharmacist prepares the prescribed medication and provides a medication schedule for caregivers. CCHS home care nurses and pharmacists collaborate with inpatient nurses to provide education on medication administration to prevent drug errors especially in the setting of polypharmacy. Lastly, the MSW ensures caregivers are mentally prepared for the transition of care from hospital to home. For CMC whose caregivers are unable to care for them in the home setting, pediatricians and CCHS home care nurses assess the CMC's suitability for placement in long-term care facilities.

Outpatient Clinics

Multidisciplinary outpatient clinics enable CMC and families to access various subspecialists, allied health professionals, and CCHS home care nurses for continued care postdischarge. One week prior to each clinic session, CCHS home care nurses consolidate caregiver concerns in order to plan the necessary consultations required. Care plans are discussed during multidisciplinary meetings to prepare all team members for the clinic session. During the session, CCHS home care nurses perform physical assessments and needed procedures such as gastrostomy button change, adjustment and checking on ventilation settings, and scheduling of appointments and processing of prescriptions.

Home Visits

Upon the discharge of a CMC, home visitations are done via physical visits or video consultations by the CCHS home care nurses. A physical visit will be conducted for newly discharged CMC 1 week postdischarge or earlier, especially when the primary caregiver requires reinforcement on care for CMC at home. Otherwise, video consultations are carried out to minimize physical interactions during the current COVID-19 pandemic. For subsequent home visits, it will be done on a 3 monthly or 6 monthly basis, depending on the patient's degree of medical complexity and technological dependence.

Roles of the CCHS Home Care Nurse

Referral of eligible patient made to the home care team are based on the following list of criteria which includes home oxygen therapy, suctioning, enteral feeding (Nasogastric tube feeding, nasojejunal tube feeding, gastrostomy feeding, gastrojejunostomy feeding), tracheostomy care, non-invasive ventilation, invasive ventilation and cardiopulmonary resuscitation. An overview of CCHS workflow for CMC is shown in Fig. 3. This illustrates the role of the CCHS home care nurses in managing the care of CMC.

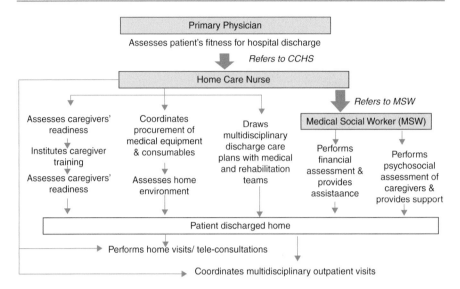

Fig. 3 Children's complex and home care service (CCHS) workflow for child with medical complexity (CMC)

Patient Assessment

Upon receiving the referral, CCHS home care nurse reviews the patient's medical history to understand the patient's background and care needs. Thereafter, CCHS home care nurse reviews the patient in the ward and introduces home care services to the caregivers. If the caregiver is unavailable, CCHS home care nurse contacts them to arrange a meet up. During the first meeting with caregivers, CCHS home care nurse explains the indication of care requirement in view of medical condition of the child and the need for the referral to the CCHS team. Identification of the primary caregivers are discussed and identified according to patient's care needs. Caregivers are also informed of the required caregiver training, competency assessment and the procurement of medical equipment as per patient's care needs. Through conversations with the caregivers, their readiness will be assessed.

Caregiver Training and Assessment

Once caregivers inform CCHS that they are ready for training, the CCHS home care nurse arranges suitable training dates with the caregivers to achieve a target discharge date. While patient is still in hospital, the list of medical supplies will be prepared by the CCHS home care nurse with a projected discharge date. Medical supplies are packed by the home care pharmacy, and caregiver is informed once it is ready for collection. Caregivers are also required to submit relevant and supporting documents to apply for government subsidies or financial assistance from philanthropic funding for the medical supplies.

Medical Equipment Procurement and Consumable Supply

For patients requiring medical equipment, CCHS home care nurse may suggest changes to patient's home to ensure that the home environment is safe with appropriate space for placement of the required equipment as well as to minimize the risk of fire hazards. If required, CCHS home care nurse and occupational therapist also do combined home visits prior to hospital discharge to provide further improvements to the home environment. Photographs of the home setup of patients with similar medical equipment may be shown to caregiver to provide visual examples.

Every equipment is required to be validated to be safe for use by BME. For new equipment, the contract agreement consists of a 5-year warranty. The first 2 years include preventive maintenance and repair cost. Subsequently, caregiver will bear the partial cost of equipment repair, based on their funding status. Caregivers are instructed to contact the vendor when they face issues with the equipment. For equipment which are no longer economical to repair, CCHS home care nurse will arrange for a replacement unit and liaise with vendor for delivery of unit to the patient.

There is an accompanying list of consumables for every medical equipment to be used by CMC for treatment (Table 2). A month's quantity of consumables will be prepared by home care pharmacist prior to their discharge date.

Table 2 Types of medical technology with their associated equipment and consumables

Medical technology	Medical equipment	Medical consumables
Oxygen therapy	• Oxygen concentrator	• Oxygen tubings
	• Oxygen cylinders	• Oximeter probes
	• Pulse oximeter	• Nasal cannulas
Home mechanical ventilation	• Ventilator	• Nasal or mask interface
	• Humidifier	• Connection tubings
	• Oxygen cylinders	• Bacterial filters
	• Bag-valve-mask equipment	• Oximeter probes
	• Pulse oximeter	
Tracheostomy	• +/− suction machine	• Tracheostomy tubes
	• Pulse oximeter	• +/− suction tubings
		• Suction catheters
		• Tracheostomy ties
		• 0.9% Normal saline
		• Sterile gauze
		• Lubricant
		• Dressing set
		• Sterile gloves
Nasogastric/ gastrostomy feeding	• +/− feeding pumps	• Nasogastric/gastrostomy tubings
		• Feeding bags/feeding syringes
		• Hyperfix tapes
		• pH papers
		• Sterile gauze
		• 0.9% Normal saline
		• Stomahesive powder

Discharge Planning

Prior to patient's discharge, post discharge home visits are arranged either through physical home visits or video consultations. The first physical home visit or video consultation is scheduled 1 week after discharge to ensure patient and caregiver are settling well or earlier if needed. A care manual prepared by the CCHS home care nurse is given to caregiver which consists of patient's brief medical history, list of medical equipment vendors, and CCHS home care nurse hotline.

On the day of discharge for patients on mechanical ventilation, CCHS home care nurses accompany them home with the caregivers. In the process of discharge, primary caregivers will be taught by CCHS home care nurses on transfer of CMC from bed to customized wheelchair, placement of medical equipment during transportation, and monitoring of CMC's condition during the travel. Upon reaching home, arrangement of medical equipment and consumable requisites are demonstrated and taught by the CCHS home care nurses.

Home Visits and Tele-Consultations

During the postdischarge and routine home visits/video consultations, the patient is assessed for his/her well-being and caregivers are again assessed on their competencies for caregiving procedures. CCHS home care nurses also review feeding regime, medications, and upcoming medical appointments. The patient's medical equipment is also assessed for its functionality and that preventive maintenance is up to date. These visits are documented and communicated to other members of the CCHS.

Looking after a CMC at home can be a daunting task for the layperson caregiver. A home care hotline manned by CCHS home care nurses is available for enquiries and support.

Training and Collaboration with Health-Care Providers

To ensure our patients have care continuity of care in the community, CCHS collaborates with private nursing agencies and community hospitals to expand their capabilities in pediatric care. CCHS team delivers talks and provides training and education for nurses and doctors on the care of CMCs. The training curricula for community nurses include didactic lectures, hands-on training, and competency checks to ensure that they are eligible to provide nursing care for CMCs in the community. This collaboration with community providers has been important to enable practice capacity for respite care and seamless transition care of these children as they grow into adults.

CCHS home care nurses conduct lectures for nursing students in tertiary institution on the services provided by the home care team. CCHS home care nurses also conduct in-service talks for the KKH's nurses on home care procedures, which might not be frequently performed in certain ward.

Liaison with Medical Equipment Vendors

CCHS home care nurses constantly keep themselves updated on home medical equipment launches from vendors and assess the need to procure new products. As part of the evaluation, CCHS home care nurses review the safety, effectiveness, ease of use, and cost.

Recruitment of Home Care Nurses

CCHS home care nurses are registered nurses under the Singapore Nursing Board and with a minimum of 2 years' experience in pediatric intensive care. Proficiency in the clinical management of children with medical high needs is imperative to the nature of work as a CCHS home care nurse. This position requires nurses to be confident in managing unanticipated, emergency situations in the home setting, which involves critical and innovative thinking. As well, CCHS home care nurses also need to be flexible and adapt to different caregiver learning styles and be responsive to their ongoing needs for support as they care for their child with CMC.

Methods of Evaluation

The effectiveness of the service is evaluated through health-care resource utilization, caregiver burden, and quality-of-life assessments. The service annually audits data on the number of visits to the Children's Emergency Department, number of unplanned hospitalizations, and the length of stay of these hospitalizations. Additionally, caregiver Patient Health Questionnaire-9 (PHQ-9) and Perceived Stress Scale (PSS) scores obtained over a longitudinal period can provide insight into the degree of caregiver burden experienced (Kroenke et al. 2001; Cohen et al. 1983). PHQ-9 and PSS are internationally recognized and evidence-based self-administered questionnaires used to screen for caregiver risk of depression and measure perceived stress, respectively. The quality-of-life assessment most applicable to the CMC population is KIDSCREEN, which provides parameters that can be answered by caregivers in the case of children with limited communicative ability (Bullinger et al. 2002).

Challenges

Lack of Community Facilities for Long-Term and Respite Care

A successful transition of a CMC from hospital to home is evidenced by a thriving child in the community who is able to achieve his/her developmental potential with minimal unplanned emergency visits and hospitalizations (Berry 2015). In situations where complex family backgrounds are unable to support the care of the CMC at home, placement in long-term care facilities or foster care may be required (Seltzer et al. 2016). However, in a country with a small CMC population, there are limited facilities equipped to support the high medical needs of these children, resulting in prolonged hospitalizations, which can be detrimental to their long-term emotional and psychological development (Davies et al. 2014).

The extensive burden of care experienced by families with technology-dependent children arises from increased stress associated with greater parental responsibility (Page et al. 2020). Caregivers can suffer from chronic fatigue and burnout, which can then compromise the quality of patient care (Chan et al. 2019; Toly et al. 2019). Respite care is a service option that provides families with a break from the demands of daily patient care and allows caregivers to attend to personal needs, rejuvenate, and recharge before continuing with the patient care journey (Breneol et al. 2019). It has been shown that respite care for caregivers is a key component in the success-ful transition of a patient from hospital to home (Elias et al. 2012). Although respite care is recognized as a key component to relieve caregiver burden, its limited acces-sibility to all technology-dependent patients and families has been identified as an international unmet need, with few available facilities catering for such patients (Sobotka et al. 2019). Additionally, despite upskilling nurses in the community sec-tor, a high staff turnover has resulted in significant staff shortage and inadequate service provision. This is evident in recent report (Tan 2021) that an increase in the number of resignation of health-care workers in Singapore have resulted in con-straints to the delivery of patient care.

With the government focusing more on the aging population, there are more community facilities such as day care activity centers and community hospitals, which are being built for the elderly to be cared for in the community and to encour-age independent living in Singapore (Ministry of Health 2019). Health-care profes-sionals should continue advocating for the unmet needs of CMC, to encourage government funding of similar facilities catered to the unique characteristics of CMCs and their families.

Responsible Care of Medical Equipment

It is assumed that the responsibility of the ongoing care and maintenance of home medical equipment lies with caregivers. However, inappropriate handling of equip-ment such as noncompliance to routine maintenance or overuse can result in reduced equipment lifespan and compromise in patient safety. Caregivers may also misplace equipment parts or entire units, resulting in increased health-care expenditure asso-ciated with equipment replacement. It is recommended that caregivers acknowledge and sign relevant agreements and indemnity documents so as to reinforce proper equipment handling, including timely maintenance and repairs.

Life support units require 24/7 maintenance and support, which is a demanding service commitment. This results in shrinking of the pool of available equipment in an already limited supply of units suitable for pediatric use that exists in Singapore. As the population of technology-dependent individuals in the country remains small, pooling of equipment among different health-care institutions with standardization of contractual agreements may provide more comprehensive options and on-demand service for patients. As medical technology advances, regular discussions with equipment vendors open up opportunities for new equipment to be brought into the market, in order to meet the changing needs of pediatric patients.

Funding

Means-tested subsidies can provide financial assistance to eligible families, but such programs often fail to acknowledge the high health-care costs of CMC (Allshouse et al. 2018). At times, means testing may also be perceived as an intrusion of privacy. Delays in approval of government subsidies can also contribute to prolonged hospitalization and conversely increase health-care resource utilization. When families are unable to afford escalating health-care costs, this may result in unwillingness to cooperate with care recommendations including compliance to routine equipment maintenance, which can result in compromise to patient safety and well-being (Baddour et al. 2021).

Caregiver's Psychological and Physical Health

In line with the country's strategy of "Beyond hospital to community" (Ng 2021), there is increased emphasis on home-based care. This has resulted in a significant increase in informal caregivers providing a high level of care within homes. The roles and responsibilities of caregivers have intensified significantly in light of their multiple duties that extend beyond just child-rearing (Woodgate et al. 2015). Caregivers of technology-dependent children experience frequent headaches, anxiety, depression, and chronic fatigue, often contributed by sleep deprivation and stress (Page et al. 2020; Woodgate et al. 2015). This could also influence the quality of care rendered to patients affecting their health and safety.

Disruption of family and day-to-day life through increased caregiver responsibilities can result in strained family relationships between parents and parent-child relationships with well siblings of CMC. The extensive time and attention spent on CMC can result in a perception of neglect among siblings and spouses (Page et al. 2020).

Facilitators

Collaboration

Ongoing collaboration with intermediate- and long-term care facilities such as community hospitals, nursing homes, and hospices provides opportunities to support the care of children within their community. This also enhances the physical and psychosocial well-being of caregivers. Provision of staff training and ongoing on-demand support can upskill community providers to care for CMC. Increased staff confidence also encourages more families to access new services to support their children, without excessive reliance on tertiary centers, significantly reducing health-care resource utilization. To date, our program has successfully engaged various private organizations to provide home-based respite care, and has provided training for nurses in a community hospital, nursing home, and hospice to support CMC.

Philanthropic Funding

Volunteer welfare organizations rely heavily on philanthropic funding to continue service provision in the community. Continued access to both government-supported grants and philanthropic funds provides health-care institutions with a greater range of services to cater for CMC. Government and philanthropic funding enables more opportunities for staff training, to empower more nurses with the skills and confidence required to care for CMC in the community.

Caregiver Support Programs (Psychosocial Counselling and Respite Care)

Caregiver support programs can reduce caregiver burden through psychosocial counseling delivered by trained personnel and enhance social network interaction between different caregivers through opportunities to gather and patient care experiences (Sung and Park 2012). Many such programs are currently supported through philanthropic funding or grants from local organizations. Through these programs, nurses are also able to engage caregivers outside of the hospital setting, while continuing to provide emotional support.

Service Adjustments Made

Medical Equipment Procurement and Maintenance

With increasing numbers of CMC with more complex medical needs, engaging a wider network of vendors has enhanced opportunities to trial new medical equipment while ensuring market competitiveness and affordability. Increased options for service and equipment provision also ensure continued high quality of technical support in the homes and, enhancing patient safety.

Funding

In the early 2000s, children who were dependent on medical technology were not discharged from the acute hospital. They remained inpatient till they were able to be weaned off technological support, or till their demise, largely due to a paucity of community-based support for pediatric home care and funding for home care equipment. As the PHCS was developed, charitable organizations and hospital endowment funds were the main sources of financial assistance for needy families, particularly to cover the cost of expensive home care equipment. However, the access to these funds was significantly limited by the need for means-testing, resulting in a large proportion of middle-class families not meeting the criteria to qualify for such financial assistance. It became evident that government-supported home care funding was imperative. The philanthropy-funded PHCS model provided data on health-care cost savings of approximately SGD 22 million in a single year for patients on home ventilation, which was an impetus for sustainable government funding.

The first government-funded model involved means-testing of patients into two tiers based on family income per-capita. Subsequently, this evolved into a modified model of reimbursement whereby funding is currently pegged to nursing home visits instead of each patient's specific equipment and consumable needs. This allows for eventual mainstreaming based on the nationwide model of intermediate- and long-term care (ILTC) funding for all citizens and permanent residents. Future plans include extending funding duration to include young adults (aged 16 and above) with home care needs, who are an emerging group of individuals with unique health characteristics and often receive limited funding from both pediatric and adult service providers.

Transition to Adult Care

The absence of a formal service to facilitate the transition of young persons to adult health-care services can result in care fragmentation and eventual loss to follow-up for many youth who are technology dependent (Zhou et al. 2016). Families also experience frustration with the lack of familiarity of adult providers with the medical issues related to CMC (Oswald et al. 2013). It has been shown that nurses can play an important role as facilitators in the transition process, as they have also journeyed with the CMC and family for many years (Li and Strachan 2021; Oswald et al. 2013). Following evidence-based guidelines on transition (Lemly et al. 2013), our program has engaged adult health-care providers to conduct combined multidisciplinary clinics for physicians and nurses from both institutions to meet the CMC and family multiple times prior to the actual transfer of care. This encourages open information exchange and provides reassurance to caregivers about the continuity of care. To date, our program has successfully transitioned an average of three young persons per year through this collaborative nurse-led model.

Lessons Learnt

A family-centered, multidisciplinary approach to the model of care for children with complex medical needs is required. However, it is only possible through collaborations between multiple medical subspecialties, allied health professionals, and community providers through sustainable financing.

Caregivers' health and well-being is also of utmost importance as the care of these children is dependent on the well-being of the caregivers and caregiving for these children is often stressful. A good social support system enables caregivers to fulfill their multiple roles and responsibilities as informal caregivers to CMC. In view of the constant contact between CCHS home care nurses and primary caregivers, the nurses have learnt to identify caregivers who may be at risk of burnout. Referring caregivers for early mental health interventions or organize respite care for support has been ongoing actively in recent years. This would positively impact caregivers' mental wellness, reduce the risk of severe depression, and ensure that CMC continue to receive quality care at home.

Children with complex care needs are characterized as having a constantly changing nature, due to the potential for clinical deterioration or improvement, and possible medical advances or challenges in care provision (Woodgate et al. 2015). Ongoing care adjustments are required as the child develops physical and psychologically. It is therefore essential for health-care providers caring for children with complex care needs to anticipate and recognize the increased complex care needs at various transition points. The various transition points include transitions from hospital to home, from children's to adult services, and from curative to palliative care (Brenner et al. 2018). These are periods whereby children and families need to adjust to changing services and care plans, and health-care providers need to render more supportive care.

Future Implications for Clinical Practice and Research

There is a lack of international integrated care system guidelines and this has resulted as a significant barrier to competent, comprehensive care delivery for children with complex care needs across all disciplines. In addition, medical, technological, and pharmaceutical advances have increased the survival and lifespan of children living with once-fatal conditions (Cohen et al. 2011b). These advances had led to the growing pediatric population living with secondary conditions and/or disabilities with complex care needs. However, there has been strong cross-disciplinary consensus that social and community service developments have not kept pace with medical progress. It was also reported that the existing provision of care at home was considered unsustainable, mainly due to structural factors relating to the availability of funding and resources that were considered scarce to meet the needs of a growing population (Brenner et al. 2018). Therefore, more evidence is needed to support the development and implementation of sustainable programs that will be able to demonstrate improvements in healthcare and psychosocial outcomes and hence reducing cost. Furthermore, more research will be helpful to countercheck if the values of the complementary therapies, which are provided to the children and parents, are considered maximized and can hence avoid misusing the therapies provided (Emond and Eaton 2004). It is also important to continually evaluate the different care systems and their sustainability.

Conclusion

With the rapid advancement of medical care, the number of technology-dependent children with chronic complex medical conditions is expected to increase. The development of a culturally adapted and holistic nursing-led home care model can be a sustainable method of care delivery, ensuring that these children are able to thrive in a caring home environment with adequately trained and supported caregivers.

References

Allshouse C, Comeau M, Rodgers R, Wells N. Families of children with medical complexity: a view from the front lines. Pediatrics. 2018;141:S195.

Avritscher EBC, Mosquera RA, Tyson JE, Pedroza C, Samuels CL, Harris TS, Gomez-Rubio A, Navarro FA, Moody SB, Beyda RM. Post-trial sustainability and scalability of the benefits of a medical home for high-risk children with medical complexity. J Pediatr. 2019;206:232–239.e3.

Baddour K, Mady LJ, Schwarzbach HL, Sabik LM, Thomas TH, Mccoy JL, Tobey A. Exploring caregiver burden and financial toxicity in caregivers of tracheostomy-dependent children. Int J Pediatr Otorhinolaryngol. 2021;145:110713.

Barnert ES, Coller RJ, Nelson BB, Thompson LR, Tran J, Chan V, Padilla C, Klitzner TS, Szilagyi M, Chung PJ. Key population health outcomes for children with medical complexity: a systematic review. Matern Child Health J. 2019;23:1167–76.

Berry JG. What children with medical complexity, their families, and healthcare providers deserve from an ideal healthcare system. Palo Alto, CA: LPFCH; 2015. http://www.lpfch.org/sites/default/files/field/publications/idealhealthcaresystem.pdf. Accessed 14 Oct 2021.

Berry JG, Agrawal RK, Cohen E, Kuo DZ. The landscape of medical care for children with medical complexity. Washington, DC: CHA; 2013. https://www.childrenshospitals.org/-/media/Files/CHA/Main/Issues_and_Advocacy/Key_Issues/Children_With_Medical_Complexity/Issue_Briefs_and_Reports/LandscapeOfMedicalCare_06252013.pdf. Accessed 14 Oct 2021.

Breneol S, King ST, Best S, Mckibbon S, Curran JA. Report summarizes home nursing study findings from IWK Health Center (Respite care for children and youth with complex care needs and their families: a scoping review protocol). Women's Health. 2019;

Brenner M, Kidston C, Hilliard C, Coyne I, Eustace-Cook J, Doyle C, Begley T, Barrett MJ. Children's complex care needs: a systematic concept analysis of multidisciplinary language. Eur J Pediatr. 2018;177:1641–52.

Bullinger M, Schmidt S, Petersen C. Assessing quality of life of children with chronic health conditions and disabilities: a European approach. Int J Rehabil Res. 2002;25(3):197–206.

Burns KH, Casey PH, Lyle RE, Bird TM, Fussell JJ, Robbins JM. Increasing prevalence of medically complex children in US hospitals. Pediatrics. 2010;126:638.

Chan YH, Lim CZ-R, Bautista D, Malhotra R, Østbye T. The health and well-being of caregivers of technologically dependent children. Glob Pediatr Health. 2019;6:2333794X18823000.

Cohen E, Patel H. Responding to the rising number of children living with complex chronic conditions. Can Med Assoc J. 2014;186:1199–200.

Cohen S, Kamarck T, Mermelstein R. A global measure of perceived stress. J Health Soc Behav. 1983;24:385–96.

Cohen E, Bruce-Barrett C, Kingsnorth S, Keilty K, Cooper A, Daub S. Integrated complex care model: lessons learned from inter-organizational partnership. Healthc Q. 2011a;14(3):64–70.

Cohen E, Kuo DZ, Agrawal R, Berry JG, Bhagat SKM, Simon TD, Srivastava R. Children with medical complexity: an emerging population for clinical and research initiatives. Pediatrics. 2011b;127:529–38.

Cohen E, Lacombe-Duncan A, Spalding K, Macinnis J, Nicholas D, Narayanan UG, Gordon M, Margolis I, Friedman JN. Integrated complex care coordination for children with medical complexity: a mixed-methods evaluation of tertiary care-community collaboration. BMC Health Serv Res. 2012;12:366.

Cohen E, Berry JG, Sanders L, Schor EL, Wise PH. Status complexicus? The emergence of pediatric complex care. Pediatrics. 2018;141:S202–11.

Davies D, Hartfield D, Wren T. Children who 'grow up' in hospital: inpatient stays of six months or longer. Paediatr Child Health. 2014;19:533–6.

Elias ER, Murphy NA, The Council on Children with Disabilities. Home care of children and youth with complex health care needs and technology dependencies. Pediatrics. 2012;129:996.

Emond A, Eaton N. Supporting children with complex health care needs and their families – an overview of the research agenda. Child Care Health Dev. 2004;30:195–9.

Glader L, Plews-Ogan J, Agrawal R. Children with medical complexity: creating a framework for care based on the International Classification of Functioning, Disability and Health. Dev Med Child Neurol. 2016;58:1116–23.

Kingsnorth S, Lacombe-Duncan A, Keilty K, Bruce-Barrett C, Cohen E. Inter-organizational partnership for children with medical complexity: the integrated complex care model. Child Care Health Dev. 2015;41:57–66.

Kroenke K, Spitzer RL, Williams JB. The PHQ-9: validity of a brief depression severity measure. J Gen Intern Med. 2001;16:606–13.

Kuo DZ. The medical home for children with medical complexity: back to basics. J Pediatr. 2019;206:8–9.

Lemly DC, Weitzman ER, O'Hare KO. Advancing healthcare transitions in the medical home: tools for providers, families and adolescents with special healthcare needs. Curr Opin Pediatr. 2013;25(4):439–46.

Li L, Strachan PH. Transitioning to adult services for youth with medical complexity: a practice issue viewed through the lens of transitions theory. Nurs Sci Q. 2021;34:301–8.

Matsuzawa A, Shiroki Y, Arai J, Hirasawa A. Care coordination for children with medical complexity in Japan: caregivers' perspectives. Child Care Health Dev. 2020;46:436–44.

Medicaid. Health Home Information Resource Center. Baltimore, MD: Medicaid; 2021. https://www.medicaid.gov/resources-for-states/medicaid-state-technical-assistance/health-home-information-resource-center/index.html. Accessed 14 Nov 2021.

Ministry of Health. Enhancing community care and caregiving. Singapore: MOH; 2019. https://www.moh.gov.sg/docs/librariesprovider5/default-document-library/cos-factsheet_enhancing-community-care-and-caregiving5b9b3cb036fa4b66992708556e8f832a.pdf. Accessed 1 Aug 2021.

Namachivayam P, Taylor A, Montague T, Moran K, Barrie J, Delzoppo C, Butt W. Long-stay children in intensive care: long-term functional outcome and quality of life from a 20-yr institutional study. Pediatr Crit Care Med. 2012;13(5):520–8.

Ng KG. Shift in emphasis from hospital to community care will help tame healthcare cost: Ong Ye Kung. Singapore: The Straits Times; 2021. https://www.straitstimes.com/singapore/health/emphasis-should-shift-from-hospital-to-community-care-in-taming-healthcare-spending. Accessed 1 Aug 2021.

Orkin J, Chan CY, Fayed N, Jia Lu Lilian L, Major N, Lim A, Peebles ER, Moretti ME, Soscia J, Sultan R, Willan AR, Offringa M, Guttmann A, Bartlett L, Kanani R, Culbert E, Hardy-Brown K, Gordon M, Perlmutar M, Cohen E. Complex care for kids Ontario: protocol for a mixed-methods randomised controlled trial of a population-level care coordination initiative for children with medical complexity. BMJ Open. 2019;9:e028121.

Oswald DP, Gilles DL, Cannady MS, Wenzel DB, Willis JH, Bodurtha JN. Youth with special health care needs: transition to adult health care services. Matern Child Health J. 2013;17:1744–52.

Page BF, Hinton L, Harrop E, Vincent C. The challenges of caring for children who require complex medical care at home: 'The go between for everyone is the parent and as the parent that's an awful lot of responsibility'. Health Expect. 2020;23:1144–54.

Peterson K, Anderson J, Bourne D, Charns MP, Gorin SS, Hynes DM, Mcdonald KM, Singer SJ, Yano EM. Health care coordination theoretical frameworks: a systematic scoping review to increase their understanding and use in practice. J Gen Intern Med. 2019;34:90–8.

Ronan S, Brown M, Marsh L. Parents' experiences of transition from hospital to home of a child with complex health needs: a systematic literature review. J Clin Nurs. 2020;29:3222–35.

Samantha. Home safety for homecare patients. Thousand Oaks, CA: Assisted Home Health, Hospice Care, and Caregiver Services; 2018. https://assistedcares.com/home-safety-for-homecare-patients/. Accessed 16 Nov 2021.

Seltzer RR, Henderson CM, Boss RD. Medical foster care: what happens when children with medical complexity cannot be cared for by their families? Pediatr Res. 2016;79:191–6.

Sobotka SA, Lynch E, Quinn MT, Awadalla SS, Agrawal RK, Peek ME. Unmet respite needs of children with medical technology dependence. Clin Pediatr. 2019;58:1175–86.

Sung M, Park J. The effects of a family support program including respite care on parenting stress and family quality of life perceived by primary caregivers of children with disabilities in Korea. Int J Spec Educ. 2012;27:188–98.

Tan C. More healthcare workers in Spore quit amid growing fatigue as Covid-19 drags on. The Straits Times. 2021. https://www.straitstimes.com/singapore/politics/more-healthcare-workers-in-spore-resigning-amid-growing-fatigue-as-covid-19-drags. Accessed 26 Nov 2021.

Toly VB, Blanchette JE, Al-Shammari T, Musil CM. Caring for technology-dependent children at home: problems and solutions identified by mothers. Appl Nurs Res. 2019;50:151195.

Woodgate RL, Edwards M, Jacquie DRB, Rempel G. Intense parenting: a qualitative study detailing the experiences of parenting children with complex care needs. BMC Pediatr. 2015;15:197.

Zhou H, Roberts P, Dhaliwal S, Della P. Transitioning adolescent and young adults with chronic disease and/or disabilities from paediatric to adult care services – an integrative review. J Clin Nurs. 2016;25:3113–30.

Affirming and Empowering Kids: Creating an Independent and Comprehensive Gender-Affirming Health-Care Center

Dallas M. Ducar

An Introduction to Transhealth

Transhealth Northampton (Transhealth) is an independent and comprehensive health-care center that opened in May 2021. Transhealth is a nonprofit that is dedicated to serving the needs of transgender and gender-diverse kids and adults. Transgender and gender-diverse individuals are those who identify with a gender different that which was assigned at birth. Cisgender individuals are those who identify with the gender they were assigned at birth. The basis of the organization was informed by a needs assessment that was responsive to the needs of the communities Transhealth served. In serving pediatric populations, Transhealth was able to offer a much-needed resource across Massachusetts and eventually New England. Transhealth was developed under a unique nurse-led model making it an exemplar for other nurse-led organizations that work with minoritized populations. While significant challenges were met, lessons were also learned including the importance of cocreating a health-care experience that is empowering, individualized, affirming,

D. M. Ducar (✉)
Transhealth, Florence, MA, USA

School of Nursing, Columbia University, New York, NY, USA

Nursing Department of Family, Community & Mental Health Systems, The University of Virginia School of Nursing, Charlottesville, VA, USA

Department of Psychiatry and Neurobehavioral Sciences, The University of Virginia School of Medicine, Charlottesville, VA, USA

School of Nursing, MGH Institute for Health Professions, Boston, MA, USA

College of Science, Interdisciplinary Affective Science Laboratory, Northeastern University, Boston, MA, USA
e-mail: dallas@transhealth.org

C. L. Betz (ed.), *Worldwide Successful Pediatric Nurse-Led Models of Care*, https://doi.org/10.1007/978-3-031-22152-1_7

and harnesses the natural resilience that children bring to the table. Overall, we at Transhealth found that our patients and clients were our greatest teachers and therefore we had to construct a health-care environment where we left assumptions at the door.

Importantly, this chapter will focus on what a dedicated group of fabulous individuals can do when they put their heads together. The drive and passion that our team brought, all founded around helping trans kids get the care they need, was the prime driver of all this. We will never forget the story of the little girl who was denied her passport because of her gender identity, and how this clinic was founded to ensure that never happened again. We will never forget the story of the kid who was first seen here and had been able to come out with his parents' support. We will never forget the young kid who finally had the chance to see themselves reflected in the folks who work here day in and day out. Transhealth is motivated, every day, by the patients we serve, by the opportunity to open up a space where kids can be seen, affirmed, and cared for. Never doubt what a group of committed and passionate people can do, indeed, they can change the world.

Background

Transgender and Gender-Diverse Kids Are Resilient and Deserve More

More transgender and gender-diverse individuals are coming out than ever before. Children discover their own gender identity around age 3–4 years of age (Rafferty 2018). It is, therefore, crucial that we create a gender-affirming environment for every child as it is likely many will explore gender for their own self. Pediatric nurses and interdisciplinary colleagues must be able to skillfully speak about gender, understand the social and clinical interventions associated with transition, and even be willing to facilitate such interventions when appropriate. This also means being able to provide the same form of healthcare that anyone would expect. A gender-affirming environment is an underlying layer for pediatric care, one that supports a child-centered and family-centered approach.

A recent needs assessment discovered that about 20,000 transgender and gender-diverse adults live in the catchment area of Western Massachusetts, Southern New Hampshire, Vermont, Connecticut, and Upstate New York (Loo et al. 2021). The needs assessment revealed that of the estimated 20,000 transgender and gender-diverse individuals in our catchment area at Transhealth, access to care issues was prominently identified. A major barrier was inadequate access to care in a rural setting that included transportation problems, and more awareness of the need for gender-affirming care. Survey respondents reported needing primary care (54%), psychotherapy (44%), and sexual and reproductive healthcare—but also, they needed a place to gather in community.

Focus groups conducted to assess areas of need during the creation of Transhealth identified specific thematic areas of need. Key areas of concern included distinct needs surrounding race and ethnicity, language, and lack of equity in the provision of health services. Other health-care barriers associated with the lack of gender-affirming care also included provider availability, provider competency, and the need for specific services like mental health care, care coordination, sexual and reproductive healthcare, holistic health, and referrals to community resources and spaces constructed to hold community gatherings (PATH Survey 2020). This model of gender-affirming care is one that was informed by the community through the needs assessment processes undertaken and was designed to be comprehensive and directly address social determinants of health.

Current evidence indicates there is a distinct need for pediatric care that is competent in serving the needs of nonbinary children and adolescents (Hastings et al. 2021). More children are identifying as nonbinary across the United States. In 2021, an investigation of high-school students from an urban school district reported that 9.2% identified as gender-diverse with one-third of these students identifying as nonbinary, significantly higher than reported in previous surveys (Kidd et al. 2021). This statistic has been consistent with percentages found in the 2015 US Transgender Survey (though this survey did not survey participants under 18 at the time) (James et al. 2016). The needs of nonbinary individuals, especially children, are best served when we as nurses, and interdisciplinary providers focus on affirming language (not using masculinizing or feminizing terminology), promote embodiment goals, and support individualized goals (Hastings et al. 2021). Our center was committed to be affirming, evolving, and holistic, in the language, interventions, environment, and actions we took.

Transgender and gender-diverse individuals have been overtly harmed by the health-care system. Children have been particularly vulnerable, unable to speak to their own needs, and oftentimes unable to have families advocate for them. This is especially harrowing as demonstrated by high rates of suicide attempts committed by transgender and gender-diverse individuals, oftentimes with little familial support (Haas et al. 2014; Bauer et al. 2015).

Nurses and interdisciplinary clinicians have the unique opportunity to speak with every patient early on about their gender identity as they undergo their own learning and development. By not engaging in early conversations and cocreating an environment of trust, nurses and interdisciplinary colleagues can inadvertently harm patients by not creating and fostering opportunities for them to be their most authentic selves. Health-care professionals have a duty to act and to provide an affirming care environment for transgender and gender-diverse individuals.

Over time, by not engaging in opportunities to open conversations, people will eventually be faced with a harmful health-care system. The system becomes the silencer. Transgender and gender-diverse patients face a cycle of discrimination that locks them out of basic health-care needs (Reisner et al. 2014). Accessible and affordable healthcare, for many, becomes a fight to be seen. This cycle leads to additional barriers including clinical paperwork, psychiatric assessments, and insurance preauthorizations, to name a few. For many children, the barriers are even more complex and require assent and consent and necessitate family support, acknowledgement, and acceptance.

Transgender and gender-diverse children and youth possess immense resilience. They are able to navigate a world that is overtly hostile, against a society that oftentimes refuses to acknowledge their existence. Resilience is defined by Hillier et al. (2020) as "bouncing back" in the face of stressful experiences protecting against harassment and discrimination. Various factors promote resilience in trans youth including peer acceptance, supportive school and parental environments, and a sense of collective and nonprescriptive trans and gender-diverse identities (Bradley et al. 2019; Meadow 2018; Travers 2022). It is imperative that any health center dedicated to caring for trans and gender-diverse children focus on ways to effectively build resilience with children and youth, rather than simply educating other communities of allies. An ally is a noun, it is someone who uses their privilege to advocate on behalf of someone else who doesn't hold that same privilege (Edwards 2006). Building a sense of collective community and focusing on what is right with rather than what is wrong will likely lead to less internalization of minority stress and instead foster resilience.

Meyer (2003) forwarded a minority stress model on how sexually diverse individuals on the margins (in addition to typical daily stress that everyone faces) contribute to a disproportionate risk for poor health compared to heterosexual populations. Hendricks and Testa (2012) adapted this model to include transgender and gender-diverse individuals. Unique stressors include distal and proximal stress, proximal consisting of internal perceptions and distal including external events such as violence or discrimination. Proximal stress may include internalized homophobia or transphobia (Hendricks and Testa 2012), while distal stress can also lead to internalizing negative societal attitudes toward oneself (Meyer 2003).

Transhealth Was Developed to Respond to Community Need

Transhealth was developed with the input of the community being an integral component. While primary and mental healthcare are both services offered in the center, there are also many additional services that are offered to build meet the needs of transgender and gender-diverse individuals. Community services continue to be developed to offer peer support, community engagement, and additional resources to expand the boundaries of gender-affirming care, based on an informed and active patient population. This community focus is the base of our organization, without it, and without listening to the community, we risk being a detached and overly rigid structure, which is antithetical to our very values.

Unfortunately, this model is rare. Even the bare minimum cannot be expected across the landscape of gender-affirming care. In many areas of the country, unnecessary paperwork, psychiatric assessments, insurance preauthorizations, and many additional barriers are constructed without any single unified standard of care guidelines. Access to care is typically predicated on the institutional views of a pre-scriber or the ad-hoc philosophy of a practice unless the organization specializes in gender-affirming care. For many children and youth, the barriers can be even more complex, as familial involvement can sometimes inhibit the patient from even dis-cussing gender. These barriers, determined strictly by the behaviors and beliefs of the providers, are accentuated by the difficulties of providing care to a community at the margins. While health-care professionals need to address the individual and family needs, they also need to address the context within which they live in, which means adding flexibility to policies, offering sliding scale, operating outside a tradi-tional work-week, and vitally, providing trauma-informed care to every individual who accesses care.

When founded, Transhealth was committed and continues to be committed to being as accessible as possible. From the beginning, Transhealth immediately began accepting all private and public insurances that it could and worked to provide lon-gitudinal care, while providing referrals to specialty and surgical networks. Care is delivered based on a holistic, dynamic, preventative, and affirming service model. Namely, all care is both patient-centered and guided by informed consent, which means that the consent for all treatment approaches and decisions are made by the patient deciding what happens and when it happens. Additionally, this comprehen-sive service model would come to mean that all needs could be met for patients across the lifespan consisting of pediatric and adult health-care services. This wrap-around framework includes medical and, mental health care, resource navigation, social services, and community-based referral support. Moreover, we specifically hired staff specialized in pediatrics to ensure children and families knew they would receive exceptional care at Transhealth.

With this in mind, we set out a course to begin to expand gender-affirming care. Our vision was ambitious and full of promise, to transform the world so that trans and gender diverse adults, children, and youth are empowered and celebrated as they work with an affirming team on own their health-care journey. Our entire team believes in our mission, feels it deep in their bones, and have worked daily to advance the commitment and mission of Transhealth. While we did not always come to agreement on every policy or procedure, we did all agree that the mission was one, which we all profoundly believed in. As a trans-led organization, we were uniquely positioned to expand the health-care possibilities for our community. Through research, expert care, and fierce advocacy, we would work to secure a healthy, affirming future for all of us. Our mission and vision have guided the care that we provide, based on a holistic model of care that recognizing identity, seeing the whole person, and approaching with a beginner's mind, one without assump-tions. Essentially, this is the ability to make new observations regardless of one's context (Bishop et al. 2004). This meant providing comprehensive, person-centered, gender-affirming care that would respond to the needs of transgender and gender-diverse individuals across the lifespan.

Description of the Nurse-Led Transhealth Model

Transhealth is a nonprofit health center serving transgender and gender-diverse individuals across the lifespan. Transhealth was founded on May 4, 2021, known by some as "Star Wars Day." It opened providing comprehensive services that includes adult primary care, pediatric primary care, hormonal care, mental healthcare, and nonclinical services such as patient advocacy and support for accessing community services. We sought to serve our communities by advancing research, education, and advocacy in the field of transgender and gender-diverse health. The origins of Transhealth first started by engaging a local trans-identified funder, who commissioned the needs assessment and envisioned the creation of the center. He was committed to caring for the various needs of the transgender and gender-diverse communities and strongly supported us and worked with us in the creation of the health-care center. We could not have done this without him. While academic medical centers may have been the easy route, the more organic and natural approach was to foster trust and organize from within our community. The entire process was based upon our vision and commitment to realize its establishment.

Initially, the health center was developed to care for those within the Northampton area and surrounding rural locations in Massachusetts. Throughout the first 12 months, the clinic was able to serve over 1500 trans and gender-diverse individuals with schedules continuing to fill in pediatric care, primary care, and psychiatric care. Psychotherapy waitlists were filled quickly, which galvanized the organization to hire more therapists to meet the mental health needs of patients. Most patients were originally from Massachusetts and in rural areas, with some commuting from Boston and other nearby urban areas such as Springfield, Massachusetts. We even saw some patients commuting across state lines, and paying out of pocket, as access to our specialized services had been so rare in their state. A couple of families literally moved across the country to be able to access care at Transhealth.

Transhealth rooted its care model in a gender-affirming philosophy rather than one based upon specific published guideline of care. Because there are multiple different models that are ever-changing, we instead base our own off of a patient-centered approach. The model of care itself is one that has been based on informed consent and harm reduction (Ashley 2019). By hiring trans and gender-diverse individuals, the center was able to not only be guided by gender-affirming protocols and policy but also the lived experience of the staff. For many patients, this meant just being seen as a human being in the fullest gender affirming sense rather than being a specific step in a workflow.

As one patient put it:

> Having a place specific to me and my unique needs is different. I like never being dead-named, or having staff who aren't familiar with me get confused with how to address me. It's especially nice to not have to explain my existence or wonder if the person across from me is an ally. There's a difference in being in an office that's working to make you feel welcome, and being in one where you never even have to consider it. There are some things that are intangible and are beyond being able to adequately explain to those, not of that experience. Other practices were okay, mostly, they checked all the boxes, but at Transhealth, I'm not a box to be checked.

This quote encapsulates the philosophy at Transhealth—one which is rooted in following the patient's lead and putting them in the drivers' seat. For children, this means being able to create a space where children and adolescents have enough time to adequately be seen not only by the team but also by their family. This means offering longer appointment times to provide space for children and caregivers to share important psychosocial aspects of their own well-being, which contextualize individualized gender-affirming treatment needs. Weighing questions surrounding gender, and having the appropriate time to explore these questions, requires time and space to do so.

Individualized care requires multidisciplinary treatment teams across the organization. We as nurses are uniquely poised to offer this care as we can serve as primary care providers, mental health providers, therapists, ambulatory clinicians, and more. While nurses can provide this care, we made the intentional choice to also hire diverse discipline team members that include medical doctors, social workers, medical assistants, community health workers, and more—to encourage a multidisciplinary model with many perspectives. Throughout this process, the CEO has been a nurse practitioner and has provided the leadership to support and promote an innovative model, one which encourages all individuals to practice within the full scope of their practice and center care based upon an inclusive, interdisciplinary model of clinical care rather than the traditional medical model of care. In this fashion, the patient is able to choose the type of care they wish to engage with rather than having one model prescribed to them. Additionally, this undoubtedly attracts clinicians who are looking for something outside of the traditional medical-industrial complex.

Transhealth has also been able to facilitate easy access to care during a time when gender-affirming care has become more difficult to attain. Specifically, the COVID pandemic made pediatric primary care difficult for many to attain as waitlists grew—this problem was only more difficult across gender-affirming services. Moreover, Transhealth allowed pediatric patients to access any service that seemed necessary and did not require primary care to access pediatric psychiatry or psychotherapy. Our community health worker allowed for capacity building and additional networking with other practices in the community. This individual is someone who is broadly aware of social determinants of health, helps to facilitate resources across the organization, assists patients in accessing community resources and works with patients to help fill in the gaps when clinical interventions are not sufficient. Our strong focus on community services also allowed for opportunities for clinicians to work with other pediatric care practices to foster clinical education.

Pediatric care is unique at Transhealth as the center sees all ages. Importantly, this means that children who have not yet encountered the concept of gender identity could still be seen if the parents or family members identified as transgender or gender-diverse. The Clinical Director position is a rotating one, every 2 years, which de-centers the notion that one discipline is poised to necessarily lead the clinical operations. This rotating model allows for the possibility of a shift in perspective thereby not necessarily rooting the leadership of the clinical operations within one discipline or philosophy. In the end, this opens up the possibility of any clinician leading the clinical operations.

The informed consent model guides pediatric care at Transhealth. This means that children and their families are able to decide what they believe is best for them and when it is best for them. The informed consent model is rooted in the ethical principle of autonomy and respect for persons, and seeks to honor the patient and their family's choices without the requirement of including another provider. Moreover, informed consent truly is a model where individuals are able to consent to every aspect of care, to where data goes, to how they are called in a public setting, to how they are addressed to others, to when and where they are touched as everything becomes based on consent. Importantly, this means that the child's voice must be the center of the conversation and that there is a focus on valuing the child for who they are now (Rafferty et al. 2018). This means that watchful waiting is not benign—choosing not to speak to a child about gender dysphoria can lead to a lifetime of trauma. While we cannot change a child's gender identity, nor should we want to, we can affect whether or not they discuss it.

Along with clinical services, we also have a large community room where we are able to host a variety of events. Within the community room, we host a variety of therapeutic groups (group therapy, art therapy, health education, etc.) along with nontherapeutic groups (peer support, makeup classes, nutrition classes) and with external partners (recovery groups, trauma survivor groups, etc.) who may also choose to engage with us. This space allows for a centering of community which reinforces the additional pillars of clinical care, research, education, and advocacy (Fig. 1).

Fig. 1 A visual representation of the Transhealth pillars being supported by the foundation that is the community

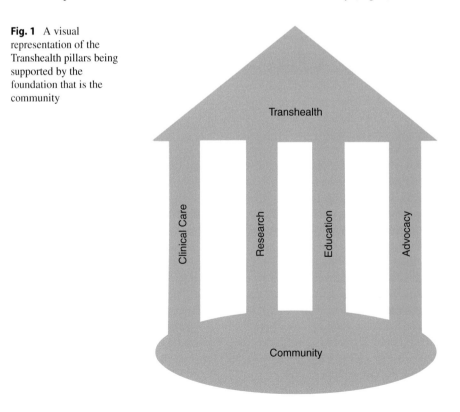

In general, we as nurses are integral to the care provided at Transhealth Northampton. Registered nurses and advanced practice nurses practice at the top of their scope of practice. This means that all nurses are encouraged to provide all services that they are deemed competent to perform and permitted to undertake. Moreover, all nurses are fully eligible to serve as the Mental Health or Primary Care Director, unlike traditional medical models. Ambulatory registered nurses are involved in all initial visits and allotted protected time for community outreach, along with all providers. Nurses and other staff members are provided time to pursue interdisciplinary education (i.e., professional development, continuing education), participate in community-building activities, engage in advocacy, and develop research projects. Ongoing and future work includes developing assessing clinical outcomes using patient-reported outcome measures that are relevant to the transgender and gender-diverse clients served by the clinic.

Challenges and Facilitators

In general, hiring individuals who have been pushed to the margins takes a substantial investment. As discussed, society disproportionately harms trans and gender-diverse individuals, possibly leading to experiences of mistrust and trauma. Some of us in the community have experienced being tokenized in a health-care system, acting as the "trans expert" which oftentimes has very harmful effects. Therefore, creating a trauma-informed workplace, especially focusing on mitigating the effects of secondary trauma and burnout prevention, becomes essential. In the formation of Transhealth, it became difficult to hire for specific roles as it would mean new staff members would have to take a leap of faith to join the organization. For many, especially coming from communities at the margins, taking this leap was risky and difficult. There was also a preconceived notion for many of what type of organization we could be, and in start-ups, the expectations did not always meet reality. Combined with intersections of race, ethnicity, ability, socioeconomic status all make this more difficult and it becomes even more crucial to create a workplace where all can show up authentically. This means creating an environment where anyone can trust their provider and therefore be more ready to engage in health-care services, decreasing morbidity and mortality in general (Ashley and Domínguez 2021).

For Transhealth, this meant being aware of how we were all feeling starting from the beginning—focusing on low retention rates and high employee satisfaction. Moreover, from the very first day, we asked the question, "What does a trauma-informed workplace look like?" To address this organizational issue, we did begin to devote substantial time to developing a culture of safety and trust. This meant starting with the assumption that others may have been traumatized in the past and creating a space that would earn trust. We recognized that people would arrive here feeling scared, worried, perhaps jaded—and we strove to create a safe space where others could be vulnerable. By getting real with people—being vulnerable—we were able to strive for a culture of love, trust, and care. One way we did this was by ensuring for a participatory environment, where all individuals from day one understood they could collaborate on new ideas. We constantly sent all policies out for comment, we ensured transparency in the budget, and we used novel technology to allow for quick collaboration and communication.

Creating this culture requires a true sense of psychological safety that inspires high-performing teams. This means ensuring that all individuals are accountable for their own performance, for the success of their stakeholders, and dedicated to the mission of expanding gender-affirming care. We had to set clear expectations and goals to understand our objectives and coming together to focus on one specific "North Star." Unfortunately, at the beginning of the organization, there was the inevitable scope creep where we wanted to solve the problems of the world when we just should have focused on building what was in front of us. Over time, we were able to focus on conversations on specific workflows and procedure, leading to a solution-oriented culture.

There also had to be a focus on developing a culture of quality. This did not just mean tasking someone with the role of measuring quality but creating a culture devoted to quality—where it was a self-reinforcing principle. We had to create a space where individuals would feel comfortable referring their family to any provider in the organization. While this may sound easy—this required a sense of mutual accountability where we all understood that we were working on the same team for the same mission. The dedication to quality care is one that remains one of our highest goals to this day. Quality care meant being able to take time and attention to be with the family and the child, and to ensure that options for multidisciplinary care were available. On an interpersonal level, this meant not turning the visit into an assessment, but rather a chance to build trust, and for our pediatric services to hold themselves accountable to a high standard of care. Each visit started with a conversation, no particular preconceived notions or hoops to jump through, just starting by knowing the child and family to understand how to best support them where they are.

We required substantial administrative support to ensure the successful delivery of clinical care. This meant having executives who were skilled in developing long-term projects and making systems scalable. Additionally, this meant robust front-end support to ensure that patients were able to be registered and scheduled efficiently while also navigating insurance and prior authorizations. At the same time, we had to operate similarly to an abortion clinic due to external threats—taking steps to hide our address or not post external pictures—making it more difficult for patients to find us. Additional administrative support was necessary for hiring and we were bringing on large groups of individuals all at once. We wanted to hire slowly to ensure that we would hire stars who had the right competency, personality, and values for the job. With every new hire and every new service line, we had to consider our marketing and communications strategy—specifically—how we would communicate our existence to communities at the margins. This meant taking more time to think about how the administrative operations interfaced with the message we were trying to convey. If a pediatric service was not able to go live and we began to market it too early, there would be a message of overpromising and underdelivery. The resources we provided were so rare that we wanted to ensure that we had adequate support prior to sending out the message that there was a much-needed resource now available.

Notably, 2021 was the year that the Commonwealth of Massachusetts passed the Nurse Practice Act. This meant that nurse practitioners were allowed to practice as independent providers. Transhealth Northampton also worked with local insurers and the local physician's group to allow for admitting privileges and primary care provider status of new nurse practitioners. Overall, this insistence on not centering the practice around one discipline, rather than creating a nurse or physician-centric practice, fostered a philosophy of patient-centered care enabling the focus on the patient. While this sounds ideal, many physicians or provider hospital organizations had to choose whether they would change their own bylaws in accordance with the changes enacted by the state to enable full practice authority for nurse practitioners. This meant that Transhealth was not only novel in our mission to provide rural gender-affirming care, but also to create a practice that would not necessarily rely on physicians as found in typical hierarchical structures in health-care organizations. While this did lead to some initial difficulties with credentialing and reimbursement, we eventually were able to work with third-party vendors to ensure the billing and insurance functioned as seamlessly as possible.

Service Adjustments Made

We endeavored to be able to accept all insurances within Massachusetts. This was especially important as there were increasingly more organizations that were dedicated to serving sexual minorities and transgender/gender-diverse communities and not taking insurance (Jones 2021). This increasing disparity can lead to a health-care landscape where some individuals have access and some are without. Despite this organizational drive, we learned that not all insurances would be able to be accepted and we had to adjust accordingly. Specifically, we primarily hired nurse practitioners as providers and strove to ensure they would be seen as a primary care provider by payors, which was much more difficult than we had anticipated, meaning that their reimbursement would be equivalent or nearly to that of physicians. Additionally, we had originally overestimated how many families and patients would be willing to engage in gender-affirming pediatric care when already having established relationships with previous pediatric providers. Instead, the biggest need demonstrated was adult primary care and this meant shifting our priorities. Regardless, we continued to invest in communications surrounding our pediatric services and focus on community initiatives to build trust in the community.

Effective strategy and planning are crucial to creating a new organization. This means acknowledging that if one wants to accept insurance, they need to build in the appropriate lag time for credentialing new clinicians. For many practices, this means embedding a 5–8-month timeline starting at the date of hire. For Transhealth, we had to decide whether we wanted to serve patients or wait until we would be able to recoup revenue. At the end of the day, we decided that our initial group of hires would be brought on without this lagtime to ensure patients were able to receive the care they need. As we were able to create redundant systems and hire more than one of the same providers, we were able to then hire providers more slowly and wait until providers would be credentialed with the appropriate insurance.

Parents and children/youth oftentimes foster deep relationships with us, as clinicians, that continue throughout their lifespan. Even when we may not be as skilled in gender-affirming care, it takes a significant commitment to build trust with a family. This means ensuring that the very first visit is one that radiates trust and connects with the child or youth. Additionally, everything from the waiting room to the exam room should be one that reflects openness and curiosity, a place where a child or youth and their entire family can explore their own relationality and the clinic can be a space of authenticity and discovery. This is why we attempted to hire trans and gender-diverse individuals across the board, to ensure that children are able to see themselves in their own provider.

Lessons Learned

Year one was full of lessons learned. When we started Transhealth, we based the budget on completely unknown numbers, estimates of what a space, medical equipment, salaries, and more, would cost. We tried our best to draw up comparable numbers but this took time, and for medical equipment, it would often be more difficult to estimate the actual value of the materials until purchased. Overall, this meant we were stepping into new territory, leading with a vision, confidence, and a whole lack of concrete experience to rely on when it came to building a health-care center. In some ways, this was an advantage, as we were able to start with a blank slate and really consider what we would want in the best health-care experience. There was a good amount of humility at this time and frequent amazement at what a group of committed queer folks could really do.

In the early days, everything rolled up to one North Star, "to get the doors open and keep them open." It was a mantra we would always come back to. Whenever new ideas and initiatives came up, there was the star, to keep us on track. Developing something new in a new field can be completely and wholly intoxicating, we had to make sure we did not "get up over our skis"; that is, that we did not advance too quickly with organizational efforts without sufficient resources. Our intense focus on this North Star, while helpful to fight against the inexorable force of scope creep, also may have been a hindrance. Our focus on one area inevitably brought us all in line with one outlook toward the future, thereby leading to one close, tight, budget. A very specific calculation on income, revenue, or anticipated losses might sound like a good estimate, but it also leads you to a space without experimentation, a place where you have to operate with little creativity or wiggle room. You need to provide some room for unexpected events to navigate uncharted waters. It's arcane to believe a business can actually estimate the budget for the year, especially in a start-up, and believe that it will be able to know the exact course for the coming year. Instead, there are many lessons to be learned and each iteration of the budget should be considered a creative learning experience that reflects the goals, mission, and values of the organization.

In a start-up, administrators need to pivot quickly and be responsive to the needs of the organization as they change. Organizational rigidity to one strategy, objective, or tactic, in the end, these are just words on a page, can be problematic if accurately assessing trends and listening to the needs of employees are not done. As we have found, there will be many challenges and unexpected changes along the way. Transhealth was founded during a global pandemic, and we had to make changes as policy and regulation continued to change. Moreover, we would constantly need to reassess our own policies and procedures. This meant responding to the needs of our patients and clinicians and to allow for flexibility at work. For example, we allowed individuals to work from home and we were able to leverage additional space and resources for those who absolutely needed to be seen in-person. We also ensured we were flexible with each other, offering grace and compassion, as we were, as our COO often said, "flying the plane while we were building it."

As mentioned before, 2021 saw unprecedented attacks on transgender youth in the United States (Ronan 2021). We had to be responsive, to work with stakeholders to help define policy, to advocate for children and youth, and as we decided to expand to other states, to be aware and possibly wary of other states like New Hampshire where some legislators sought to advance restrictions on gender-affirming care or even talking about gender in school settings (An act relative to the propagation of divisive concept 2021). Proponents of this act would restrict what educators can say about race, gender, gender identity, sexual orientation and has been challenged in court (DiStaso 2021). Critics of transgender and gender-diverse issues have focus on politically charged issues to disrupt advances for transgender and gender-diverse children and youth; therefore, it was critical for organizations like Transhealth to be advocates to advance science-driven policy. This also meant developing a flexible business model that would retain strategy, advance advocacy, and be flexible in changing political landscapes.

Future Implications

We learned that it was possible to provide care for communities at the margins while guided by ethics and still remain financially sustainable. Importantly, creating a nonprofit organization, without any initial organizational foundations, was possible by developing a mission, a vision, and values—and employing a specific strategy. As mentioned before, it would not have been possible without the gracious support we received from our primary funder, and the communities we serve. We had to develop one guiding principle that we could always come back to, to guide our organizational development. Oftentimes as a group of new individuals working together, there would be differing opinions and one guiding mission was central to this.

We will expand care across rural settings. Moving forward, we endeavor to create a spoke-and-hub model, one in which we can reach underserved individuals in hard-to-reach settings. This model has been shown to be especially useful for working with other community partners and galvanizing resources across settings with little access to care (Elrod and Fortenberry 2017). Moreover, the recent expansion of availability and reimbursement of telehealth services by the Commonwealth of Massachusetts permits an increase in access to care for many in rural settings. We saw no-show rates that were lower than the national average and reduced barriers to care for those who often travel great distances to be able to access culturally responsive care. To this day we continue to advocate for an expansion of telehealth services as we build out a spoke-and-hub approach to improve access to care across New England (Ducar 2021a, b). This underlines the importance of ensuring that all individuals have the time and space to be able to advocate for the rights of the most marginalized and be actively involved in shaping the landscape of care.

Many parents view endocrinologists as experts in gender-affirming care. Additionally, some insurances view gender-affirming care as a form of specialty care. It is essential to dispel this myth, endocrinologists are not essential to providing gender-affirming care. In fact, guidelines illustrate the importance of a primary care provider providing gender-affirming hormones (Deutsch 2016). It is essential, as gender-affirming care progresses, that more pediatric and primary care providers are willing to discuss and provide access to gender-affirming care (Shires et al. 2018). We are just one example of where this has been done successfully.

Transhealth has also illustrated the need for interdisciplinary care. We are able to provide an all-inclusive approach where one can access primary care, psychotherapy, psychiatry, gender-affirming hormonal therapy, community services, and more, all under one roof. Moreover, the leveraging of technology and licensing across state lines allows Transhealth to provide clinical services in novel and innovative ways. This model is founded upon the belief of patient-centered care: those at the margins should be able to be in the driver's seat and define what they need for their own selves. This requires having access to multimodal forms of treatment that give people options and allow them to be self-directional.

Conclusions

Our modern health-care system has been created by those in power who have historically reduced access to care. Cisgender people, in particular, have created systems that inevitably reduce access to care, which has resulted in the medicalization of identity. The development of gender is part of the human story, it is who we are, and should never be subject to those who are in positions of power. Instead, we should strive to reflect on their own identity, and positionality, and how they can make healthcare a liberatory and emancipatory space. This means actively talking about gender, actively working to see the whole child and their family, and reducing any barriers to care. We should be welcoming the child for who they are and giving them the opportunity to explore their own selves. Some may call this an extension of the "trans agenda." We will not be forcing any children into anything. Advancing affirming care means affirming each human being for who they are. It is a rebuke to those who tell others how they need to act and behave, and instead, we say, "we value you for who you are." Our mission is not prescriptive but one of acceptance.

The current health-care system is one that generally requires privilege and sacrifice to become a key player. Executives frequently tell clinicians that we should be valued for our resilience rather than the system's resilience. A system that arises from diversity and inclusion allows for a more generative and creative approach to care. Transhealth is unique. We are led by the trans community and for the trans community. We focus on expanding gender-affirming care in a rural landscape. We as an organization have placed all our chips in one basket, to advance quality clinical care and commit to meaningful research, education, and advocacy.

We believe our victories will extend far beyond our community. Gender-affirming care offers a model for all of healthcare. It is a profound expression of patient-centered care, one based on the human story. One that has been shaped by an active, informed, and vocal patient population that has had to learn, out of necessity, to demand rights, be seen and be cared for. It is time that the transgender community shows America what healthcare can be.

Useful Resources

The resources below are additional resources on caring for transgender and gender-diverse individuals across the life-span.

- https://transhealth.org/
- https://transcare.ucsf.edu/guidelines
- https://www.ustranssurvey.org/
- https://pointofpride.org/get-support/
- https://www.transhealth.org/wp-content/uploads/2021/06/6.16_Trans-Youth-Foster-Care.pdf
- https://www.transhealth.org/wp-content/uploads/2021/06/6.16_Toomey-Minority-Stress-and-resilience-in-Gender-minority-youth.pdf
- https://www.transhealth.org/wp-content/uploads/2021/06/6.16_Fenway-Resource-Sheet-for-Parents-of-Transgender-Youth-V3.pdf
- https://interactadvocates.org/
- https://www.lgbtqiahealtheducation.org/wp-content/uploads/2020/08/Neurodiversity-and-Gender-Diverse-Youth_An-Affirming-Approach-to-Care_2020.pdf
- https://www.lgbtqiahealtheducation.org/
- https://www.rainbowhealthontario.ca/TransHealthGuide/pdf/QRG_full_2020.pdf

References

An act relative to the propagation of divisive concepts. H.R. 544 NH 2021. http://www.gencourt. state.nh.us/legislation/2021/HB0544.html.

Ashley F. Gatekeeping hormone replacement therapy for transgender patients is dehumanising. J Med Ethics. 2019;45(7):480–2.

Ashley F, Domínguez S. Transgender healthcare does not stop at the doorstep of the clinic. Am J Med. 2021;134(2):158–60.

Bauer GR, Scheim AI, Pyne J, Travers R, Hammond R. Intervenable factors associated with suicide risk in transgender persons: a respondent-driven sampling study in Ontario, Canada. BMC Public Health. 2015;15(1):1–15.

Bishop SR, Lau M, Shapiro S, Carlson L, Anderson ND, Carmody J, Devins G. Mindfulness: A proposed operational definition. Clinical psychology: Science and practice. 2004;11(3):230

Bradley E, Albright G, McMillan J, Shockley K. Impact of a simulation on educator support of LGBTQ youth. Journal of LGBT Youth, 2019;16(3):317–39.

Deutsch MB. Initiating hormone therapy. Initiating hormone therapy | Gender Affirming Health Program. 2016. https://transcare.ucsf.edu/guidelines/initiating-hormone-therapy. Accessed 24 Dec 2021.

DiStaso J. Lawsuit challenges constitutionality of 'divisive concepts' law passed by GOP Legislative majority. WMUR. 2021. https://www.wmur.com/article/lawsuit-challenges-constitutionality-of-divisive-concepts-law/38505123#. Accessed 6 Jan 2022.

Ducar D. Expanding telehealth is vital to the Trans Community. The Hill. 2021a. https://thehill. com/opinion/healthcare/566488-expanding-telehealth-is-essential-to-the-trans-community. Accessed 11 Nov 2021.

Ducar D. How to expand health care coverage for trans and gender diverse populations. The Boston Globe. 2021b. https://www.bostonglobe.com/2021/11/20/opinion/how-expand-health-care-coverage-trans-gender-diverse-populations/?event=event12. Accessed 23 Dec 2021.

Edwards KE. Aspiring social justice ally identity development: a conceptual model. NASPA J. 2006;43(4):39–60.

Elrod JK, Fortenberry JL. The hub-and-spoke organization design revisited: a lifeline for rural hospitals. BMC Health Serv Res. 2017;17(4):29–35.

Haas AP, Rodgers PL, Herman JL. Suicide attempts among transgender and gender nonconforming adults. Findings of the National Transgender Discrimination Survey, vol 50; 2014. p. 59.

Hastings J, Bobb C, Wolfe M, Amaro Jimenez Z, Amand CS. Medical care for nonbinary youth: individualized gender care beyond a binary framework. Pediatr Ann. 2021;50(9):e384–90.

Hendricks ML, Testa RJ. A conceptual framework for clinical work with transgender and gender nonconforming clients: an adaptation of the Minority Stress Model. Prof Psychol Res Pract. 2012;43(5):460–7. https://doi.org/10.1037/a0029597.

Hillier A, Kroehle K, Edwards H, Graves G. Risk, resilience, resistance and situated agency of trans high school students. Journal of LGBT youth. 2020;17(4):384–407.

James S, Herman J, Rankin S, Keing M, Mottet L, Anafi MA. The report of the 2015 US Transgender Survey; 2016.

Jones I. Healthcare open season for trans people [Podcast]. 2021. https://open.spotify.com/episode/6b0C9232Gk71JOfHeaGhDh?si=Sgq9A8xES1iy9X0iGO4xLg&nd=1. Accessed 9 Dec 2021.

Kidd KM, Sequeira GM, Douglas C, Paglisotti T, Inwards-Breland DJ, Miller E, Coulter RW. Prevalence of gender-diverse youth in an urban school district. Pediatrics. 2021;147(6):e2020049823.

Loo S, Almazan AN, Vedilago V, Stott B, Reisner SL, Keuroghlian AS. Understanding community member and health care professional perspectives on gender-affirming care—A qualitative study. PloS one. 2021;16(8):e0255568.

Meadow T. Trans Kids: Being Gendered in the Twenty-First Century (1st ed.). University of California Press. 2018.

Meyer IH. Prejudice, social stress, and mental health in lesbian, gay, and bisexual populations: conceptual issues and research evidence. Psychol Bull. 2003;129(5):674–97. https://doi.org/10.1037/0033-2909.129.5.674.

Rafferty J. Gender identity development in children. 2018. healthychildren.org.

Rafferty J, Yogman M, Baum R, Gambon TB, Lavin A, Mattson G, Wissow LS, Breuner C, Alderman EM, Grubb LK, Powers ME. Ensuring comprehensive care and support for transgender and gender-diverse children and adolescents. Pediatrics. 2018;142(4):e20182162.

Reisner SL, White JM, Dunham EE, Heflin K, Begenyi J, Cahill S, Project VOICE Team. Discrimination and health in Massachusetts: a statewide survey of transgender and gender nonconforming adults. Boston: Fenway Health; 2014.

Ronan W. Officially becomes worst year in recent history for LGBTQ state legislative attacks as unprecedented number of states enact record-shattering number of anti-LGBTQ measures into law. HRC. 2021. https://www.hrc.org/press-releases/2021-officially-becomes-worst-year-in-recent-history-for-lgbtq-state-legislative-attacks-as-unprecedented-number-of-states-enact-record-shattering-number-of-anti-lgbtq-measures-into-law. Accessed 6 Jan 2022.

Shires DA, Stroumsa D, Jaffee KD, Woodford MR. Primary care providers' willingness to continue gender-affirming hormone therapy for transgender patients. Fam Pract. 2018;35(5):576–81.

Travers A, Marchbank J, Boulay N, Jordan S, Reed K. Talking back: Trans youth and resilience in action. Journal of LGBT Youth. 2022;19(1):1–30.

Caring for Patient on Extracorporeal Membrane Oxygenation (ECMO) in the Pediatric Intensive Care Setting

Angela Hui Ping Kirk, Qian Wen Sng, Pei Fen Poh, Chandra Sekaran Pethaperumal, Yee Hui Mok, and Yoke Hwee Chan

Introduction

Extracorporeal membrane oxygenation (ECMO) provides respiratory and/or cardiac support for patients with cardiac and respiratory failure as a bridge to recovery, organ transplantation, or ventricular assist device implantation. Since the first published case of pediatric ECMO in 1972 followed by neonatal cases in 1976, subsequent decades witnessed an increased utilization of ECMO in neonatal and pediatric critical care settings. The deployment of this form of extracorporeal life support therapy is lifesaving, complex, and often time critical. While advancements in technology have improved and simplified ECMO circuit design over the years, the need for multidisciplinary stakeholder input and rapid and seamless team coordination remains crucial. A successful ECMO program incorporates a multidisciplinary team, clear and concise operations workflows, policies and procedures as well as quality assurance measures. A key component of an ECMO program is the team of ECMO-trained specialists with the necessary skills and expertise to manage both the critically ill patient and the extracorporeal circuit. ECMO programs across the

A. H. P. Kirk (✉) · Q. W. Sng · P. F. Poh · C. S. Pethaperumal
Division of Nursing, Children's Intensive Care Unit, KK Women's and Children's Hospital, Singapore, Singapore
e-mail: angela.kirk.hui.p@kkh.com.sg

Y. H. Mok · Y. H. Chan
Department of Paediatric Subspecialties, Children's Intensive Care Unit, KK Women's and Children's Hospital, Singapore, Singapore

Yong Loo Lin School of Medicine, National University of Singapore, Singapore, Singapore

Duke-NUS Medical School, Singapore, Singapore

C. L. Betz (ed.), *Worldwide Successful Pediatric Nurse-Led Models of Care*,
https://doi.org/10.1007/978-3-031-22152-1_8

globe recruit these specialists from diverse backgrounds of perfusion, respiratory therapy, physiotherapy, or critical care nursing, based on local needs and available resources.

Globally, nursing manpower accounts for majority of the health-care professionals (World Health Organization 2020). This profession has expanded rapidly in scope of practice beyond basic nursing care into advanced practice nursing in various specialties as well as in academia. Intensive care nurses in pediatric intensive care units (PICU) and neonatal intensive care units (NICU) are highly specialized. These specialized intensive care nurses require sound understanding of pediatric and neonatal physiology and quick critical thinking in times of emergencies. They are also attuned to teamwork in complex situations such as during cardiac arrest codes. These qualities make them suitable candidates to take on the expanded role as ECMO specialists. Hence, in many ECMO programs, ICU nurses have taken on leadership roles in ECMO programs and invested interest in ECMO specialist training and learning, development of ECMO policies and procedures as well as quality and risk management measures.

This chapter provides an overview of a multidisciplinary nurse-led ECMO program for critically ill children in a PICU in Singapore. It includes the contextual background from which the program was conceptualized, the planning and evaluation of the program including the theoretical framework that was used to develop the model, a description of the nurse-led model of care, the challenges and facilitators faced in the development and implementation of the model, the service adjustments made, the lessons learned, and the future plans for this program.

Background

ECMO is an advanced life-support that utilizes a modified heart-lung machine to provide temporary support for patients with severe cardiorespiratory failure refractory to conventional management. ECMO is not a curative but a supportive therapy that can stabilize the patient as a bridge to organ recovery, organ transplantation, device implantation, or decision. Currently, ECMO is utilized in more than 492 medical facilities worldwide and was successfully used to treat more than 46,000 neonatal and pediatric patients (ELSO 2020).

KK Women's and Children's Hospital (KKH) is an 830-bedded tertiary institution for women and children. As the largest pediatric hospital in Singapore, KKH caters to the majority of pediatric emergency cases in the country. It is both a local and regional tertiary referral center with about 26,000 pediatric admissions per year. KKH has a 16-bedded multidisciplinary PICU and a 40-bedded NICU. Both the PICU and NICU have about 700 admissions each annually, with the PICU admitting all postoperative cardiac patients and pediatric patients weighing more than two kilograms.

ECMO was first introduced to KKH PICU in 2002 and KKH NICU in 2006. In the first decade after the first case of ECMO was instituted for a child with postcardiotomy syndrome with low cardiac output state at KKH, ECMO was initiated on an ad hoc basis with an average of less than 10 cases per year. The decision to initiate ECMO on a patient was mainly undertaken by the cardiothoracic surgeons and the circuits were managed by perfusionists who used the same knowledge base and billing practices of the intraoperative cardiopulmonary bypass for the management of these bedside ECMO circuits. Over time, the increase in demand for ECMO beyond cardiac indications posed a strain on the capacity of perfusionists to manage bedside ECMO circuits. It was also evident that it was not a cost-effective and sustainable model of care with the limited supply of highly trained perfusionists in Singapore. This was especially so as the perfusionist manpower at KKH was centrally managed at the National Heart Centre, an adult specialty center within the same regional health-care cluster that KKH also belongs to. Besides the workload from open heart surgeries, the adult center was also experiencing increased demand for ECMO in adults, which posed additional strain on perfusionist manpower. When there were competing needs for perfusionist support for both ECMO and elective cardiac surgeries at KKH, the latter were occasionally postponed or canceled. In the absence of trained in-house ECMO specialists, the ICU team also anticipated a potential risk where there would be no perfusionist expertise for the emergency activation of ECMO or to troubleshoot acute ECMO complications.

Furthermore, ECMO is a highly specialized, time-critical, and complex therapy involving collaboration between multiple health-care professionals. The ECMO service requires nurses, cardiothoracic surgeons, cardiologists, perfusionists, and intensivist care physicians to be ready for the deployment of ECMO 24 h a day. Before 2012, there was no multidisciplinary coordinated program or an ECMO committee dedicated to review the ECMO service at KKH. With the rising volume of ECMO cases (Fig. 1), unstructured system, and lack of perfusionists, a team of intensive care physicians and nurses felt a strong impetus for the need of a formal ECMO program with trained in-house ECMO specialists at KKH.

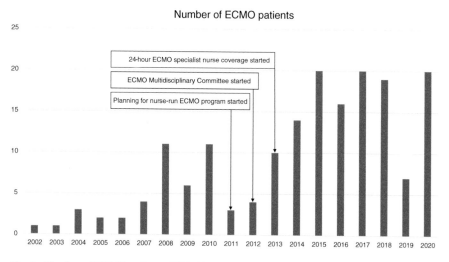

Fig. 1 Number of ECMO patients, 2002–2020

The Extracorporeal Life Support Organization (ELSO) defines the ECMO specialist as "the technical specialist trained to manage the ECMO system and clinical needs of the patient on ECMO under the direction and supervision of a licensed ECMO trained physician" (ELSO 2010, Page 2). The ECMO specialist should also have a strong critical care background in neonatal, pediatric, and/or adult critical care (ELSO 2010). The role of ECMO specialists is to manage patient-circuit interaction and the clinical needs of the patient, ensure the safety of the ECMO circuit through continuous surveillance, assessment, and troubleshooting, as well as prevent and manage circuit emergencies. These duties include the titration of ECMO blood flow and sweep gas to achieve adequate oxygen delivery and gas exchange targets, and titration of anticoagulation to achieve a balance the risks between thrombotic and bleeding events. The absence of a bedside ECMO specialist may increase the incidence of major technical complications and result in the need for emergent change in ECMO circuits (Padalino et al. 2017).

A nurse-led ECMO program has been shown to reduce cost with no difference in the rate of ECMO complications or survival to discharge and allow an increase in ECMO capacity as compared to a perfusionist-run ECMO program (Odish et al. 2021). In the study, the patient to ECMO specialist nurse ratio was reported as 3:1 and was in addition to existing ICU nursing care ratio.

The ECMO specialist nurses are skilled with precannulation responsibilities, patient and equipment management and assessment, managing ECMO complications and emergency, documentation, and weaning and decannulation (Table 1). Perfusionists continue to be activated during initiation or discontinuation of ECMO and circuit changes; perfusionists are always available by phone to provide

Table 1 Responsibilities of ECMO specialist nurse

• Prepares and assembles dry ECMO circuit for circuit change or emergency use
• Ensures appropriate blood products are available according to the ECMO protocol
• Primes ECMO circuits and assists perfusionist in the initiation of ECMO therapy
• Provides direct patient care by implementing, operating, and managing ECMO system, assembles back-up system, completes the prepump checklist prior to the start of ECMO
• Performs other patient care and related activities including continuous monitoring of patient during ECMO procedures, managing the circuit, preventing potential complications, and troubleshooting equipment when necessary
• Performs hemofiltration setup when necessary
• Performs activated clotting time (ACT) and administers/titrates anticoagulation according to ECMO protocol
• Identifies and diagnoses complication and makes recommendation for changes in patient's care in consultation with perfusionist and physician
• Ensures standby circuit, supplies, and equipment are always ready for emergency use and ECMO transport service
• Ensures safe inter- and intra-hospital transfer of ECMO supported patients, collaborating with other health-care personnel, managing the patient and the circuit
• Provides guidance and ensure safety during turning and repositioning patient on ECMO
• Provides wound care and dressing of the cannula site
• Assists surgeon and perfusionist in the process of decannulation

Table 1 (continued)

• Ensures strict infection control protocols are adhered to
• Performs monthly check and maintenance of stocks for ECMO cart and machine
• Participates in writing and reviewing ECMO policies and procedures
• Participates in three monthly ECMO multidisciplinary meeting
• Contributes to case presentation of individual ECMO cases during ECMO meeting
• Provides psychological support to patient and their families

expertise when needed. In this new model, ECMO specialist nurses are the primary ECMO resource person in the ICU, coordinating care and collaborating closely with other ECMO multidisciplinary team members. ECMO specialist nurses are primarily responsible for around-the-clock care of the ECMO circuit at bedside. They are also responsible for preventive maintenance of ECMO equipment, maintenance of inventory for ECMO consumables, coordination of ECMO transport, and quality assurance initiatives. The implementation of this new ECMO specialist nurse care model has enabled service expansion, increased ECMO capacity, and decreased costs.

Process Undertaken to Implement the Model

Acquiring ECMO Knowledge and Skills from Established ECMO Centers

In 2011, a team of two physicians, four ICU nurses, and one perfusionist was awarded the Health Manpower Development Program (HMDP) team award from the Ministry of Health, Singapore, to acquire knowledge and skills from established ECMO centers in North America, namely, the Children's Hospital of Michigan, Duke Children's Hospital, Boston Children's Hospital, and The Hospital for Sick Children, Toronto. The team studied the structure of these ECMO programs including the operations planning, training, and education as well as quality assurance measures. The team was also exposed to clinical care of ECMO patients through clinical observations and participated in ECMO workshops. The team also established useful and enduring links with international ECMO leaders. While the ECMO specialist teams in these centers consisted of respiratory therapists, the HMDP team returned with plans to establish a nurse-led, perfusionist-supported ECMO program at KKH.

KKH Pediatric-Neonatal ECMO Committee

The KKH Pediatric-Neonatal ECMO committee was set up in January 2012 with the aims of establishing an ECMO program with a multidisciplinary ECMO team with defined roles and responsibilities, as well as to formalize workflows, establish policies and procedures, formulate training and education, and make decisions on equipment selection and accreditation requirements for ECMO specialist nurses. Currently, the ECMO committee is comprised of the program director and an ECMO nurse coordinator with members from the PICU and NICU medical and nursing teams, cardiothoracic surgeons, ECMO specialist nurses, cardiologists, and hematologists. The ECMO committee is responsible for every issue related to ECMO in the hospital and strategizes how the institutional ECMO capacity can be maintained or increased.

During the development phase, the committee embarked on plans to establish evidence-based clinical guidelines, policies and procedures, training and an accreditation program for ECMO specialist nurses as well as budget planning and equipment acquisition (Table 2). Subcommittees were formed and assigned to work on different aspects of the ECMO program. As part of change management, all stakeholders were involved in the planning of this new model of care and ICU nurses

Table 2 Components of program planning	Clinical guidelines
	Indications for ECMO
	Initiation of ECMO
	Maintenance and daily monitoring
	Troubleshooting of acute complications
	Weaning and decannulation
	Hemofiltration and continuous renal replacement therapy
	Anticoagulation and monitoring
	ECMO transport
	Policies and procedures
	Team composition
	Roles and job descriptions
	Quality assurance
	Training and accreditation

	Training
	  – Didactic lectures
	  – Simulations
	  – Wet labs
	  – Bedside preceptorship

	Accreditation
	  – Competency checks
	  – Bedside hours
	  – Yearly logbook review

	Budget planning

	Capital equipment
	  – ECMO machine and monitors
	  – Thermoregulator
	  – Transport equipment

	Operating expenditure
	  – Manpower (ECMO specialist nurses)
	  – ECMO consumables
	  – Point-of-care test consumables

played critical roles as leads or members in each of the subcommittees. The ECMO committee met fortnightly to discuss, amend, and approve the work of the subcommittees. The committee sought consensus from best practices and also through simulations for workflow-related issues. The ELSO guidelines were instrumental in the development of our institutional nurse-led ECMO model (ELSO 2021).

Working with Stakeholders

The ECMO committee also worked with numerous other stakeholders in the hospital to facilitate change (Table 3). To standardize medication and laboratory orders, the team worked with the health informatics team to create medication and laboratory order sets in the electronic medical record (EMR) for ECMO initiation and daily ECMO management. Documentation templates were created in the EMR for daily ECMO goals for physiological, laboratory, and anticoagulation parameters as well as ECMO monitoring charts. The ECMO committee also worked with the Children's Hospital Emergency Transport Service and radiology department to streamline ambulance service and diagnostic imaging service for patients on ECMO. ECMO transport timeout and equipment checklists were also created in the EMR to facilitate systematic preparations of the patient, equipment, and medications before transportation of an ECMO patient.

When emergency ECMO initiation is required, particularly in extracorporeal cardiopulmonary resuscitation (eCPR), a quick and effective way to activate the multidisciplinary team of cardiothoracic surgeon, operating theater staff, ECMO specialist nurse, and ICU attending is crucial. The committee decided to utilize the

Table 3 Interdepartmental collaboration

Collaboration roles and responsibilities include
Health informatics department   – Medication order sets for ECMO initiation

Biomedical engineering and finance departments
  – Tender for equipment acquisition and review
  – Equipment maintenance contract

Laboratory   – Acquisition of additional point-of-care tests, e.g., plasma-free hemoglobin, activated clotting time
Blood bank   – Readily available fresh and O+ blood products in "ECMO packs"

ECMO "code"
  – Operating room staff, e.g., scrub nurses
  – Cardiothoracic surgeons and cardiologist
  – Perfusionists

Transport service
  – Trained ambulance service personnel for transporting ECMO patient
  – Availability of ambulance

Radiology service   – Diagnostic imaging services

existing system for "code" activation via the hospital's public address system, manned by the hospital security team, for emergency deployment of the ECMO team. This system had been tested and effected for cardiopulmonary arrests and obstetric emergencies in the hospital for years. The ECMO specialist nurse, operating theater staff, ICU attending and junior medical staff, cardiothoracic surgeon, anesthetist, and cardiologist were allocated preassigned roles during such "ECMO codes." The availability of blood products for "ECMO codes" was also a key consideration for the priming of ECMO circuits. As the national maternal and child hospital in the country with a large population of vulnerable neonates and young children, it was decided that fresh and leuco-depleted blood products in "packs" ready for ECMO initiation, defined by weight range, should be on standby in the blood bank for such emergency requests in agreement with the hospital's blood bank service. To test the feasibility of the various workflows from ECMO team activation to execution, the committee conducted simulations through mock "ECMO codes."

Recruitment and Training of ECMO Specialist Nurses

Another challenge in the development of this nurse-led ECMO program was the recruitment and training of ECMO specialist nurses. The pioneer cadre of ECMO specialist nurses were the four senior registered nurses from NICU and PICU who took part in the HMDP study trips. The HMDP committee agreed that ICU nurses in the hospital would be the most appropriate candidates to take on the expanded role of ECMO specialists based on the following considerations: (1) familiarity with the physiology of critically ill neonates and children, (2) familiarity with multidisciplinary teamwork in complex settings as they play key roles as first responders in hospital "codes" for cardiopulmonary arrests and trauma, (3) expertise in the initiation and maintenance of continuous hemodialysis, which also involved extracorporeal circuits, and most importantly (4) support from the hospital nursing leadership. The ECMO committee acknowledged that the success of this nurse-led ECMO program leveraged strongly on the successful implementation of this expanded role of the ICU nurses. The process took three phases: (1) engagement, (2) enablement, and (3) empowerment. In the *engagement* phase, the ECMO committee engaged the ICU medical and nursing teams in this new initiative and collected feedback. The eligibility for recruitment into the ECMO specialist nurse team was based on the agreed criteria of the individual's ability to work in a team, communication skills, experience in ICU nursing, and critical thinking skills. *Enablement* took the form of a structured ECMO course designed by the perfusionist and medical teams consisting of didactic lectures, wet laboratory, and simulation sessions. Completion of the ECMO course was followed by bedside preceptorship and accreditation by the perfusionists. Policies and procedures to guide nursing practice were compiled and prepared by the ECMO committee and ICU nursing team. After one year of training, the pioneer cohort of ECMO specialist nurses completed their didactic and clinical hands-on training in 2012. They achieved 50 h of experience each before being qualified as an ECMO specialist nurse. The planning phase to the first independent nurse-led ECMO run took about 24 months. The committee *empowered* this pioneer group of ECMO specialist nurses to lead and further expand the pool of ECMO specialist nurses. One of the four ECMO specialist nurses subsequently became an ECMO nurse coordinator in the committee. By 2013, KKH had eight ECMO specialist nurses (Fig. 1). With the eight ECMO specialist nurses, the team was then able to provide round-the-clock bedside coverage for ECMO patients, with perfusionists providing support during ECMO initiation, decannulation, transport, and ECMO emergencies.

Theoretical Framework

We used the intensive care unit team performance framework to guide development of this new ECMO team model within the ICU (Reader et al. 2009). This framework outlines how team outputs such as patient outcomes, adverse events, teamwork, and morale are influenced by team processes relating to team communication, leadership, coordination, and decision making within the ICU.

In developing the ECMO team model, ECMO committee members and ECMO specialist nurses were chosen based on their experience and knowledge as well as personal characteristics such as resilience, communication skills, and collaborative mind-set. Roles and responsibilities of the committee members and specialist nurses (Table 1) were clearly defined within the program. The ECMO committee also developed clear policies and procedures and worked with stakeholders (Table 3) to streamline processes relating to ECMO support. In defining the leadership within the ECMO team model, the committee identified recognized leaders from within the medical and nursing professions who had both the required knowledge and expertise as well as the drive for change.

Managing ECMO patients involves a comprehensive, systematic assessment of patient and circuit-related factors and skilled multidisciplinary team input and management. Therefore, effective communication and collaboration is a core requirement for the provision of high-quality care for the ECMO patient (Key 2020). While the ECMO program director is a physician, the care and maintenance of the ECMO circuit is primarily nurse-led. To inculcate team inclusiveness and multidisciplinary decision-making, the program director and deputy directors encourage all team members to express their concerns and ideas freely. Junior team members are encouraged to speak up if there are any concerns. During an emergency, a directive leadership approach is used, where team members have clear, delegated tasks assigned to them by the ICU team leader, and are encouraged to follow and acknowledge the team leader's instructions with closed loop communication.

The ECMO committee also set up multiple channels of communication to facilitate multidisciplinary collaboration and co-ordination. This included the creation of mobile instant messaging chatgroups for ease of dissemination of information; implementation of a hospital wide "ECMO code," as well as standardized documentation of ECMO support and daily management goals in the EMR. The use of a standardized template for daily goals tool enables better communication and collaboration and guides patient care (Key 2020). Transporting patients on ECMO is high-risk, with the potential of catastrophic mechanical and clinical complications. As part of the risk management measures, the team used the failure mode and effects analysis (FMEA) method to identify and analyze processes to mitigate the risk of adverse events for high-risk activities such as the transportation of patients on ECMO. FMEA is a systematic method of identifying and preventing product and process problems before they occur (Liu et al. 2020). It offers a proactive approach to detecting failures in contrast to incident analysis and root cause analysis which are performed retrospectively. The six steps in FMEA process are as follows: (1) Define the topic. (2) Assemble the interdisciplinary team. (3) Identify potential failure modes. (4) Conduct the analysis. (5) Determine high-risk failure modes. (6) Identify actions and outcome measures. Through this process, the ECMO team recognized 4 stages of processes and 18 subprocesses when transporting patient on ECMO (Fig. 2): 28 failure modes were identified and their risk priority number ranges from 60 to 280. Proposed solutions were applied to 20 failure modes that had a risk priority number of more than 100. Findings and proposed solutions from the FMEA process were used to develop a hospital-based guideline for the safe transport of a patient on ECMO.

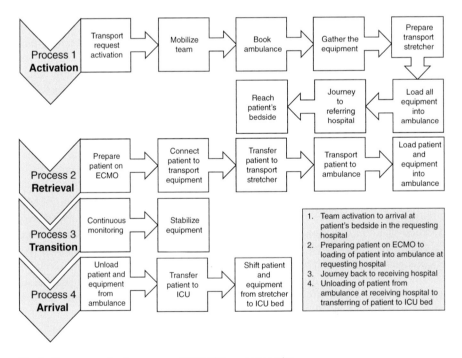

Fig. 2 Processes and subprocesses of ECMO transport service

As part of quality assurance, regular audit meetings with clinical stakeholders are held quarterly, where each case is discussed and learning points identified. Patient and team-related outcomes are tracked and presented to the committee on a yearly basis.

Organizational Component

The organizational component of the nurse-led ECMO model is presented in Fig. 3. The ECMO nurse coordinator is a senior ECMO specialist nurse who works closely with the ECMO director to develop and maintain guidelines, implement training, maintain competency, and conduct equipment evaluations and procurement. During ECMO treatment, the ECMO specialist nurse is the technical specialist in charge of the ECMO circuit, whereas the ECMO bedside nurse is responsible for the primary care of the patient. In addition to being a technical specialist, the ECMO specialist nurse also has the necessary skills and knowledge on patient-circuit interactions to maintain physiological goals on oxygen delivery, gas exchange and anticoagulation as well as to troubleshoot acute complications related to ECMO.

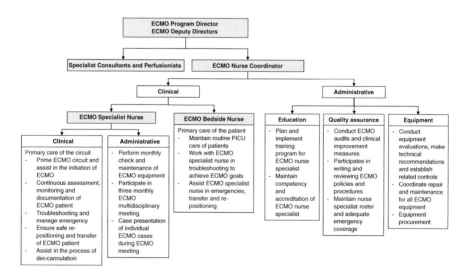

Fig. 3 Organizational component of the nurse-run ECMO program

Service Components

The ECMO service consists of three phases: (a) ECMO initiation, (b) ECMO maintenance, and (c) post-ECMO management.

ECMO Initiation

Prior to the initiation of ECMO, the pediatric intensivist will review the clinical condition of the child to assess if the child is a suitable candidate for ECMO support. Clinical indications for veno-arterial (VA) and veno-venous (VV) ECMO, contraindications of ECMO and the hemodynamic, respiratory, and metabolic parameters that may guide the decision to institute ECMO, are available in an ECMO guideline document.

Once a decision for ECMO cannulation has been made, the ECMO specialist nurse is instrumental in facilitating the smooth precannulation preparation. The ECMO specialist nurse delegates tasks such as the activation of the perfusionist, collection of blood products for ECMO circuit priming, positioning and preparation of the patient while getting ready to prime the ECMO circuit. The ECMO specialist nurse, with the help of the perfusionist, aims to complete clear priming of the ECMO circuit within 30 minutes of activation. After successful completion of ECMO cannulation by the cardiothoracic surgeons, the ECMO specialist nurse monitors blood gases and activated clotting time (ACT) to determine the timing of initiation of anticoagulation, as well as titration of ECMO blood flow, oxygen, and gas sweep.

Where ECMO initiation is required for patients outside of KKH, the ECMO specialist nurse co-ordinates the necessary equipment and consumables required to be brought along by the transport team, and assists with the initiation process by the bedside together with the transport team.

ECMO Maintenance

ECMO therapy is managed in accordance with daily ECMO goals set by the managing physicians, based on recommended targets in the ECMO guidelines. ECMO specialist nurses' role in the daily management of patients on ECMO support include close monitoring of the physical health of the ECMO circuit, titration of anticoagulation based on ACT targets, adjustment of the ECMO variables including gas sweep, oxygen content and blood flows in response to patient condition in consultation with the managing physician. In the event that patient transportation is required, a large multidisciplinary team comprising the pediatric intensivist, cardiothoracic surgeon, perfusionist, ECMO specialist nurse, ICU nurse, and security officers is required. The ECMO specialist nurse also plays a central role in the co-ordination and physical transfer process.

Post-ECMO Management

Follow-up of ECMO patients includes doppler ultrasound studies of the vessels used for ECMO cannulation, to document and manage any post-ECMO cannulation complications such as vessel thrombosis and stenosis. Where applicable, neonatal and pediatric ECMO patients up to eight years of age will be offered follow-up with a developmental pediatrician for neurodevelopmental assessment and interventions. In addition, neonatal ECMO patients will receive a referral for early intervention with high-risk hearing screening upon home discharge. ECMO data for each ECMO run will also be reported to ELSO registry.

Roles of the Nurses

ECMO Nurse Coordinator

The ECMO nurse coordinator is a senior ECMO specialist nurse who serves as the primary liaison between the ECMO committee and perfusion services, nursing, pharmacy, laboratory, transfusion services and the respective vendors. The nurse coordinator serves as liaison between the ECMO team and the patient and their families on all ECMO related patient issues, such as providing education and psychological support.

Logistically, ECMO nurse coordinators work with respective vendors and our hospital's biomedical engineers to ensure that the ECMO equipment and point-of-care testing machines are valid and safe for use. They are also responsible for the ordering, storing, and using of equipment, and ensuring availability of equipment at all times. In terms of human resources management, the nurse coordinator develops and maintains training and accreditation for the ECMO specialist nurses under the guidelines put forth by the ELSO Registry, and is responsible for the ongoing education and continual assessments of the ECMO specialist nurses. The nurse coordinator also plans the ECMO specialist nurse roster, oversees recruitment and manpower planning. As part of ECMO team recruitment, the ECMO nurse coordinator will also invite bedside nurses who exhibit exemplary work and interest during the care of an ECMO patient to join the team as an ECMO specialist nurse.

ECMO Specialist Nurse

ECMO specialist nurses are PICU/NICU nurses with over 2 years of senior-level experience nursing critically ill neonates and children. They have demonstrated high levels of independence, critical thinking and resilience to stressful events, are decisive, and exhibit excellent teamwork and communication skills. The ECMO specialist nurse is central to the care of the patient and facilitates communication between the multidisciplinary team and the patient's family. The ECMO specialist nurse oversees up to three patients supported on ECMO with a bedside nurse allocated to each patient.

The overarching responsibilities (Table 1) of the ECMO specialist nurse includes facilitation of cannulation, management of the extracorporeal circuit, troubleshooting, accessing the circuit (hemofilter or continuous renal replacement therapy), ensuring optimal function of the oxygenator by monitoring blood gases from both the pre- and post-oxygenator limb, wound care and dressing of the cannula sites, titration of support (blood flow, sweep gas, oxygen and anticoagulation) according to stipulated ECMO goals, and to ensure patient safety during patient movement and transport. The ECMO specialist nurse serves as the person of reference, especially after-hours to facilitate swift multidisciplinary coordination, blood requisition and patient preparation simultaneously, while other respective specialists such as the perfusionist, cardiologist and cardiac thoracic surgeon travel on-site. The ECMO specialist nurse is also trained to manage emergencies, for example, able to recognize the need to emergently isolate patient from the ECMO circuit and transition the pump head from primary motor to back-up motor and console, when indicated.

During an off-site ECMO activation, the ECMO specialist nurse, who is also well-versed in transportation of a critically ill pediatric patient, will travel on-site with the pediatric intensivist and transport team. While on-site, the ECMO specialist nurse will work with the pediatric intensivist to facilitate circuit priming, medication, and anticoagulation administration. This teamwork allows seamless collaboration during a highly stressful and high-stake procedure at an external setting.

As part of quality assurance, the ECMO specialist nurse performs an audit of each ECMO run and presents the findings at the quarterly ECMO audit meeting. The audit includes discussion on the duration from activation to initiation of pump flow, challenges encountered with personnel or equipment during initiation, review of the use of anticoagulation, rationale for blood product transfusion, adequate documentation, and adverse events and complications during the ECMO runs. The review of all ECMO runs via the audit meetings has helped to continually improve the ECMO services over time to improve patient outcomes. As a member of the ELSO Registry, we contribute to the collective database of neonatal and pediatric ECMO runs. The ECMO specialist nurses are responsible of the data-entry of ECMO run information and participation in ELSO surveys.

Bedside Nurse

The bedside nurse, although not as qualified as an ECMO specialist nurse, are nurses of a senior level who are confident in nursing pediatric patients with high acuity. They do not have the skills to troubleshoot or access the extracorporeal circuit. Bedside nurses receive on-the-job training regarding ECMO physiology, treatment goals and monitoring. The ECMO specialist nurse also regularly provides tutorials to bedside nurses to ensure safe care and to educate them on signs for concerns that should be communicated to the ECMO specialist nurse promptly. The bedside nurse training program includes the knowledge and indications for various ECMO support, safe handling and movement of the patient, point-of-care monitoring, such as ACT monitoring and the understanding of the role and responsibilities of the bedside and ECMO specialist nurse. The involvement of highly skilled bedside nurses has been especially helpful during episodes of concurrent ECMO runs.

Multidisciplinary Team

The main ECMO care team includes the pediatric intensivist, cardiologist, cardiothoracic surgeons, perfusionist, ECMO specialist nurse, and bedside nurse. In addition, there is a multidisciplinary team of health-care professionals inclusive of the hematologist, anesthesiologist, dietician, physiotherapist, respiratory therapist, medical social worker, and child life therapist, who also contributes to the overall management of the patient on ECMO to optimize care.

Child-centered and family-centered care initiatives are integrated into the daily care of patients on ECMO. Our PICU has adopted 24-hour open visiting policies for parents, to promote family presence and involvement in care. The ECMO specialist nurse and bedside nurse are always at the bedside, and will update parent on child's status or attend to parents' queries. Depending on the patient's condition and level of sedation, child life specialist, music therapist, and art therapist can be engaged to assist in patient care. These trained professionals can help to minimize patient's anxiety, increase understanding, and provide support and age-appropriate coping strategies while the child is on ECMO therapy. All health-care professionals attending to patient are encouraged to address the child by his/her preferred name.

Family members are encouraged and supported in participating in care and decision-making at the level they choose. The medical social worker regularly follows up with parents, conducts psychosocial assessment, and provides counseling and financial assistance if required. Together with the ECMO specialist nurse or bedside nurse, family members are encouraged to do simple things such as touch, talk, read, or sing to the child as the familiarity of their voice and face, as well as comfort of their touch will help ease the anxieties of the child. Family members are also encouraged to play the child's favorite music and bring in their favorite toy to make the environment more familiar and reassuring. Participation in basic care such as changing diapers, applying lotion, and performing passive range-of-motion exercises are also allowed and encouraged. Lastly, as part of family-centered care initiatives, family conferences are regularly conducted in a private room with the family members, ECMO team, and, at times, the palliative team. These meetings allow for the sharing of information, reassurance, and an opportunity for parental feedback. Mutual understanding, agreement on treatment plan, and shared decisions making based on the best clinical evidence and consistent with patient and family values are goals, which the ECMO team strives to achieve with the family.

ECMO is an invasive intervention focused on curative or life-prolonging therapy, it can help bridge patient to recovery or to definitive therapies like device implantation or organ transplantation. However, there are times when prolonging ECMO therapy will not change outcome and death may be expected despite maximum therapies or when organ transplantation is not available. In these situations, the goal of care will shift from curative to ECMO decannulation and end-of-life care.

Together with the palliative team, the ECMO team may recommend that ECMO be discontinued. As Singapore is a multicultural and multiracial county, end-of-life discussions with the family will be done in a respectful, empathetic, and culturally sensitive manner when shared end-of-life goals of care with patient and family are established. The team facilitates and encourages the family to participate in the end-of-life care if desired. Prior to decannulation, the patient is transferred to a single room where family members visit and activities such as memory-making (e.g., family photographs, handprints) and performance of religious rituals will be offered. The ECMO nurse, with the bedside nurse and palliative team, ensures adequate symptom control for pain, dyspnea, or anxiety before, during, and after decannulation. After the patient's death, the bereavement team consisting of the nurses and the medical social workers continue to offer and provide the family psychological, social, and spiritual support. A multiprofessional mortality debrief session will be held among the health-care providers to address the emotional needs of staff through sharing of personal impressions of the process.

Training for ECMO Specialist Nurses

ECMO is a low occurrence and high-risk therapy. We adopted a multimodal approach in the delivery of ECMO training for the ECMO specialist nurses. The initial training consisted of three main components: a didactic ECMO specialist course, hands-on sessions in the wet-laboratory or simulation sessions, and on-the-job training precepted by senior ECMO specialist nurses. The wet-laboratory session includes the revision of the circuit configuration and function, priming and circuit setup, and the change of pressure monitors.

The didactic ECMO course is held over 2 days and is conducted by the perfusionists, intensivists, specialist consultants, and senior ECMO specialist nurses. The course includes both the theoretical and practical aspects of ECMO. The theoretical part of ECMO includes the introduction and history of ECMO, physiology of the illness related with ECMO, criteria and contraindications for ECMO, and physiological of VA and VV ECMO. Pre-ECMO preparations, management of anticoagulation, handling of ECMO equipment, daily management of the patient and ECMO circuit, troubleshooting, ECMO emergencies and complications, weaning from ECMO, decannulation procedures, post-ECMO complications, and monitoring are practical aspects of ECMO, which are included in the course.

Each trainee ECMO specialist nurse also undergoes hands-on training in the selection of the appropriate circuits, oxygenator, and cannulas for patient as well as priming of the ECMO circuits. Simulated ECMO scenarios such as pump failure, circuit change, deairing the circuit, power failure, cannula dislodgement, loss of venous output, and emergency ECMO cannulation or ECPR are conducted regularly. ECMO transport scenarios are also performed to familiarize the specialist with ECMO emergencies as well as the transport stretcher setup and limitations of cannulation in an unfamiliar location. These sessions provide the trainee ECMO specialist nurse with a full understanding of the function of the circuit and all circuit-related emergencies.

After completion of the ECMO specialist course, ECMO specialist nurses are required to fulfill 50 h of clinical time caring for an ECMO circuit, complete an annual skills competency, exhibit appropriate clinical experience, and receive a satisfactory evaluation by the ECMO nurse coordinator to fulfill the annual recertification requirements. For nurses who are unable to fulfill 50 h of clinical time due to the low number of ECMO cases, they are required to attend a one-day wet-laboratory session before recertification.

Methods of Evaluation

In 2012, KKH's pediatric and neonatal ECMO program joined the ELSO registry, which maintains the largest registry of ECMO cases worldwide. Being a member of ELSO allows us access to the registry and international benchmarking with other centers listed in the registry.

Our ECMO program also holds quarterly audit meetings that are open to all multidisciplinary team members involved in the care of ECMO patients. Individual cases are presented by ECMO specialists for discussion with the multidisciplinary team. Adverse events and learning points were captured for each case. Statistics, including caseload, benchmarking with the ELSO Registry, and future directions for the year ahead, are presented on an annual basis.

Since the introduction of the nurse-run ECMO model in 2012, our average number of ECMO cases in KKH per year has increased from 4.4 to 14.4 cases (Fig. 1). To date, we have trained 31 ECMO specialist nurses (Fig. 4).

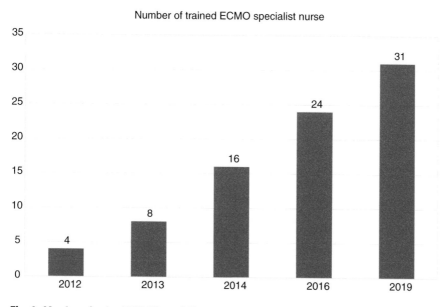

Fig. 4 Number of trained ECMO specialist nurses

Challenges and Facilitators

During the initial implementation period of the program, it was challenging to recruit nurses to be part of the ECMO specialist nurse team. Nurses felt hesitant to take on the new role as the nurse-led, perfusionist-supported ECMO program was novel in the local context. It is the first and only ECMO center in Singapore to deviate from the "traditional" perfusionist-led model. In addition, nurses recognized the inherent risks of ECMO and the heavy responsibilities of the ECMO specialist nurse. To overcome these barriers, the perfusionists provided robust on-the-job training with the pioneering ECMO specialist nurses. Close guidance and supervision were provided during the transition period to help the pioneer ECMO specialist nurses build confidence and technical expertise. Even after the transition to the new ECMO specialist nurse-led program, perfusionists are required to be present for high-risk procedures such as ECMO cannulation, decannulation, and intra- and inter-hospital transfers.

The maintenance of skills and competence remains an ongoing challenge for ECMO specialist nurses. Although KKH is the largest pediatric hospital in the country, we are considered a low volume ECMO center with an average of less than 20 cases per year. It remains challenging to improve technical skills and experience due to the low volume of such cases. Hence, an accreditation process was introduced to ensure the competency of ECMO specialist nurses. Accreditation includes a yearly competency assessment of all advanced care procedures, point-of-care tests, and pharmacologic agents used in ECMO management. Wet-laboratory training was provided for ECMO specialist nurses who did not meet the minimal number of practice hours. In situ simulations were also conducted on a regular basis and served as valuable training opportunities to help ECMO specialist nurses repeatedly practice technical skills and become proficient in high-risk, high-complexity, low-volume procedures.

Over time, several ECMO specialist nurses expressed that they were shouldering too much responsibility especially during emergencies. ECMO specialist nurses are often the first to respond to ECMO technical crises or complications and need to intervene independently. ECMO specialist nurses were sometimes overwhelmed with anxiety about making mistakes, which may lead to catastrophic outcomes. This was especially so among newer ECMO specialist nurses, whose lack of experience exacerbated their anxiety in new and challenging clinical scenarios. Regular formal and informal meetings were organized by ECMO committee leaders to discuss specific ECMO cases and evaluate their outcomes with the ECMO specialist nurses. Mistakes and difficulties were shared openly as learning points for all team members to improve their care. Such candidness improves team learning and creates a feeling of psychological safety (Wellman 2017). Although the model of care had shifted away from perfusionist-led management, perfusionists remain critical members of the team and provide their services readily in times of need. The perfusionists' support helped to allay some anxiety for the ECMO specialist nurses. Frequent words of appreciation were given by senior leadership to maintain morale among team members, especially after challenging ECMO cases. Timely group debriefs are conducted to address distress especially for ECMO mortality.

There was also initial apprehension among ECMO specialist nurses when they presented cases at audit meetings before an audience comprising of various medical personnel and perfusionists. Steps were taken to boost their confidence and these included the creation of a presentation template that was easy to use, and preview of the case presentations with the ECMO committee deputy director before the audit meetings to refine and rehearse the case presentations. The ECMO committee also made efforts to support and encourage ECMO specialist nurse presentations at regional and international ECMO meetings. Over the years, ECMO specialist nurses' confidence has strengthened as the content experts and resource persons for other health-care professionals.

Address Financing/Reimbursement

In Singapore, government subsidies for hospital bills are provided through the "3M" system—Medisave, Medishield, and Medifund. Parents can utilize their Medisave and Medishield to pay for their children's hospital bills. The former is a savings account within the central provident fund of all working adults where monthly contributions are provided to the account by both the working adult and his employer. Medishield is government medical insurance program wherein the premium is collected from the Medisave account to help to cover the costs of large hospitalization bills. Medifund is a safety net provided by the government to all Singaporeans who cannot afford the balance. From the hospital end, funding to public hospitals is given as a block budget. As ECMO is a costly but life-saving procedure, this new model of training ECMO nurse specialists from existing PICU nursing manpower to replace perfusionists in routine bedside care offers manpower cost savings without compromising quality of care in a sustainable manner.

Service Adjustments Made

Several adjustments were made after stabilizing the nurse-led, perfusion-supported ECMO service. This included (1) provision of off-site ECMO initiation and transport, (2) expansion of clinical indications of ECMO, (3) centralization of ECMO care to the PICU, and (4) pandemic preparedness planning for patients requiring ECMO support.

In 2014, with the ECMO team's increasing experience and technical expertise, initiation of ECMO outside the hospital for stabilization and transport back to KKH was added as part of the program's capabilities for children referred for severe cardiac or respiratory failure. Within Singapore, only two public hospitals have ECMO capabilities for pediatric and neonatal patients. Pediatric and neonatal patients presenting in other hospitals or emergency departments did not have easy access to the life-saving ECMO treatment. Patients requiring high ventilatory and inotropic support are often also too unstable to be transported safely. Prior to the development of this ECMO transport service, no other institutions could provide transport of pediatric and neonatal ECMO patients in Singapore. Recognizing the need for pediatric and neonatal off-site ECMO initiation and retrieval, a protocol was created to provide this service. The service leveraged on the hospital's existing transport service for retrieval of critically ill children. With the new transport service, new equipment was purchased. It remains a vital service for pediatric and neonatal patients, whom in the past would have had no access to this life-saving treatment.

In the initial period, ECMO support was limited to myocarditis and postcardiotomy cases. The transition to a nurse-led, perfusionist-supported ECMO program mitigated the issue of insufficient perfusionist manpower, allowing us to expand our services to deploy ECMO for severe sepsis, respiratory failure, and ECPR.

When the ECMO program was first set up, neonatal and pediatric patients requiring ECMO were managed in the NICU and PICU, respectively. These units were housed on the same floor of the hospital but across a long corridor. As the program's caseload increased, it was not feasible for rostered ECMO specialist nurses to care for ECMO patients in two different locations. Furthermore, neonatal patients only comprised less than a third of the ECMO runs in the hospital. The issue of unfamiliarity for the NICU medical staff due to the low numbers of neonatal ECMO patients also posed a challenge. ECMO cases were subsequently centralized in the PICU to facilitate ease of ECMO specialist nurse deployment as well as to consolidate clinical expertise and resources.

The ECMO program was also involved in the hospital pandemic planning for novel respiratory virus outbreaks after our experience with the severe acute respiratory syndrome (SARS) outbreak in 2003. This was ramped up to full preparatory mode in 2020. The novel human coronavirus disease COVID-19 was first reported in Wuhan, China, in December 2019 and subsequently spread globally. Singapore reported its first patient with COVID-19 in January 2020. While Singapore did not yet have any pediatric patients with severe COVID-19 infection, in anticipation of the possible need for ECMO in pediatric patients with COVID-19-related respiratory failure, in situ simulations of ECMO activation were conducted within the hospital's isolation ICU to familiarize the ECMO team members with the modified workflow including need for full PPE and isolation precautions during ECMO cannulation and space constraints within the isolation ICU. Findings and learning points from the simulation were incorporated into a new ECMO workflow for infectious patients requiring ECMO in isolation ICU.

Lessons Learned

The ability to provide effective and safe ECMO care takes the dedication of a comprehensive, multidisciplinary team. A centralized, dedicated multidisciplinary team with a robust service delivery model and mechanisms for quality improvement is likely to make the provision of ECMO safer and feasible in low-volume centers. Key factors for program success include a clear clinical governance structure, ongoing training, accreditation, maintenance of standards, sustainable program delivery, and consideration of caseload required to maintain proficiency (McCaffrey et al. 2016).

Being the 24/7 bedside health-care specialist, the ECMO specialist nurse has a comprehensive knowledge of the patient's overall status during ECMO therapy. The multidisciplinary team values the contributions of the ECMO specialist nurse to the patient's plan of care as they are able to provide details of the patient's response to therapy and actively collaborate with the team in the development of the care plan. ECMO physicians are trained in the ECMO process but will often look to the ECMO specialist nurse to perform technical tasks necessary to troubleshoot a problem. In a nurse-led ECMO program, nursing staff play an integral role within the ECMO team. Apart from acquiring and maintaining appropriate accreditation, nurses must ensure both initial and ongoing clinical competence. Additionally, support from the hospital senior management with commitment to provide access to continuing education is also essential to help maintain the clinical competence of the multidisciplinary team.

An implementation that builds in continuous quality improvement methodology is essential in new models of care. With the advancement of ECMO technology and increase in ECMO cases and experience, the team needs to regularly evaluate its services and outcomes. All ECMO cases are routinely and critically reviewed in a multidisciplinary meeting after each ECMO run. The ECMO specialist nurses regularly update the ECMO database that includes patient data and ELSO registry information. Collected data are analyzed and used for quality improvement initiatives, research projects, and benchmarking against international and national standards. Throughout the years, the team has successfully implemented multiple quality improvement initiatives such as neurodevelopmental follow-up and an early mobilization program for ECMO patients. Early mobilization is defined as the initiation of safe, appropriate mobility activities for patients within 48–72 h of admission to the PICU, with the aim of improving functional and clinical outcomes and reducing ICU-related morbidities (Table 4). All ICU patients, including ECMO patients, are evaluated from Monday through Friday for their suitability for participation in physical therapy. Patients are systematically assessed by a multidisciplinary team involving physiotherapists, nurses, nurse practitioners, respiratory therapists, and intensive care physicians, for clinical stability and suitability for mobility activities.

Table 4 Early mobilization and ICU liberation

• Early mobilization is the initiation of safe and appropriate physical activities within 48–72 h of ICU admission
• Critically ill patients in the ICU are at risk of developing postintensive care syndrome, which is a collection of health problems that can remain after the critical illness, and can affect physical, psychological, cognitive, and social functions
• Early mobilization is part of an ICU liberation bundle, with the aim of improving functional and clinical outcomes and reducing ICU-related morbidities
• Other elements of the ICU liberation bundle include adequate analgesia, prioritizing analgesia over sedation, spontaneous awakening and breathing, screening for and managing delirium, and family-centered care
• Early mobilization requires multidisciplinary team planning and implementation, including nurses, physiotherapists, respiratory therapists, occupational therapists, speech and language therapists, child-life therapists, doctors, and families

Mobility activities are categorized according to their level of intensity. As a relatively new initiative, mobility activities for ECMO patients have been limited to less intense activities, such as active-assisted limb ranging while in bed. In time, we hope to achieve greater degrees of mobilization for our ECMO patients, including activities such as sitting out of bed, standing, and ambulation.

Future Implications

There are currently no agreed standards of practice or certification for ECMO specialists in Singapore nor internationally. ECMO specialist accreditation in each institution is dependent on the institution's internally developed standards. Each ECMO center, depending on the center's need and the availability of resources, such as finances and manpower, has developed its own ECMO specialist role, staffing arrangements, and training program. There are also no internationally agreed frameworks of service provision or defined competencies for ECMO specialists and the specific roles within the multidisciplinary clinical team (Daly et al. 2017). Different models have been used for bedside ECMO care and future research is required to better understand the risks and benefits of ECMO specialist nurses versus other care-provider models. With individual institutions granting accreditation to their ECMO specialists, Singapore should work toward national practice standards and certification process for ECMO specialists, as well as establishing an ECMO specialist's career development plan.

In our ICU, we adopted the manpower-intensive "two carers" approach to staffing, where each ECMO patient is supported by an ECMO specialist nurse as well as a bedside nurse. If there is more than one ECMO patient in the unit, the ECMO specialist nurse will manage up to 3 ECMO patients with a bedside nurse allocated to each patient. The bedside nurse is usually not qualified as an ECMO specialist and does not have the skills to access or troubleshoot the ECMO circuit. Since the start of ECMO nurse-led program in 2012, the number of ECMO specialist nurses in our unit has been steadily increasing (Fig. 4). With the advancement of simpler circuit designs and anticoagulation protocols, there is potential for all PICU nurses to be trained as ECMO specialists and have ECMO competency as part of core PICU nurse competency training. As the demand for ECMO increases and the number of ECMO specialist nurses increases, the unit can consider a 1:1 nurse-to-patient ratio whereby the bedside nurse assumes primary care of the patient and the circuit. The single care-giver model is currently being practiced in other centers (Cavarocchi et al. 2015; Connelly et al. 2012) and can help in cost reduction and manpower planning. However, the nurse-to-patient ratio should be increased for high acuity patients, such as those on ECMO and continuous renal replacement therapy (Connelly et al. 2012).

ECMO is a short-term mechanical circulatory support that can support patients for weeks, whereas a ventricular assist device (VAD) can support patients for months. VADs have been available since the early 1980s for adult use and have been approved for use in children in the United States in 2011. VADs are used as a bridge to transplant or as chronic therapy until either myocardial recovery is achieved, or a decision is made regarding transplant eligibility. After the approval of the first pediatric Berlin Heart EXCOR VAD, VAD has become an available treatment option for chronic heart failure (Stiller and Buchholz 2014). Our institution is in the planning phase for introducing a VAD program in our hospital and ECMO specialist nurses have been identified as potential technical specialists who can assist with management of patients on VAD. With this possible role expansion, ECMO specialist nurses will have greater responsibilities and new skills to develop as they care for patients on mechanical circulatory support.

Conclusion

ECMO is a time-critical, life-saving, and life-sustaining support for critically ill patients with severe respiratory and/or cardiac failure. A successful ECMO program requires a multidisciplinary approach and a team of competent ECMO specialists. The model of care will differ according to the capability and capacity of the ECMO center. This chapter chronicles the journey of the establishment of an ECMO specialist nurse program in a PICU in Singapore.

References

Cavarocchi NC, Wallace S, Hong EY, Tropea A, Byrne J, Pitcher HT, Hirose H. A cost-reducing extracorporeal membrane oxygenation (ECMO) program model: a single institution experience. Perfusion. 2015;30:148–53.

Connelly JT, Weaver B, Seelhorst A, Beaty CD, McDonough M, Nicolson SC, Tabbutt S. Challenges at the bedside with ECMO and VAD. World J Pediatr Congenit Heart Surg. 2012;3:67–71.

Daly KJ, Camporota L, Barrett NA. An international survey: the role of specialist nurses in adult respiratory extracorporeal membrane oxygenation. Nurs Crit Care. 2017;22:305–11.

ELSO. ELSO guidelines for ECMO for training and continuing education of ECMO specialists [Online]. 2010. Available https://www.elso.org/portals/0/igd/archive/filemanager/97000963d6-cusersshyerdocumentselsoguidelinesfortrainingandcontinuingeducationofecmospecialists.pdf. Accessed 9 August 2021.

ELSO. ECLS registry report, international summary [Online]. 2020. Available https://www.elso.org/Registry/Statistics/InternationalSummary.aspx. Accessed 24 August 2021.

ELSO. ELSO guidelines [Online]. 2021. Available https://www.elso.org/Resources/Guidelines.aspx. Accessed 29 September 2021.

Key AE. Enhancing interdisciplinary communication and collaboration in the management of adult ECMO patients: a quality improvement project. D.N.P., The University of Arizona. 2020.

Liu HC, Zhang LJ, Ping YJ, Wang L. Failure mode and effects analysis for proactive healthcare risk evaluation: a systematic literature review. J Eval Clin Pract. 2020;26:1320–37.

McCaffrey J, Orford NR, Simpson N, Jenkins JL, Morley C, Pellegrino V. Service delivery model of extracorporeal membrane oxygenation in an Australian regional hospital. Crit Care Resusc. 2016;18:235–41.

Odish M, Yi C, Tainter C, Najmaii S, Ovando J, Chechel L, Lipinski J, Ignatyev A, Pile A, Yeong Jang Y, Lin T, Tu XM, Madani M, Patel M, Meier A, Pollema T, Owens RL. The implementation and outcomes of a nurse-run extracorporeal membrane oxygenation program, a retrospective single-center study. Crit Care Explorat. 2021;3:e0449.

Padalino MA, Tessari C, Guariento A, Frigo AC, Vida VL, Marcolongo A, Zanella F, Harvey MJ, Thiagarajan RR, Stellin G. The "basic" approach: a single-centre experience with a cost-reducing model for paediatric cardiac extracorporeal membrane oxygenation. Interact Cardiovasc Thorac Surg. 2017;24:590–7.

Reader TW, Flin R, Mearns K, Cuthbertson BH. Developing a team performance framework for the intensive care unit. Crit Care Med. 2009;37:1787–93.

Stiller B, Buchholz H. Uni and biventricular assistance (LVAD-RVAD). In: Da Cruz EM, Ivy D, Jaggers J, editors. Pediatric and congenital cardiology, cardiac surgery and intensive care. London: Springer; 2014.

Wellman J. An exploration of staff experiences of extracorporeal membrane oxygenation (ECMO). 2017.

World Health Organization. Nursing and midwifery: key facts. World Health Organization [Online]. 2020. Available https://www.who.int/news-room/fact-sheets/detail/nursing-and-midwifery. Accessed 28 September 2021.

Transitioning from Pediatric to Adult Care in Sickle Cell Disease: An Innovative Nurse-Led Model

Barbara Speller-Brown

Introduction

Transitioning from pediatric to adult health care can be a difficult and challenging process. Having a chronic illness makes that process even more challenging. In this chapter, we present the need for a nurse-led model of transition and how it was developed and implemented. We also address the issues associated with transitioning and how to help patients make it a smooth process. The core elements of readiness assessment, education, and self-care management are presented. In each section, the critical roles and responsibilities of an interdisciplinary team will be highlighted.

Background

Advances in medicine, disease-modifying therapies, and research are helping individuals with chronic illnesses like sickle cell disease live longer, well into adulthood. In the early 70s, the expected life expectancy for those with SCD was less than 20 years (NHLBI 2022) with a mean age of about 14 years. Individuals are now living well into adulthood, into their 40s and 50s (Hamideh and Alvarez 2013). SCD affects approximately 100,000 individuals in the USA (Centers for Disease Control and Prevention 2016). SCD is an inherited blood disorder and is the most common, severe hemoglobinopathy worldwide (Cappelli and Gluckman 2019). It is characterized by multisystem disorders, namely, painful episodes (the hallmark of the

B. Speller-Brown (✉)
Children's National Hospital, Washington, DC, USA
e-mail: BSbrown@childrensnational.org

disease), infections, and end-organ damage. However, with over 95% of children now surviving into adulthood (Chaturvedi and DeBaun 2016) and this increase in life expectancy, there is a need for transitional care from child-centered to adult-centered health care. There needs to be a coordinated, comprehensive approach for this population, as with many chronic illnesses, given that the literature shows that transition is a time of increased morbidity and mortality (Blinder et al. 2013), particularly between 18 and 24 years of age. A longitudinal study of 940 youth with SCD found that 85% of deaths occurred after transitioning to adult health care, with a mean time to death of 1.8 years after transition (Quinn et al. 2010). In addition, post-transition has been shown to be a time of increased complications, such as increased hospitalizations and emergency room visits (Brousseau et al. 2010) and not locating to a new medical home.

Transition has been defined as the "purposeful planned movement of adolescents with chronic medical conditions from child-centered to adult-oriented health care" (Blum et al. 1993, p. 570). Adolescents and young adults (AYAs) have described the transition period as difficult and often challenging, provoking anxiety and fear (de Montalembert and Guitton 2014). Transition readiness is vital in preparing AYA for transition to adult-centered care. Providing adequate preparation and equipping AYA with the tools and skills needed to self-manage (defined as a key to successful transition) is critical (de Montalembert and Guitton 2014). Adult primary care providers and emergency care providers may not be comfortable caring for patients with SCD; therefore, disease education and knowledge are also critically important (Bemrich-Stolz et al. 2015). Older age does not necessarily translate to disease management knowledge, and healthcare providers should continue to assess knowledge levels overtime and not make assumptions based on age (Speller-Brown et al. 2018).

Process

As survival rates continue to improve, there needs to be a systematic, coordinated process for transition to be effective. There is limited research on transition readiness, disease-specific knowledge, and self-management skills needed for successful transition. The author embarked on a doctoral path to undertake a project to address patient and parent concerns at the time of transition and identify the barriers, expectations, and needs of the AYA population. The goal was to develop a clinical transition pathway that would enable AYA to complete a successful transition and, once developed, could translate to other chronic illnesses. A nurse-led innovation model was developed to address these transitional issues and ensure AYA are equipped with the disease knowledge and self-management skills needed to help them navigate and assimilate into the adult healthcare world.

Theoretical Framework

Studies have shown that self-care management (SCM) and transition readiness are essential to improved health outcomes (Cerns et al. 2013). SCM ability was defined as the capability to engage in therapeutic behaviors to maintain and/or improve health status and quality of life (Jenerette and Murdaugh 2008, p. 256) and the use of self-regulation skills to manage chronic conditions or risk factors (Ryan and Sawin 2009). Activities such as self-monitoring, goal setting, decision-making, self-evaluation, and reflective thinking are a part of the process (Ryan and Sawin 2009). Transition readiness has been defined as the specific decisions made and the actions taken for building the capacity of the adolescents, parents, and the providers to prepare for, begin, continue, and finish the process of transition (van Staa et al. 2011, p. 296). Consequences due to the lack of readiness for transition have been demonstrated in the literature to include increased emergency room visits and hospitalizations and a decrease in routine outpatient utilizations. Investigations of transition practices found that well-planned transitions increased the likelihood for continuity of care and patient compliance with medical regimens and contributed to independence and self-advocacy (Saulsberry et al. 2019). Individual and family self-management and transition readiness of both AYA and caregiver are essential in preparing AYA to transition from child-centered to adult-centered care.

A descriptive, midrange theory, *The Individual and Family Self-management Theory Framework* (IFSMT) (Fig. 1), has been used successfully in research on transition of youth with chronic illnesses. IFSMT suggests that the development of optimal knowledge and self-management is a combination of active and purposeful

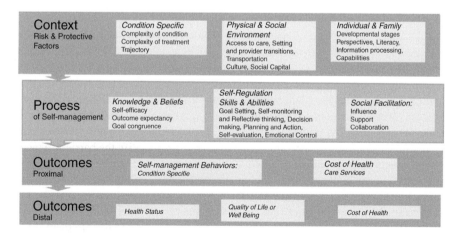

Fig. 1 Model of the individual and family self-management theory

involvement by the AYA and caregiver dyads (Ryan and Sawin 2009). The theory explains how the development of self-management occurs in the context of families and the environment and is influenced by a variety of risk and protective factors, which influence AYAs' involvement in health behaviors required for successful transition to the adult healthcare setting. The theory also explains the complexity of SCM in three dimensions, context, process, and outcomes. The context dimension is centered risk and protective factors such as individual and family characteristics and physical and social environments. Process dimension addresses knowledge and beliefs and how they impact self-efficacy and self-regulation (goal setting, decision-making, reflective thinking). Lastly, the focus of the outcomes dimension includes health status, quality of life, and cost of health. Outcomes are proximal and distal. For example, SCM of SCD resulting in therapy adherence and decrease painful crisis results in improved morbidity and mortality. This theory focuses on individual and family self-management, and utilizing this theory offers new opportunities for expanding knowledge of SCM and how transition readiness can be incorporated for both patient and caregiver.

Nurse-Led Module Description

Many components are needed to have a successful transition program. A multidisciplinary approach is essential, as services and healthcare are needed from other subspecialties as there may be other comorbidities associated with the chronic illness. For SCD, every organ can be affected, and care from many subspecialties is often required. Healthcare providers caring for chronic illnesses like SCD must assess and implement various components of the transition process. These should include transition planning, preparation, healthcare system design, implementation, and AYA and caregiver views on transition. These components play a major role in a successful transition program. Transition programs that address medical, educational, and vocational needs of patients are also essential components (Betz et al. 2013). The Six Core Elements of Health Care Transition (2021) is a widely adopted approach that defines the basic components for a structured transition process. The process timeline includes (1) policy/guide, (2) tracking and monitoring, (3) readiness, (4) planning, (5) transfer of care, and (6) transition complete. Included are guidelines to help healthcare providers integrate the six core elements into their practice, beginning in early adolescence and continuing into adulthood. A detailed summary of each approach and timeline can be found at gottransition.org/six-core elements (2021).

A summary of the organization components used to guide the SCAT program was as follows:

1. Readiness assessments for patient and caregiver (American Society of Hematology (ASH) 2021; GoT transition 2021).
2. Transition medial summary (complete by the primary pediatric hematology provider prior to the first SCAT visit and updated by the NP Director of the pro-

gram). A paper copy is given to the patient. This medical summary is sent to the new adult hematology provider. The AYA request the complete medical records from the hospital's medical records department.

3. Notes to the new adult hematology provider as applicable include:
    (a) Last transition clinic visit note sent to adult hematology provider
    (b) Last medical hematologic visit note and any pertinent inpatient note
    (c) Last subspecialty notes (i.e., pulmonary, neurology, cardiology, etc.)
    (d) Most recent imaging (hip X-ray, brain imaging, ultrasounds, etc.)
    (e) Pain clinic summary (if AYA attend the clinic)
    (f) Immunization record
    (g) Recent laboratory results
    (h) Medication list
    (i) Blood bank summary

The SCAT clinic has team members specifically dedicated to transition, to include the Director Nurse Practitioner, Scheduler/RN Nurse Coordinator, and Social Worker. Each member's roles and responsibilities are outlined in Table 1. The SCAT visit is for 1 h. The NP is allotted 30 min with the AYA to conduct the medical clinic visit, review readiness assessments (AYA and caregiver), update the medical summary, and provide disease education. The RN coordinator is primarily

Table 1 SCAT clinic sessions: team member roles and responsibilities

Transition sessions 1–6
St. Jude module 1: pathophysiology (sickle cell and me)
Pretest, modules, posttest: Accessed at: https://www.stjude.org/treatment/disease/sickle-cell-disease/step-program.html
Team member roles
Nurse practitioner
• Meets with AYA/caregiver (explains transition process/expectations)
• Reviews completed "Readiness Assessment" (AYA/Caregiver) at each SCAT visit
• Reviews transition policy
• Reviews and updates AYA medical summary
• Review transition notebook components and educational materials
• Complete medical visit
• Completes SCAT checklist
• Request pain clinic summary and Blood Bank Summary (when applicable)
RN nurse coordinator
• Sends medical summary to providers via REDCap and ensures summary completion
• Update AYA Registry
• Gives AYA transition education binder (in-person or via email)
• Ensures AYA is up to date on appointments and assist with scheduling any needed follow-ups
• Administers pretest, education modules, and posttest for Modules 1–6
• Obtains medical release
• Sends medical records to new adult hematology provider
• Provides additional AYA education

(continued)

Table 1 (continued)

Social worker
• Review insurance details (member portal access, create profile, find adult PCP, change insurance)
• Review and assist with AYA completion of advance directives
• Review education/vocation goals
• Address academic/vocational challenges
• Assist with supportive decision-making needs
• Review advocacy scenarios
Research assistant
• Maintain clinic registry/update database
• Monthly report on who's turning 22 years of age
• Monthly report on post-assessment calls

responsible for the education, using the St. Jude's Education Modules (2021), which includes a pretest, module video education, and a posttest. The nurse coordinator is allotted 15 minutes and is also responsible for sending a request for the AYA to be scheduled in the SCAT Clinic. This is done to ensure the medical summary is completed prior to scheduling. The medical summary form is sent to the primary hematologist, who completes the form in REDCap (a secure electronic database) where all surveys and assessment are stored. The social worker addresses insurance issues and assists the AYA in accessing the insurance carrier's website and creating a patient profile, completing advance directives, addressing education and vocation goals and school accommodations, and providing information on community resources. The social worker is allotted 15 min and, when time permits, reviews scenarios that allow the AYA to think through and process how to respond in certain healthcare situations.

We request AYA and caregivers complete a readiness assessment at each SCAT visit. This assessment identifies where they both are in the process and what interventions are needed to move them through preparing to transition. This also allows the caregiver the opportunity to know what is expected of them and how they can help their AYA self-manage, become more independent, and voice any concerns they have concerning the transition process. One of the goals for the SCAT clinic is to request and encourage the AYA's caregiver to attend the first and last clinic session to ensure the caregiver is aware of the process and can express any concerns they may have, help their AYA in the transition process, and is aware of the final transition date. We have found that when the caregiver is an active participant, this helps in making the transition more successful by increasing self-care management competencies of the AYA. A study by Speller-Brown et al. (2015) showed strong positive correlations between caregiver involvement in AYA responsibility and perception of overall transition readiness from the caregiver perspective.

We often find when completing the readiness assessment, AYA initially report they think transitioning by age 22 is important, and they feel a certain confidence in doing so (reporting a 10 on a scale of 1–10). When they are approaching the age for transition, we find they now may rate their confidence level lower, as they now fear leaving pediatric care. This is an opportunity to address their fears or concerns and renew a sense of confidence in their ability to self-manage. We require the AYA to visit their identified adult hematologist at least once before transitioning. This will help to build confidence, become acquainted with the new adult hematology provider, and address any concerns of the AYA, caregiver, and new adult provider. This is also an opportunity to change adult provider, if desired, while time permits before transitioning. We also advise AYA to visit the adult emergency departments of the adult facility at least once, as this seems to be an area of most concern for transitioning to adult care, as wait times are longer; they feel stigmatized and labeled as drug seekers (Bulgin et al. 2018) and are afraid the providers will not understand their disease and what treatments work best for them.

Most adult hematology providers now have infusion centers that patients can access for pain control, often preventing visits to the ED, and AYA are encouraged to use these centers. The literature shows there is a paucity of hematology providers willing and comfortable caring for patients with SCD (Whiteman et al. 2013). We are fortunate to have identified several adult hematology providers willing, knowledgeable, and comfortable in this setting. We compiled a list of adult hematology providers, which is included in the AYA's notebook. In preparation, a letter was sent to each adult hematologist with a questionnaire (Table 2) soliciting how they operate their clinic for new adult patients. This information is also included in the AYA notebook. As new adult hematologists are identified, they also complete the questionnaire, and the information is updated in the AYA notebook (Table 3).

Transition can be anxiety-provoking and difficult for many young adults. Our transition clinic aims to teach practical skills, such as filling prescriptions, making appointments, obtaining referrals, etc., in addition to promoting disease knowledge and independence in healthcare management. All team members can be contacted by phone for concerns after transition. We hope that through this clinic, our patients will be better prepared as they transition to adult health centers. For this reason, we are soliciting the adult hematology provider to provide answers to the questions

Table 2 Adult provider transition questionnaire

1. How do we refer patients to your clinic, how do patients make appointments? (i.e., scheduling number, fax number, email)
2. Will patients receive a primary hematologist or do several team members follow each patient?
3. What happens if a patient needs a prescription when they run out of medication?
4. Do you keep adult patients on penicillin prophylaxis?
5. Are most of your sickle cell patients maintained on hydroxyurea?
6. Do you continue to transfuse patients who were on chronic transfusions for abnormal TCD or ischemic stroke?
7. Do you have a pain clinic? If so, what services are offered?
8. Do you have a day hospital/infusion center? If so, what are the criteria to be seen?
9. Are there active research studies at your facility?
10. What insurances do you accept? Are there any types of insurance that you do not accept?
11. Do you have support staff? (i.e., social work, RN, case manager, NP or PA)

Table 3 SCAT notebook components	1. Transition policy
	2. Adult providers list
	3. Advance directives
	4. Authorization for release of information
	5. Six core elements of health care transition 2.0
	Transition flow sheet
	Transition registry
	Transition readiness assessment (TRA)—youth/parent—(Got transition/ASH)
	Medical summary and emergency care plan
	Transition checklist
	Portable health summary
	Health and transition summary/transfer summary letter
	Feedback survey (last clinic visit)
	6. College preparation worksheet
	7. Pharmacy sheet
	8. Community resources
	Education materials
	St. Jude education modules
	Got transition information: www.GotTransition.org
	Living well with sickle cell disease: self-care toolkit (CDC)
	Children's PATH Hydroxyurea info
	Insurance fact sheet
	CDC: Nine steps to living well with SCD in college
	APHON: a sickle cell disease handbook for families
	Hope and destiny or hope and destiny Jr. (books)
	How to make appointments
	Pregnancy in SCD fact sheet
	Listing of education/community websites

about their practice so that our patients can make an informed decision when choosing a new treatment center.

AYAs and caregivers are surveyed at the last SCAT visit utilizing the "Sickle Cell Adolescent Transition Health Care Transition Feedback Survey" developed by the Got Transition protocol (GoT transition 2021). This survey addresses the AYA and caregiver's experience changing from pediatric to adult health care. It evaluates valuable information about the effectiveness of the SCAT program and their experiences. One important question for the caregiver is "How could your child's health care provider have made the move to an adult health care provider better for you and your child? This information is useful to strengthen the program by incorporating the feedback from caregivers and reinforce what is effective or address what needs modifications. Another question, "Did your previous health care provider have information about community resources?" This prompted our team to develop a list of community resources and websites to assist AYA with accessing other transition

Table 4 SCAT clinic post-assessment follow-up questionnaire

Questions	Yes	No
Have you seen your identified adult provider since you left children's? If no, why not?		
Since leaving children's, have you changed your adult provider? If yes, why?		
What is the name of your adult hematology provider?		
What is the name of the adult hematology facility?		
When was your last adult hematology appointment?		
Are you satisfied with the care you've received? If no, why not?		
Are you on hydroxyurea therapy? If yes, do you take as prescribed? If no, why not?		
Were you prescribed hydroxyurea at children's hospital?		
Were you on chronic transfusion therapy at children's?		
If yes? Are you currently on transfusion therapy?		
Have you been hospitalized since transferring to adult care?		
If yes, how many times and for what reason?		
Have you been to the ER since transitioning? If yes, how many times?		
Are you in school? If no, why not?		
Are you working? If no, why not?		

*Administered to all AYAs regardless of attending SCAT clinic (Survey developed by the Sickle Cell Team at Children's National Hospital)

and adult-related services. A full list of the questions can be accessed on the Got Transition website.

All team members participate in the post-assessment follow-up of and feedback from the AYA. This program survey was developed by the team (Table 4). The AYA is called every 3 months for the first year after transitioning, every 6 months the second year, and annually thereafter. We are now in the 6th year of this service and will be evaluating whether to continue this follow-up practice.

Methods of Evaluation

It is important to evaluate a program's effectiveness. Evaluation of the SCAT program was done several ways. We administered the GoT transition feedback surveys at the final SCAT visit with both AYA and caregiver. We often use this feedback survey results to improve the program. Essential for a successful transition program is the follow-up experience and outcomes reported after they are in the adult healthcare system. We follow up with AYAs after transition to adult care to assess if they are continuing to follow-up with their new adult provider. A study by Travis et al. (2020) reported that transition may be improved if pediatric hematology centers assist and verify adult provider contact. Nearly 90% of our young adults reported establishing an adult hematology home. Our program assisted AYA in identifying an adult hematologist and provided a comprehensive medical summary for the adult provider, regardless of whether the AYA attend the SCAT clinic.

We conducted an IRB-approved, descriptive study that evaluated AYAs' and caregivers' feedback of the healthcare transition experience after transition by feedback transition surveys (GoT transition 2021) and post-assessment transition surveys (developed by the SCAT Team) (Table 4). We surveyed AYA 20–21 years of age at CNH who transitioned to adult care. Post-assessment surveys were also conducted with AYA who did not attend SCAT. Data were analyzed using descriptive statistics. Fifty-seven AYA with SCD attended SCAT and 15 did not attend, from January 2018 to January 2021. Of those who attended SCAT, 53% ($n = 25$) felt very prepared to change to an adult provider, 40% ($n = 19$) felt somewhat prepared, and 4% ($n = 2$) felt unprepared, with 78 % having seen their identified adult healthcare provider since leaving pediatric care. Due to the ongoing communication between the AYA in our program after transition, we were able to support them during a crucial time to prevent lost to follow-up, regardless of SCAT attendance.

We found there were AYA who did not return to their adult provider after the first clinic visit. During our program's follow-up, we were able to identify them and assist to reconnect them with their adult provider or help them gain access to another adult hematologist. Under these circumstances, we provide outreach to the adult hematologist if they are having issues in establishing continuity of care for the AYA. We have team meetings with our largest adult hematology center monthly to obtain reports on patients who are having difficulty with transition and provide reports to the adult provider of impending transitions. We have found this communication helpful and hope to expand to other adult receiving hematology providers.

Challenges and Facilitators

There were challenges in the development and implementation of this nurse-led model. The first was obtaining dedicated space (pre-COVID pandemic) to see patients. It was decided the SCAT clinic could be held 3 days a month for a half day to accommodate four patients each clinic. Each visit would last an hour. Another challenge was deciding how much time each team member was allowed to spend with the AYA/caregiver, as everyone felt their position was equally important. However, it is was decided that the medical healthcare provider (Director) needed the most time to conduct the medical portion of the visit in addition to updating the SCAT medical summary and providing SCD education. Attendance at appointments, although improved with telemedicine remains a challenge. We continue to work with AYA to improve adherence.

There were facilitators that enabled this program to be implemented. The process undertaken to develop and implement this model/service required and accomplished buy-in from the healthcare system at Children's National Hospital, a large urban center in Washington, DC, that manages over 1500 patients with SCD. Buy-in from administration, the SCD Director, and Hematology Division Chief and the willingness and cooperation of the SCAT team members made this possible. A social worker and RN nurse coordinator were dedicated to this clinic, which helped to develop and implement the process. The AYA's insurance is billed for services like any other clinic visit. Education materials used (i.e., AYA Notebook, education pamphlets, handouts, etc.) are provided by the hematology department.

Service Adjustments Made

Modifications continue to be made as the program is a "work in progress." Team members assume more responsibilities as the clinic continues to expand. The RN coordinator coordinates clinic visits with the AYA's work and school schedule, helps optimize AYA compliance, and sends the surveys via email. The social worker adds community resources and scholarship information as they become available. She also has the AYA access the insurance website and walks them through how to create a member profile. Modifications were also necessary due to the COVID pandemic. Since the COVID pandemic, all SCAT clinic visits converted to Telemedicine visits, still requiring an hour-long session, but all services are provided virtually. This has allowed flexibility for the AYA and caregiver and has increased appointment adherence and AYA and caregiver satisfaction.

We also added two research assistants to our team, which have proven valuable. Responsibilities include (1) maintain clinic registry/update database (for all AYA regardless of SCAT attendance); (2) generate a monthly report on who's turning 21 and 22 years of age; (3) generate a monthly report on when post-assessment calls are due; and (4) maintain/update the REDCap database. Readiness assessments and feedback surveys are sent to the AYA and caregiver via email link, and the completed, submitted forms populate in REDCap. The post-assessment surveys are completed by phone call to the AYA and entered into REDCap by the SCAT team. The team understands the need for flexibility and teamwork if the SCAT clinic is to be successful and is committed to the process.

When the clinic was held in person, at the last clinic visit, the AYAs ring the "Victory Bell" signifying transition completion. This was adopted having witnessed this ceremony performed by cancer patients who entered remission. This was deemed important as the message we wanted the AYA to receive was viewing transition as another developmental milestone (similar to high school or college graduation) not a "kicking out" from pediatric care. With virtual attendance, certificates are sent electronically.

Lessons Learned

Developing and implementing a nurse-led model of transition require dedication, patience, and compassion. This SCAT clinic was born out of a need to make a difference in the lives of patient with SCD, as the literature demonstrates this is a time of increased morbidity and mortality for AYA with SCD. We found that including the parents in some SCAT visits and having them complete readiness assessments as helpful. Some AYA still need the support and guidance of their caregivers, so we encourage them to work with us in the best interest of the AYA. Establishing and maintaining collaborations with adult hematology providers are important. Our team meets regularly with one main hematology provider to obtain updates on those AYAs who have transitioned and provide information on future transitions. The SCAT team continues to add to the adult hematology providers' list those willing to accept patients with SCD.

Future Implications for Clinical Practice and Research

Studies show that AYAs often lack the needed skills to successfully transition from pediatric to adult health care (Jenson et al. 2017). Disease knowledge and self-care management have been identified as key in the process. Future plans for our program include starting transition planning at an earlier age. The literature suggests starting at least by age 12 (Saulsberry et al. 2019). We have begun to institute actively engaging the young patient in communications, having the caregiver allow the patient to speak on their own behalf and answer questions directed to them. This will help the patient becomes comfortable talking to their provider and help him to articulate how SCD affects them. The Health Care Transition Timeline for parents/caregivers, developed by GoT transition (2021), is a useful tool for caregivers to work with their child to gain the needed skills to self-manage. We are also developing a transition clinic for younger patients, titled "Sickle Cell Adolescent Education and Readiness" (SCALE). It is targeted for SCD patients 12–17 years of age and will address what we think is needed at different stages of maturity to include disease knowledge basics and SCM skills.

It would also be helpful to expand the clinic to accommodate more patients, which would require staffing changes that include an additional NP, nurse coordinator, and social worker. Additionally, if the program is to develop to its full potential and each AYA can be seen in the six visits as we suggest, it would allow completion of the education modules developed by St. Jude. Each module deemed important to SCD knowledge.

The research shows there is increased morbidity and mortality after transition (American Society of Hematology (ASH) 2019). Increased staffing will also allow the follow-up that is so important after transition to enable long-term surveillance of AYAs for longitudinal data purposes. Currently, AYAs are followed for 6 years after transitioning. If expansion of follow-up can continue annually for at least 10 years, this may be more helpful and inform future treatment approaches. More research is needed to validate this hypothesis.

Another essential aspect of transition is ensuring AYAs have an adult primary care provider (PCP) and emphasizing they are seen by their PCP at least annually. When transitioning to adult care, an adult PCP is often needed to provide needed referrals to the new adult hematologist.

Telemedicine has proven to be helpful in health care. Having the pediatric provider attend the first adult hematology clinic virtually can serve as an introduction to the new adult service and serve to put the AYA at ease at the first adult clinic visit. Future research is needed in areas of recommendations to ensure successful transition and AYAs outcomes.

Conclusion

Transitioning from child-centered to adult-centered care can be challenging and is a process that requires many moving parts and a dedicated team to be successful. We hope this nurse-led model for transition can help in that process. There are several websites that can serve as useful educational and community resources in the transition process. These include but are not limited to the following websites listed below.

Useful Resources/Websites

https://www.stjude.org/treatment/disease/sickle-cell-disease/educational-resources.html

https://www.stjude.org/content/dam/en_US/shared/www/patient-support/hematology-literature/plan-of-care-visits.pdf

https://www.youtube.com/watch?v=FuelQDBOxXI

https://www.youtube.com/watch?v=H9IPkTg4pBA

https://www.youtube.com/watch?v=D0SjptWfBeE

ASH resources on transition

http://www.hematology.org/Clinicians/Priorities/5573.aspx

http://www.hematology.org/Advocacy/Policy-News/2016/5581.aspx

Transition summit—keynote address "next steps: planning with confidence to move from pediatric to adult healthcare": https://www.youtube.com/watch?v=iYexjQZt5Ek

Transition summit—provider panel: https://www.youtube.com/watch?v=Uhb0ceQn8u4

Transition summit—patient/family panel: https://www.youtube.com/watch?v=ZdEu_rXW0Hg

Transition summit—discussion: https://www.youtube.com/watch?v=ZdEu_rXW0Hg

http://www.medikidz.com/flipbooks/preview/sickle-cell-2016/

Pain video

https://www.youtube.com/watch?v=FuelQDBOxXI

What is SCD?

http://www.youtube.com/watch?v=6DGrmaCtR0g

https://www.youtube.com/watch?v=H9IPkTg4pBA –

Hydroxyurea

https://www.youtube.com/watch?v=2a7FXibkubQ

Passport

www.sickkids.ca/myhealthpassport/Default.aspx

Social media

https://www.cdc.gov/ncbddd/sicklecell/links.html (Social Media Resources-Sickle Cell Disease—CDC)

https://www.nhlbi.nih.gov/education/sickle-cell-month/social-media

References

American Society of Hematology (ASH). Fragmentation of care among young adults with sickle cell disease. ASH Annual Meeting and Exposition. 2019.

American Society of Hematology (ASH). SCD transition readiness assessment. 2021. Available at https://www.hematology.org/education/clinicians/clinical-priorities/pediatric-to-adult-care-transition. Accessed 1 Jan 2022.

Bemrich-Stolz CJ, Halanych JH, Howard TH, Hilliard LM, Ledensburg JD. Exploring adult care experiences and barriers to transition in adult patients with sickle cell disease. Int J Hematol Ther. 2015;1(1):1–5. https://doi.org/10.15436/2381-1404.15.003.

Betz CL, Lobo ML, Nehring WM, Bui K. Voices not heard: a systematic review of adolescents and emerging adult's perspectives of health care. Nurs Outlook. 2013;61:311–6.

Blinder MA, Vekeman F, Sasane M, Trahey A, Paley C, Duh MS. Age-related treatment patterns in sickle cell disease patients and the associated sickle cell complications and healthcare costs. Pediatr Blood Cancer. 2013;60:828–35. https://doi.org/10.1002/pbc.24459.

Blum RW, Garell D, Hodgman CH, et al. Transition from child-centered to adult health-care systems for adolescents with chronic conditions: a position paper of the Society for Adolescent. J Adolesc Health. 1993;14:570–6.

Brousseau DC, Owens PL, Mosso AL, Panepinto JA, Steiner CA. Acute care utilization and rehospitalizations for sickle cell disease. J Am Med Assoc. 2010;303:1288–94. https://doi.org/10.1001/jama.2010.378.

Bulgin D, Tanabe P, Jenerette C. Stigma of sickle cell disease: 'a systematic review'. Issues Ment Health Nurs. 2018;39(8):675–86. https://doi.org/10.1080/01612840.2018.1443530.

Cappelli B, Gluckman E. Hemoglobinopathies (sickle cell disease and thalassemia). In: Carreras E, Dufour C, Mohty M, Kroger N, editors. The EBMT handbook. Cham: Springer; 2019. https://doi.org/10.1007/978-3-0303-02278-5_79.

Centers for Disease Control and Prevention. Data and statistics on sickle cell disease. 2016. Available at https://www.cdc.gov/ncbddd/sicklecell/data.html. Accessed 12 November 2021.

Cerns S, McCraken C, Claire R. Optimizing adolescent transition to adult care for sickle cell disease. Med Surg Nurs. 2013;22:255–7.

Chaturvedi S, DeBaun M. Evolution of sickle cell disease from a life-threatening disease of children to a chronic disease of adults: the last 40 years. Am J Hematol. 2016;91:514.

de Montalembert M, Guitton C. Transition from pediatric to adult care for patients with sickle cell disease. Br J Hematol. 2014;164:630–5.

GoT transition. Health care transition timeline for parents and caregivers. 2021. Available at https://www.gottransition.org/resource/?hct-timeline-parents-caregivers. Accessed 16 February 2022.

Hamideh D, Alvarez O. Sickle cell disease related mortality in the United States (1999-2009). Pediatr Blood Cancer. 2013;60:1482–6. https://doi.org/10.1002/pbc.24557.

Jenerette CM, Murdaugh C. Testing the theory of self-care management for sickle cell disease. Res Nurs Health. 2008;31:355–69.

Jenson PT, et al. 'Assessment of transition readiness in adolescents and young adults with chronic health conditions. Pediat Rheumatol Online. 2017;15(1):70. https://doi.org/10.1186/s12969-017-0197-6.

NHLBI. Century of progress: milestones in sickle cell disease. 2022. Available at nhlbi.nih.gov/files/docs/public/blood/Tagged2NHLBISickleCellTimeline.pdf.

Quinn CT, Rogers ZR, Mccavit TL, Buchanan GR. Improved survival of children and adolescents with sickle cell disease. Blood. 2010;115:3447–52. https://doi.org/10.1182/blood-2009-07-233700.

Ryan P, Sawin KJ. 'The individual and family self-management theory: background and perspectives on context, process, and outcomes. Nurs Outlook. 2009;57:217–25. https://doi.org/10.1016/j.outlook.2008.10.004.

Saulsberry AC, Porter JS, Hankins JS. A program of transition to adult care for sickle cell disease. Hematology. 2019;2019(1):496–504.

Speller-Brown B, et al. Measuring transition readiness: a correlational study of perceptions of parent and adolescents and young adults with sickle cell disease. J Pediatr Nurs. 2015;30(5):788–96. https://doi.org/10.1016/j.pedn.2015.06.008.

Speller-Brown B, Varty M, Thaniel L, Jacobs M. Assessing disease knowledge and self-management in youth with sickle cell disease. J Pediatr Oncol Nurs. 2018;36(2):143–9.

St. Jude's Education Modules. Sickle cell transition E-learning program (STEP) for teens with sickle cell disease. 2021. Available at: https://www.stjude.org/treatment/disease/sickle-cell-disease/step-program.html. Accessed 2 December 2021.

Travis K, et al. Pediatric to adult transition in sickle cell disease: survey results from young adult patient. Acta Haematol. 2020;143(2):163–75. https://doi.org/10.1159/000500258.

van Staa A, et al. Readiness to transfer to adult care of adolescents with chronic conditions: exploration of associated factors. J Adolesc Health. 2011;48:295–302.

Whiteman LN, Feldman L, McQuire A, Haywood C. Primary care providers comfort levels in caring for patients with sickle cell disease. Am J Hematol. 2013;88(12):E32–3. https://doi.org/10.14423/SMJ.0000000000000331.

The Sierra Leone National ETAT+ Programme: Delivering Nurse-Led Emergency Paediatric Care

Christopher Hands, Sandra Hands, Jacklyn Bangura, and Kadiatu Sankoh

Introduction

This chapter describes how Sierra Leonean nurses develop the skills to undertake the initial assessment and treatment of acutely unwell children presenting to hospital. The programme includes a core timetable of education based on the World Health Organisation (WHO)-approved Emergency Triage Assessment and Treatment+ (ETAT+) package, as well as process modifications to improve patient flow through the hospital and to improve the availability of essential equipment and medications where acutely unwell patients are being treated. It also describes some of the challenges involved in implementing this programme in a resource-limited setting, including utilities, equipment, medication and institutional policies.

Background

Need for the Model and the Target Population

Sierra Leone faces urgent challenges in improving rates of newborn and under-five mortality if the country is to meet Sustainable Development Goal (SDG) 3 by 2030. The country has seen a prolonged recovery phase following the end of a decade-long civil war in 2001, which was interrupted by the 2014–2015 Ebola epidemic in

C. Hands (✉)
Paediatric Intensive Care Unit, Starship Hospital, Auckland, New Zealand

S. Hands
Department of Anaesthesia, Auckland City Hospital, Auckland, New Zealand

J. Bangura · K. Sankoh
Ola During Children's Hospital, Freetown, Sierra Leone

Guinea, Liberia and Sierra Leone, and then again by the global COVID-19 pandemic in 2020–2022. Sierra Leone continues to have high rates of deprivation and high rates of preventable under-five mortality, including from malnutrition, malaria, tuberculosis and pneumonia (SSL and ICF 2020).

Despite these challenges, Sierra Leone has been making gains in under-five mortality which is more rapid than the wider West and Central Africa region (Hands et al. 2021). As more children are treated effectively at the primary care level, the proportion of under-five deaths that would be preventable with hospital-level care is increased. Access to health care has also improved following the launch of the Free Healthcare Initiative in 2010, and there has been an increase in the demand for facility-based care (Witter et al. 2018). This increase in care-seeking means that more acutely unwell children requiring emergency treatment arrive at hospital; this can be seen in data collected at the national paediatric referral hospital in the period immediately following the Ebola epidemic (Hands et al. 2020) and from national data from government hospitals in subsequent years (Hands et al. 2021).

Whilst it is welcome that more children present to hospital to access a higher level of care, this represents a demand which is challenging for medical staff to meet. In 2017, there were 122 doctors in Sierra Leone with few working in rural districts (MoHS 2017). There are 13 government referral hospitals outside of the capital, Freetown, and these are divided into 3 regional referral hospitals (for the 3 regions of Sierra Leone, North, South and East) and 10 district hospitals. The district hospitals have one doctor allocated as the medical superintendent and may have one additional medical officer to assist in covering clinical duties across the whole range of medical and surgical adult, paediatric and maternity services. In some centres, they are supported by one or two community health officers who have undergone a different training pathway which is comparable to that undertaken by a physician's assistant. In the regional hospitals, there may be up to three medical officers and between three and six community health officers supporting the medical superintendent.

There are also challenges in facilitating the clinical processes that underpin paediatric emergency care such that hospitals can deliver a good service. In an assessment of emergency paediatric services at all 13 government hospitals outside Freetown in 2016, only 4 hospitals had access to a consistent electricity supply and to running water on the paediatric ward, whilst only 3 hospitals had a resuscitation area for children, and no hospital had a process to support the clinical triage of acutely unwell children.

Impetus for the Development of This Model

In the wake of the Ebola epidemic in Sierra Leone, there were fewer members of hospital staff available to treat patients. Members of medical and nursing staff had died from Ebola; many surviving staff members were traumatised or demoralised. At Ola During Children's Hospital (ODCH, Sierra Leone's paediatric referral centre), most of the medical cover was provided by the five house officers on rotation at the hospital. In a hospital which often had 150 inpatients, it was difficult for the doctors to provide service coverage across all the clinical areas, and this sometimes led to long waits for children arriving at the emergency department. Some of the necessary changes made during the epidemic had also undermined the clinical processes that had previously existed. The triage of acutely unwell patients was not working well; patients faced long journeys around the hospital to the laboratory, the pharmacy and the ward before treatment could be initiated; and the treatment initiated often did not follow WHO guidelines (Hands et al. 2020).

There was an opportunity to trial an alternative model of care to make urgently needed improvements to a system under strain. The Ebola epidemic was ending, and there were many fewer suspected and proven cases. However, nurses who had been assigned to the Ebola isolation unit at the hospital had not yet been redeployed, and many amongst them were enthusiastic to be part of a new initiative to improve care for children arriving at the hospital under these circumstances.

The Process Undertaken to Develop and Implement the Model

The WHO-approved ETAT guidelines and training materials provide a framework for health workers in limited-resource settings quickly to become competent in assessing for signs of serious illness in infants and children and to provide prompt treatment for deranged physiology using a symptom-based approach. The ETAT teaching has been expanded in some settings to include the management of patients during the first 24 h of admission and to include detailed aspects of the management of premature or sick neonates. This training is known as ETAT+. There is some evidence that ETAT+ training may rapidly improve the quality of paediatric and neonatal care in hospitals in low-resource settings (Molyneux et al. 2006; Irimu et al. 2012; Ayieko et al. 2011; Crouse et al. 2016).

In collaboration with the medical superintendent of ODCH, a pilot project was organised in the hospital based on a nurse-led model of paediatric emergency care using ETAT+ from December 2015 to June 2016. The nurses who had previously been assigned to the holding unit for children with suspected Ebola virus were released to undergo training in ETAT+ protocols. The teaching programme was an expanded version of the existing ETAT+ course, with more extended discussion of the anatomical and physiological principles underpinning the approaches to treatment and more time to coach the candidates on the treatment protocols in simulated scenarios. At the end of the training period, the candidates underwent written and clinical assessments, with a third of the written questions focused on prescribing. Those candidates who passed both elements of the assessment were given the authority to manage the resuscitation of acutely unwell children and give the first dose of emergency medications according to the ETAT+ protocols. The successful nurses were deployed to the outpatient department.

In partnership with two external facilitating physicians and the hospital medical superintendent, the team of nurses made changes to the clinical processes and environment to improve the timing and quality of triage and treatment. All patients

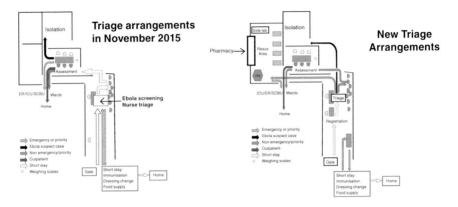

Fig. 1 Changes to patient flow in the ODCH pilot project

would now undergo clinical triage by one of the trained nurses immediately on arrival at the outpatient department. Patients presenting with ETAT+ 'emergency' or 'priority' signs would be transferred to a dedicated resuscitation area, where essential equipment and consumables were available. A side pharmacy was also established in the resuscitation area so that there was no wait for essential medications. The changes to patient flow through the outpatient department are shown in Fig. 1.

Before the changes were implemented, and at 3 and 6 months following implementation, the quality of triage and the time taken for children presenting with emergency and priority signs to be assessed and treated were measured by a team made up of two external physicians and nurses working elsewhere in the hospital (Hands et al. 2020). These initial data were reviewed by representatives from the MoHS and WHO. The MoHS decided to implement a national programme implementing the same model across all government hospitals with the support of WHO and the UK Royal College of Paediatrics and Child Health (RCPCH).

In late 2016, assessment visits were undertaken to all government hospitals outside Freetown to review the status of infrastructure and utilities, the availability of essential medicines and utilities and the management of common clinical presentations at each institution. At every hospital, the programme team discussed with the hospital management and the staff working in the paediatric ward what improvements could be made to the existing clinical processes and established the basis of a quality improvement process grounded in a shared endeavour to improve paediatric emergency care.

In 2017, mentors were deployed to all 13 hospitals. Each hospital received a pair of mentors: one international paediatrician or paediatric nurse and a Sierra Leonean nurse from ODCH who had received supplementary training to develop the skills to teach and mentor their colleagues. Training in ETAT+ principles and processes was offered to all clinical members of staff working on the paediatric ward. In practice, this was taken up almost exclusively by members of nursing staff.

Theoretical Framework

This model of care was framed as a task-sharing initiative, building on the evidence of related initiatives in Sierra Leone and other West African countries. As the nurses involved had been working in the acute care service of the hospital and had long experience of assessing sick children, the model aimed to capitalise on their knowledge of the signs of critical illness and of clinical deterioration and to allow them to use those skills to their fullest potential, working in an integrated way with the medical team.

Description

Organizational Components

The key principle of the model is that nurses, who would usually need to wait for a prescription from a doctor before administering medication, were authorised to undertake a full assessment of the patient and administer the first doses of relevant emergency medication if they had passed the ETAT+ assessment. A referral would be made to the doctor on call at the time of assessment so that the patient would also receive a medical review when the doctor was next available. Infrastructural changes frequently had to be made to facilitate triage processes, which provide a clear path for the sickest children to be triaged efficiently and seen quickly in a resuscitation area with appropriate supplies.

Services

The programme aims to deliver timely and high-quality paediatric emergency care, with the initial assessment and treatment being provided by nurses who have undergone supplementary training in the ETAT+ theory and practice. In every government hospital outside Freetown, the 2017 national rollout established the key elements of this service, staffed 24 h/day by nurses who had successfully completed the ETAT+ training course:

- An easily accessible triage station close to the main access to the hospital where every child is reviewed at presentation using the ETAT+ triage framework (Fig. 2)
- A paediatric resuscitation area within easy reach of the triage point which has electricity and running water and is stocked with essential equipment, diagnostics and medications

Triage of all sick children

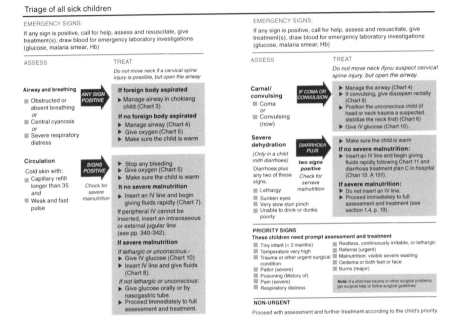

Fig. 2 ETAT+ triage framework

- Written one-page treatment protocols for the most common paediatric presentations, displayed on the wall of the resuscitation area (see Fig. 3)
- Standard one-page pro formas to document the child's status at triage, full assessment and resuscitation of each child (see Fig. 4)
- A national ETAT+ manual, setting out the pathological basis of each major disease process, and the rationale and protocols for treatment for each disease process

The delivery of this service is underpinned by a training programme describing the principles and processes of ETAT+. The programme is based on the pilot programme described above which was updated and revised to function as a course for the whole country. Training takes place over 3 months, with sessions taking place immediately before or after clinical shifts. Knowledge must be complemented by appropriate processes of care, and the 2017 national rollout entailed an initial quality improvement process to situate the triage station in an optimal location, standardise the triage processes so that sick children are not missed, and standardise resuscitation so that it follows an ABC systems format and is documented on the national pro forma.

The service is further supported by an ongoing quality improvement approach. In each hospital, a core group was convened to address operational and logistical challenges to delivering high-quality care. These included issues of staff motivation and commitment, stock-outs of essential medications, non-availability of laboratory tests, and interruptions to the electricity supply.

Early Detection in Hospital

> All babies in hospital shoved be observed at least every 6 hours
>
> Review should include: full set of vitals; review of cord; review of activity and breastfeeding

Treatment of Suspected Neonatal Sepsis

if you notice any of the danger signs:

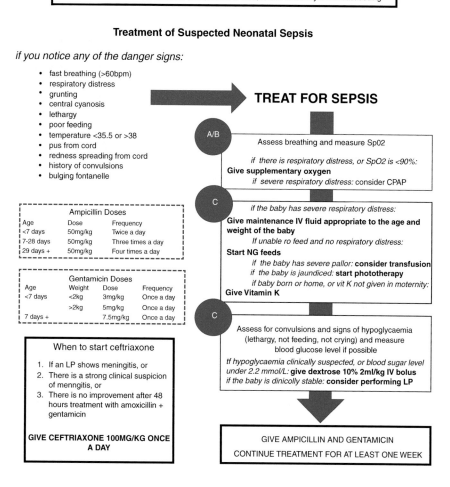

- fast breathing (>60bpm)
- respiratory distress
- grunting
- central cyanosis
- lethargy
- poor feeding
- temperature <35.5 or >38
- pus from cord
- redness spreading from cord
- history of convulsions
- bulging fontanelle

TREAT FOR SEPSIS

A/B
Assess breathing and measure SpO2

if there is respiratory distress, or SpO2 is <90%:
Give supplementary oxygen
if severe respiratory distress: consider CPAP

C
if the baby has severe respiratory distress:
Give maintenance IV fluid appropriate to the age and weight of the baby
If unable ro feed and no respiratory distress:
Start NG feeds
if the baby has severe pallor: **consider transfusion**
if the baby is jaundiced: **start phototherapy**
if baby born or home, or vit K not given in moternity:
Give Vitamin K

C
Assess for convulsions and signs of hypoglycaemia (lethargy, not feeding, not crying) and measure blood glucose level if possible

tf hypoglycaemia clinically suspected, or blood sugar level under 2.2 mmol/L: **give dextrose 10% 2ml/kg IV bolus**
if the baby is dinicolly stable: **consider performing LP**

Ampicillin Doses

Age	Dose	Frequency
<7 days	50mg/kg	Twice a day
7-28 days	50mg/kg	Three times a day
29 days +	50mg/kg	Four times a day

Gentamicin Doses

Age	Weight	Dose	Frequency
<7 days	<2kg	3mg/kg	Once a day
	>2kg	5mg/kg	Once a day
7 days +		7.5mg/kg	Once a day

When to start ceftriaxone

1. If an LP shows meningitis, or
2. There is a strong clinical suspicion of menngitis, or
3. There is no improvement after 48 hours treatment with amoxicillin + gentamicin

GIVE CEFTRIAXONE 100MG/KG ONCE A DAY

GIVE AMPICILLIN AND GENTAMICIN

CONTINUE TREATMENT FOR AT LEAST ONE WEEK

Fig. 3 Example of an ETAT+ treatment protocol—neonatal sepsis

Team Members

In every hospital, most of the members of the original ETAT+ team were from the State-Enrolled Community Health Nurse (SECHN) grade. These nurses had been trained in a cadre which was originally designated for work in community settings, but many of them had been employed by hospitals. The State-Registered Nurse (SRN) grade, which requires more academic qualifications for entry and involves a longer training pathway, was intended to provide nurses to work in hospitals. In 2017, the total number of nurses with an SRN qualification was small, but the

Staff Name_____　　　Signature _____

National ETAT+ Paediatric Admission Triage and Screening Form

Name:		Date: _____	Time:	
Date of birth:		Age: _____	Patient ID:	
Address:		Caregiver's name/number :		

Ebolavirus Disease Screening Questions	Yes	No
1.　Fever >2 days with no response to treatment	☐	☐
and		
2.　Signs of bleeding *(bloody diarrhoea/urine, bleeding gums, bleeding into skin, red eyes)*	☐	☐
or		
3.　Clinical suspicion *(excessive crying, irritable, restless, drooling, hiccups, abdominal pain, Sore throat, Pain swallowing, intense fatigue)*	☐	☐

If patient has **2 of the above isolate and notify clinician**, if not proceed to triage

Triage Questions

Reason for presentation: _____

Emergency signs

Airway	☐ patent	☐ obstructed	
Breathing	☐ normal	☐ resp. distress ☐ cyanosis	Resp rate_____/min SpO2 _____ %
Circulation	☐ warm	☐ skin cold ☐ CRT >3 s ☐ pulse weak/ fast	heart rate_____/min
Coma/Convulsion	☐ alert	☐ convulsing ☐ coma	AVPU　A　V　P　U
Dehydration	☐ hydrated	☐ sunken eyes ☐ lethargy ☐ v. slow skin pinch ☐ unable to take 　 oral fluid	

Temp _____　Kg_____

Priority signs

| ☐ Tiny infant
　<2month
☐ Temp. very
　high (>39) or
　low
☐ Trauma/urgent
　surgical cond. | ☐ Pallor (severe)
☐ Poisoning
　(history)
☐ Pain (severe) | ☐ Respiratory
　distress
☐ Restless,
　irritable,
　lethargic
☐ Referral (urgent) | ☐ Malnutrition:
　visible severe
　wasting
☐ Oedema of both
　feet or face
☐ Burns (major) |

Emergency or priority sign ☐ ⟶ **Resuscitation area**

No emergency or priority sign ☐ ⟶ **Waiting area**

Fig. 4 ETAT+ triage, assessment and treatment pro forma

Staff Name_____ Signature _____

Patient Name_____ Date of birth_____ Time of arrival_____

ASSESSMENT   ## TREATMENT

Airway Patent ☐ Obstructed ☐

	Dose	Time	Sign
☐ Open airway		___	___
☐ Oxygen		___	___
☐ Dexamethasone	___	___	___

Breathing Normal ☐ Respiratory ☐ Distress

SpO2_____   RR_____

☐ Antibiotics:	Dose	Time	Sign
Drug name: _____	___	___	___
Drug name: _____	___	___	___
☐ Salbutamol:	___	___	___
☐ Hydrocortisone:	___	___	___

Circulation Normal ☐ Impaired
CRT >2sec ☐
Cold hands ☐
Weak/rapid pulse ☐

HR _____ Time_____

Hb _____ Time_____

Malaria positive ☐   Malaria negative ☐   Time_____

☐ Antibiotics:	Dose	Time	Sign
Drug name:_____	___	___	___
Drug name:_____	___	___	___
☐ Artesunate	___	___	___
☐ Fluid Bolus	___	___	___
☐ Adrenaline	___	___	___
☐ Blood	___	___	___

Temp: **Weight:**

MUAC:

Disability Alert ☐   Coma ☐
Convulsion ☐

Blood sugar level:_____

AVPU :_____

	Dose	Time	Sign
☐ Diazepam	___	___	___
	___	___	___
☐ Phenobarbital	___	___	___
☐ Ceftriaxone	___	___	___
☐ Paracetamol	___	___	___
☐ 10% Dextrose	___	___	___

Dehydration Hydrated ☐   Some Dehydration ☐

Severe Dehydration ☐

☐ IV Fluid	Volume	Duration	Time	Sign
Fluid:_____	___	___	___	___
☐ ORS/ReSoMal	___	___	___	___

Transfer Destination_____ Time of transfer_____

Fig. 4 (continued)

number of SRNs involved with the ETAT+ programme at each hospital has gradually begun to increase. No cadre limitations have been imposed for the participation of nurses in the ETAT+ programme; the only requirement for participation in the programme is successful completion of the ETAT+ training programme and its final written and clinical assessment.

Recruitment and training have also continued for a smaller group of nurse mentors, whose role is to teach and train their peers across the different hospitals. These team members undergo further coaching on adult learning, classroom and small group teaching methods and the principles of mentorship in a clinical setting. In 2017 and 2018, the mentors supported learning and quality improvement during 6-month implementation periods at each hospital site, and they continue to offer top-up interventions over shorter time periods.

Evaluation

The 2017 national rollout was subject to a detailed evaluation that measured the timing of triage and treatment, adherence to key aspects of the ETAT+ treatment protocols and hospital mortality. Timings were measured by the mentor teams who undertook a week of observation at the beginning and end of the implementation period and documented the time at which every child was triaged and when they received the first treatment relevant to their presenting problem. Adherence to the treatment protocols was assessed by review of the national triage and treatment pro formas and/or the clinical notes for every patient admitted to the paediatric ward. Mortality was evaluated by the mentor teams who individually reviewed the outcome for every patient who was admitted to the paediatric ward. This was necessary because during the assessment phase, large discrepancies had been observed between the mortality rates submitted to the Sierra Leone Ministry of Health and Sanitation (MoHS) and the true number of deaths on the ward. The scale of the discrepancy in relation to ODCH has been described by Ragab et al. (2020).

The evaluation of the 2017 rollout showed large improvements in the process measure of time from triage to treatment at the larger regional hospitals (Fig. 5). Adherence to ETAT+ treatment protocols also improved over the 6 months of the national rollout (Fig. 6). Mortality on the paediatric wards also improved over the 6 months falling from a mean of 14.5% to 9.7% (Fig. 7).

Ongoing evaluation of the nurse-led emergency paediatric care service remains a challenge, most obviously because of the issues of access to reliable data on potential indicators of care quality, as information on treatment and outcomes is often inconsistently collected and reported. There is also a more fundamental issue of how individual indicators can account for the quality and impact of one aspect of a

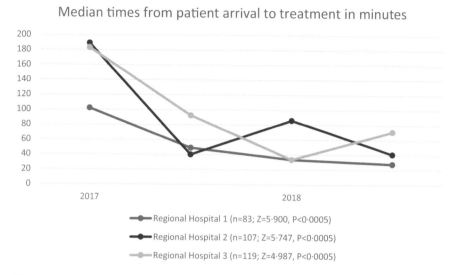

Fig. 5 Time from triage to treatment for children with ETAT+ emergency or priority signs at the three regional hospitals in 2017–2018

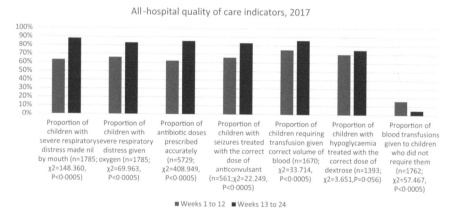

Fig. 6 Trends in adherence to ETAT+ treatment protocols during the 2017 national rollout

complex adaptive system such as a hospital (English M et al. 2021); there are many other factors that may impact on a patient's journey, and whilst it may be possible to design an evaluation system that could begin to account for these factors, it would be difficult to justify the amount of resource that would need to be allocated to gathering such a large dataset.

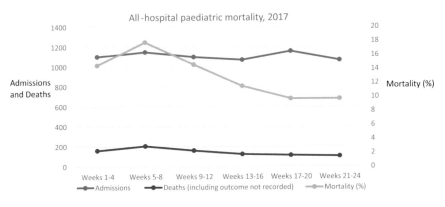

Fig. 7 Paediatric admissions and mortality rate during the 2017 national rollout

Challenges and Facilitators

The challenges and facilitators that have affected the implementation of this nurse-led program are described in this section. The challenges associated with implementation include operational issues with the free healthcare initiative, destabilising effect of the rotations of nurses to different wards and medical staff and NGO resistance. Facilitation of nurse-led efforts has been met with some limited support as presented below.

Challenges

Free Healthcare Initiative: The national free healthcare initiative aims to offer treatment free of charge to children under 5, and it is clearly advertised to the public that treatment for the under-fives is free in government facilities. However, operational challenges mean that there are frequent stock-outs of essential medications and consumables. When this happens, the treating team is forced to ask parents to buy the essential items from outside pharmacy, as under the free healthcare initiative rules, the hospital is unable to buy in stock and sell it on to parents. The journey to the pharmacy introduces delays to treatment, and the non-availability of medicines and the need for payment when the service had been advertised as free disrupt the concordance between staff and families.

Rotation of Nurses: One of the standard processes of nurse management in Sierra Leonean hospitals is the regular rotation of nurses across different ward environments to facilitate a wider range of clinical experiences for all nurses working in an individual hospital. This process had a destabilising impact on the implementation of the ETAT+ programme, as nurses who had built shared experience in delivering emergency paediatric care and were involved in further refining the clinical processes were moved to other wards. They were replaced by nurses who had no paediatric experience and who required the training package to be recommended from the beginning. In some hospitals, it was possible to defer the rotation of staff, sometimes indefinitely, but this was dependent on discussions with the matron at each institution.

Medical Staff: Although agreement had been reached at a national level to allow nurses to undertake the initial full assessment and give the first dose of medication in accordance with the ETAT+ protocols, at some hospitals, there was resistance from medical staff to allowing nurses this degree of autonomy in delivering emergency care. In some cases, this resistance was enough to disrupt the effective implementation of the service.

Non-governmental Organisation (NGO) Partners: Several of the hospitals involved in the programme were working with NGO partners at the time of implementation. Whilst some outside organisations welcomed the approach of developing the skills of the ward staff, others were resistant to any training initiative that was not their own and pushed back against the full implementation of ETAT+ processes in the hospital in which they were working. In one setting, an outside NGO set up a parallel hospital to which ETAT-trained staff from the government hospital were recruited with the incentive of higher salaries, which further undermined the sustainability of the service.

Facilitators

Improving quality in paediatric emergency care in resource-limited settings depends on adjusting multiple interlocking factors and being able to find pragmatic solutions to frequent challenges. Empowering staff on the paediatric ward to identify those challenges and work towards solutions led to successes at many of the government hospitals, but this was dependent on the collaboration of the hospital management. Where the management team has not been actively supportive of the ward staff in making improvements, progress has been limited. This is consonant with previous research investigating the facilitators of quality improvement work based on ETAT+ (Nzinga et al. 2009).

Lessons Learned

The evidence from the Sierra Leone national ETAT+ programme suggests that building a quality improvement approach around nurse-led emergency paediatric care can be an effective way to improve the timelines and quality of care, but only where the relevant enablers are in place. Plotting the paediatric mortality rates at individual Sierra Leonean hospitals in 2017 and 2018 suggests that there is great inter-institution variability in the impact of the intervention (Fig. 8).

Many similar programmes in comparable settings deliver training courses over several days at a separate site and offer incentives (often a monetary payment) for staff to attend. This approach has multiple costs: staff are taken away from the clinical environment, meaning their absence must be covered by other members of the

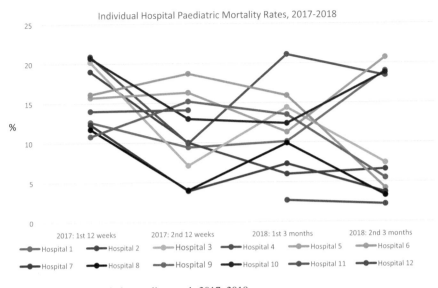

Fig. 8 Individual hospital mortality trends 2017–2018

team; knowledge is gained over a short period of time, meaning that if it is not implemented immediately and regularly, it is likely that much of it will be lost. There is some evidence to suggest that short standalone courses may have a limited impact on knowledge acquisition and clinical outcomes (Cancedda et al. 2015; Musafili et al. 2013; Smith et al. 2008). There is also an extra financial burden associated with delivering the course, as transport costs and incentive payments need to be funded for participants. The active and successful participation from many nurses (410 passed the end-of-course assessment in 2017 and 317 in 2018) suggests that in situ delivery of relevant training on a timetable built around the participants' shift patterns over a longer (3-month) period without financial incentives for attendance may represent a successful approach if the skills being taught are recognised as valuable and likely to make a difference to clinical practice.

The extended ETAT+ course continues to be taught in Sierra Leonean government hospitals, and nurse-led emergency paediatric care continues to work well where the programme and staff are well-supported. Sierra Leone's judicious approach to continuing professional development for nursing staff and to sharing time-critical tasks amongst appropriately trained members of the clinical may offer a model for other countries in the sub-region and further afield to consider.

Future Implications for Clinical Practice and Research

In Sierra Leonean hospitals in 2017, there were rapid gains to be made in paediatric emergency triage and treatment. The obvious improvements in care quality and outcomes made by a short training course and simple changes to process were hugely encouraging. This likely gave impetus to an initial honeymoon period, enhanced by the perceived novelty of the programme, where staff felt increased motivation to contribute to the success of the initiative. Five years after the beginning of the national rollout, a further evaluation of how the programme is embedded and maintained in clinical practice in Sierra Leonean hospitals would be beneficial.

Whilst the results of the initial evaluations of this service have been promising, gold-standard evidence for this approach is lacking. The next step in developing the evidence base is a randomised controlled trial of nurse-led emergency care in West African hospitals. In tandem, further research should be directed towards how hospital management in limited-resource settings can be supported to enable such a system to thrive, given the other competing pressures on the institution.

Conclusion

Nurse-led paediatric emergency care in Sierra Leone has been shown to be feasible and acceptable. Initial evaluations of the service suggest that its implementation may lead to improved clinical outcomes due to improved timeliness of care and adherence to clinical protocols. Grounding the service in a quality improvement approach has allowed clinical teams to make ongoing improvements to the functioning of the service, as nursing staff are engaged in the details of service implementation from patient arrival to discharge. Follow-up evaluation of how the service functions would be beneficial to broaden understanding of the advantages this design could have for Sierra Leone and other settings, although the development of adequate systems of data capture and a relevant approach for assessment of the complex adaptive system of the hospital remains an important challenge.

Useful Resources

WHO Pocketbook of Hospital Care for Children
   World Health Organization. ETAT: manual for participants. 2005. Available from: https://www.who.int/maternal_child_adolescent/documents/9241546875/en/

References

Ayieko P, Ntoburi S, Wagai J, et al. A multifaceted intervention to implement guidelines and improve admission paediatric care in Kenyan district hospitals: a cluster randomised trial. PLoS Med. 2011;8:e1001018.

Cancedda C, Farmer PE, Kerry V, Nuthulaganti T, Scott KW, Goosby E, et al. Maximizing the impact of training initiatives for health professionals in low-income countries: frameworks, challenges, and best practices. PLoS Med. 2015;12:e1001840.

Crouse HL, Torres F, Vaides H, et al. Impact of an emergency triage assessment and treatment (ETAT)-based triage process in the paediatric emergency department of a Guatemalan public hospital. Paediatr Int Child Health. 2016;36:219–24.

English M. Improving emergency and admission care in low-resource, high mortality hospital settings - Not as Easy as A, B, C. Health Policy Plan. 2021;22:128.

Hands S, Verriotis M, Mustapha A, Ragab H, Hands C. Nurse-led implementation of ETAT+ is associated with reduced mortality in a children's hospital in Freetown, Sierra Leone. Paediatr Int Child Health. 2020;40(3):186–93.

Hands C, Hands S, Verriotis M, Bunn J, Bailey E, Samuels RJ, Sankoh K, Mustapha A, Williams B, Taylor S. Emergency triage assessment and treatment plus (ETAT+): adapting training to strengthen quality improvement and task-sharing in emergency paediatric care in Sierra Leone. J Glob Health. 2021;11:04069.

Irimu GW, Gathara D, Zurovac D, et al. Performance of health workers in the management of seriously sick children at a Kenyan tertiary hospital: before and after a training intervention. PLoS One. 2012;7:e39964.

MoHS. Government of Sierra Leone. Human resources for health policy, 2017-21. Freetown: Sierra Leone; 2017.

Molyneux E, Ahmad S, Robertson A. Improved triage and emergency care for children reduces inpatient mortality in a resource-constrained setting. Bull WHO. 2006;84:314–9.

Musafili A, Essen B, Baribwira C, Rukundo A, Persson LA. Evaluating helping babies breathe: training for healthcare workers at hospitals in Rwanda. Acta Paediatr. 2013;102:e34–8.

Nzinga J, Ntoburi S, Wagai J, Mbindyo P, Mbaabu L, Migiro S, Wamae A, Irimu G, English M. Implementation experience during an eighteen month intervention to improve paediatric and newborn care in Kenyan district hospitals. Implement Sci. 2009;4:45.

Ragab H, Mclellan A, Bell N, Mustapha A. Making every death count: institutional mortality accuracy at Ola During Children's Hospital, Sierra Leone. Pan Afr Med J. 2020;37:356.

Smith KK, Gilcreast D, Pierce K. Evaluation of staff's retention of ACLS and BLS skills. Resuscitation. 2008;78:59–65.

SSL and ICF. Sierra Leone demographic and health survey 2019. Freetown: SSL and ICF International; 2020.

Witter S, Brikci N, Harris T, Williams R, Keen S, Mujica AM, et al. The free healthcare initiative in Sierra Leone: evaluating a health system reform. Int J Health Plann Manag. 2018;33:434–48.

Interactional Model of Caring for Families of Children with Chronic Conditions

Maria Angélica Marcheti ⓘ, Myriam Aparecida Mandetta ⓘ,
Beatriz Rosana Gonçalves de Oliveira Toso ⓘ,
Eliane Tatsch Neves ⓘ, Fernanda Ribeiro Baptista Marques ⓘ,
Neusa Collet ⓘ, Patrícia Kuerten Rocha ⓘ,
and Lucila Castanheira Nascimento ⓘ

M. A. Marcheti · F. R. B. Marques
Universidade Federal de Mato Grosso do Sul. Instituto Integrado de Saúde, Clínica Ampliada
em Pesquisa e Intervenção Familiar, Mato Grosso do Sul, MS, Brasil
e-mail: fernanda.marques@ufms.br

M. A. Mandetta
Universidade Federal de São Paulo. Departamento de Enfermagem Pediátrica, Escola Paulista
de Enfermagem, Collaborating and Cooperating Centre for ANVISA-Brazilian National
Health Surveillance Agency, São Paulo, SP, Brasil

B. R. G. de Oliveira Toso
Universidade Estadual do Oeste do Paraná, Departamento de Enfermagem, Cascavel, PR,
Brasil

E. T. Neves
Universidade Federal de Santa Maria, Departamento de Enfermagem, Rio Grande do Sul,
RS, Brasil

N. Collet
Universidade Federal da Paraíba, Departamento de Enfermagem, Paraíba, PB, Brasil

P. K. Rocha
Universidade Federal de Santa Catarina, Departamento de Enfermagem, Florianópolis,
SC, Brazil

L. C. Nascimento (✉)
Universidade de São Paulo, Escola de Enfermagem de Ribeirão Preto, Rho Upsilon Sigma
Theta Tau International, WHO/PAHO Collaborating Centre for Nursing Research
Development, Ribeirão Preto, SP, Brazil
e-mail: lucila@eerp.usp.br

© The Author(s), under exclusive license to Springer Nature
Switzerland AG 2023
C. L. Betz (ed.), *Worldwide Successful Pediatric Nurse-Led Models of Care*,
https://doi.org/10.1007/978-3-031-22152-1_11

Introduction

Brazil is the largest country in Latin America in terms of territory and population. Currently, the country has 213.3 million inhabitants, and of these, 69.8 million are children and adolescents from birth to 19 years of age, which represents 33% of the country's total population. Data (Instituto Brasileiro de Geografia e Estatística 2012) show that among 9% of children and 11% of adolescents have a chronic condition.

In Brazil, children are supported by the legal guarantee of the right to life and health through various regulations that protect and support their citizenship rights, such as the Federal Constitution of 1988 and the Child and Adolescent Statute of 1990 (Constituição da República Federativa do Brasil 1988; Lei No. 8.069 de 13 de julho de 1990). These rights are consolidated in several public policies and health programs that specifically target care for children, adolescents, and the family. The focus is the maintenance of favorable living conditions for full healthy development. The aforementioned policies are based on the principles of the Brazilian Unified Health System (SUS), which includes equity, universality, and integrality, developed in an integrated care network, covering primary health care, specialized and hospital care (Lei No. 8.080, de 19 de setembro de 1990; Lei No. 8.142, de 28 de dezembro de 1990).

However, it is observed that families of children with chronic health conditions experience situations in their daily lives that affect their family functioning. This requires a series of adjustments and transitions in the family system to manage the child's health problem. To meet the unique demands of this population, it is fundamental that a greater investment in the contributions by healthcare professionals, changes in public policies, and proposition of nursing care models is needed to assist them. In this chapter, we will discuss the process of developing and implementing a nurse-led family care model for children with a chronic health condition.

Background

The practice of nursing with families' needs is to be based on theories and models, considering that no theoretical or conceptual framework can adequately describe the complex relationships between family structures, function, and process (Wright and Leahey 2012). Family care models provide a basis for nursing practice with families based on theoretical perspectives from Social Sciences, Family Therapy, and Nursing. Some examples of available models are the Calgary Family Assessment Model (CFAM) and the Calgary Family Intervention Model (CFIM) (Wright and Leahey 1984); Family Health System Approach (Anderson and Tomlinson 1992); Friedmann Family Assessment Model (Friedman et al. 2003); Family Assessment and Intervention Model and Family Systems Stressor-Strength Inventory (Mischke-Berkey and Hanson 1991); Illness Beliefs Model (Wright and Bell 2009); Development Model of Health and Nursing (McGill Model); Concentric Sphere Family Environment Model—CSFEM (Hohashi and Honda 2011); Family

Adjustment and Adaptation Model (Patterson 1988); and the Family Management Style Framework (Knafl and Deatrick 1990).

In the international literature, there are studies on the application of theoretical models with families of children with chronic health conditions (An and Palisano 2014; Tomlinson et al. 2012; Grey et al. 2006), to support research (Clark 2003; Svavarsdottir et al. 2012) and for the development of measurement instruments (Jones et al. 2011; Han et al. 2018; Knafl et al. 2013; Nemati et al. 2021; Minooei et al. 2016). In the Brazilian literature, studies use international models as a theoretical and methodological framework in research (Mendes-Castillo et al. 2014; Dias et al. 2020; Neves et al. 2013; Oliveira et al. 2017, 2018; Lôpo et al. 2020). However, their application in practice with families is still doubtful, considering that they are not developed for the Brazilian reality, making the clinical application process difficult for many professionals unfamiliar with the theory and its instruments.

Furthermore, Brazilian nurses have not been fully prepared to assist families and do not have a theoretical base to guide their actions. Thus, a model of care to guide their practice with families of children with chronic conditions was needed. The Interactional Family Care Model (IFCM) provides a basis for nursing practice with the Brazilian family in this context, promoting empowerment to deal with adversities along the trajectory of the child's chronic health condition. The focus is on the Brazilian family as a care system, considering vulnerability, resilience, and the interactions and meanings that the family attributes to the illness experience (Marcheti 2012; Marcheti and Mandetta 2016).

The impetus to develop the model began initially with the provision of care to children with disabilities and their families. During encounters with families of children with intellectual disabilities in a nongovernmental organization in Brazil, we observed their lack of empowerment to manage the illness experience. Their voices were not heard, and they were not cared for in their needs and demands. They presented emotional, relational, and functional demands on a daily basis. Historically, Brazilian children with disabilities and their families have faced difficulties regarding societal inclusion because of the disability itself, prejudice, and poverty. Hence, care provided to these children depends entirely on their families' efforts. Therefore, we realized that these families suffered deeply when taking care of the children under these conditions. The process of social inclusion requires transformations in society and public policies to improve the care provided to these families. Therefore, the aim of the IFCM is to include the families of children with chronic conditions in their care, hearing their voices, and strengthening the family's ability to cope with the situations fulfilling their needs and demands.

The target population of IFCM services is families of children with chronic conditions in primary healthcare settings, specialized outpatient clinics, and hospital settings. The implementation of the IFCM first began at a specialized ambulatory program for families of children with an intellectual disability and cerebral palsy. Eventually, the IFCM services were expanded to other children with chronic conditions such as cancer, sickle cell disease, chronic kidney diseases, and autism spectrum disorder.

Description of the Nurse-Led Model

The description of the nurse-led model will begin with an overview of the theoretical basis of the Interactional Family Care Model (IFCM), followed by an explanation of the dimensions of IFCM. The assumptions upon which the IFCM are based are presented as well as the eligibility for families who receive IFCM services.

Theoretical Foundations of the Model

The development of the Interactional Family Care Model (IFCM) was influenced by the theoretical models of Symbolic Interactionism (Blumer 1969), Family Vulnerability (Pettengill and Angelo 2005), and the Family Resilience Model (Walsh 2015). According to IFCM, the family is considered a system that interacts with situations and defines them based on its experiences, vulnerability, and resilience to deal with the demands and challenges caused by the chronic health condition of one of its members (Marcheti and Mandetta 2016). The focus of care in the IFCM is based on the identification of the symbolic definition of the family and the provision of interventions that help it to resignify and relieve suffering, so that it can develop its sense of empowerment to make decisions and modify patterns of functioning in the face of situations experienced (Marcheti and Mandetta 2016). The theoretical influences that guided the development of IFCM are described below which include Symbolic Interactionism (Blumer 1969), Family Vulnerability (Pettengill and Angelo 2005), and Family Resilience (Walsh 2015).

Symbolic interactionism (SI) is the theoretical basis for understanding the way the family acts when faced with situations and defines them. It is a useful perspective for understanding human action as it focuses on individual and group human behavior, having as its principle the understanding of the lived process. Interactionism sees the individual as being unpredictable and active in the world. Such meanings can be common and different for each family group and for each family member, due to each person's internal process, guided by feelings, values, attitudes, and experiences with previous interactions. According to Blumer (Blumer 1969), SI seeks to study the nature of interactions and actions performed by the individual and is based on three basic premises: human beings act in relation to things based on the meaning they have for them; such things include all that individuals can perceive in the world; the meanings of things derive from the social interactions they have with each other; and these meanings are modified in an interpretive process used by the person her/himself in dealing with the things they encounter.

The lived experiences of the children with chronic conditions and their families are highly individualized. The provision of services for this population of children and their families will require acknowledgment of their individualized reactions, behaviors, and aspirations in order to be responsive to their ongoing needs for services and support.

Family vulnerability (Pettengill and Angelo 2005) refers to the family's experience in the context of the child's chronic health condition, as vulnerability is perceived as a threat to their autonomy. The family's vulnerability develops in response to the accumulation of care demands required by the situation, by the family's previous experiences with illness and with health care, and by the imbalance in the functioning of the family that the presence of the chronic condition causes. Vulnerability is identified in the family's interactions with the child's own health condition, with the nuclear and extended family, and with the healthcare team and the healthcare system.

Family resilience (Walsh 2015) refers to the family's ability to withstand difficulties and the unexpected in the face of adversity, recover, and become strong and organized. It is characterized by its ability to respond positively to the demands of everyday life, despite the adversities it faces throughout its development. The conceptual framework of resilience comprises three domains: belief systems, organizational patterns, and communication processes. Family belief systems provide coherence and organize experience to enable family members to make sense of crisis situations. A family resilience approach allows us to move from viewing families as damaged to understanding how they are challenged by adversity and affirms the family's potential for self-repair and growth from crisis.

The Interactional Family Care Model (IFCM) Dimensions

IFCM is composed of six interrelated dimensions that guide the understanding of the symbolic definition of the family's experience of suffering and vulnerability with the child's chronic condition, such as their resilience, and to guide interventions with the aim of helping them find potentialities to deal with the situations arising from the child's condition. The six dimensions of the IFCM are represented in the diagram presented below:

Symbolic definition represents the meaning that the family attributes to the experience and guides the family's actions and reactions to this experience. It is influenced by the interactions of the family with the child with the chronic condition, with the other actors in this process (healthcare team, extended family, community, among others) and with the symbols, self, and mind of the family. Understanding the symbolic definition given by the family is central, as it allows nurses to propose interventions that help the family in the process of resignification, in which the family sees a potential for transformation.

The six dimensions as depicted in Fig. 1 are dimension 1, interaction with the child's chronic condition; dimension 2, interaction with family members; dimension 3, interaction with the healthcare team and social facilities; dimension 4, system beliefs; dimension 5, organizational patterns; and dimension 6, communication processes.

Dimension 1 refers to the family's vulnerability in the *symbolic interaction with the child's chronic health condition*. Its understanding makes it possible to identify the elements that contribute to the intensification of the family's vulnerability. In this context, the elements that contribute to the family's vulnerability are triggered by the diagnosis or even the suspicion of it, including the following: uncertainty, powerlessness, real or imaginary threat, exposure to harm, fear of the result, submission to the unknown, and expectations of returning to the previous life.

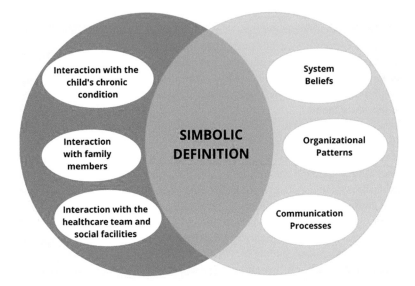

Fig. 1 Diagram of the interactional family care model dimensions (IFCM). Source: Marcheti and Mandetta (Marcheti and Mandetta 2016)

Dimension 2 refers to the family's vulnerability in the *symbolic intrafamily interactions* due to the child's chronic health condition. Its understanding provides evidence about the way the family deals with the situation in the intrafamily environment. In this interactional context, the vulnerability of the family is manifested through the imbalance in the ability to function, lack of structure, distancing, changes in family life, and conflicts that arise.

Dimension 3 refers to the vulnerability of the family in the *symbolic interaction with the health team and social facilities*. Recognition of these interactions provides an understanding of how the processes of information acquisition, reception, participation in care, and decision-making occur. When this interaction is marked by conflicts due to a lack of dialogue, a lack of respect and the family's distance from its role, the family's vulnerability is intensified.

Dimension 4 refers to the *family's belief system*, providing clues about what the family believes and values in the lived context and the elements that influence their perceptions. The identification of facilitating beliefs can be fundamental to develop and strengthen the family's potential to face the challenges emerging from the context of the child's chronic health condition. The family's beliefs encompass their values, convictions, attitudes, and assumptions that form a set of basic premises that trigger reactions and emotions that inform decisions and guide family actions.

Dimension 5 refers to the *family's organizational patterns*. Acknowledgment of their organizational patterns facilitates understanding of how the family of the child with a chronic health condition can mobilize resources, resist stress, and reorganize itself to adapt to the context and to efficiently deal with crises and the persistent adversity arising from this condition.

Dimension 6 refers to the *family's communication processes* that are established, which are fundamental for understanding how it deals with adversity. Effective communication processes can facilitate family functioning by improving the competence of its members to express feelings and emotions that emerge from the context of the child's chronic condition. These communication processes can assist the family to meet new demands in the crisis caused by the child's chronic condition and to negotiate the processes of change within the family.

Understanding of the family's responses to these dimensions enables the nurse to identify the family's symbolic definition of the lived situations and to address the needs and suffering of the family. Based upon this needs assessment, nursing interventions can be implemented to help the family to reframe their definitions of the lived situations changing their responses to them. Assisting and supporting the family to access the key points of resilience are fundamental to strengthening their ability to cope with the difficulties and demands imposed by the situation.

IFCM Assumptions

Assumptions, upon which a model is based, can be defined as beliefs about a phenomenon and based on accepted knowledge or on individual beliefs and values. The assumptions for the *IFCM* are:

- Welcome the family, recognizing their feelings of vulnerability and suffering, and identify individual and family beliefs and strengths.
- Recognize the symbolic definition attributed by the family to the experience and establish interactions based on respect, empathy, open communication, and attentive listening.
- Promote the strengthening of the family's resilience, proposing interventions that help them to restructure or change their pattern of functioning and give new meaning to the situation.
- Value interactions with the family so that interventions are proposed together with the family.

Based upon these assumptions, the Interactional Family Care Model guides interventions with families of children and adolescents with chronic health conditions. The IFCM recognizes that families are in a situation of vulnerability triggered by interactions in dealing with the child's condition, with the family members, with healthcare professionals, and with the healthcare services.

IFCM Practice

The IFCM practice is located within the expanded Clinic for Research and Family Intervention, which is linked to the Research Group: Laboratory of Studies and Research in Family Intervention (LEPIF). LEPIF is located at the Integrated School

Clinic of the Federal University of Mato Grosso do Sul, which is in the Central-West region of Brazil. Families who meet the following eligibility criteria receive IFCM services:

- Families of children and adolescents diagnosed with chronic diseases such as diabetes, cancer, sickle cell disease, kidney disease, and mental disorder; families undergoing difficulties in managing the treatment of children with chronic health conditions; families facing situations that threaten their interactions and relationships among their members or that are experiencing disruptions due to conflicts caused by the chronic health condition of the child or adolescent; and families with difficulties in establishing routines and adaptations for the care and inclusion of children and/or adolescents in school, family, and social environments.

IFCM Service Components

IFCM services begin with a thorough assessment process. The comprehensive family assessment process based upon the Calgary Family Assessment Model is described. A focus on family suffering is provided that involves an in-depth exploration of its meaning and behavioral manifestations.

Assessment Dynamics An interview is scheduled to receive the family and to establish a commitment with the family members and also to perform an initial assessment of the hypothesis of family suffering. Confidentiality of information is ensured for each family, who attend meetings individually.

First Meeting: Engagement It is essential that the nurse establishes a bond of trust and cooperation with the family. The environment needs to be private and welcoming. This first meeting is designed to engage the family as it is a moment of attentive listening to the reasons why the family considers that they need help with their demands and challenges.

Subsequent Encounters The aim of subsequent encounters is to get to know the family's experience in depth and explore the family's interactional processes in order to elaborate upon the hypotheses of suffering and guide the development of the intervention plan.

The Family Assessment Process

The family assessment is based on The Calgary Family Assessment Model (CFAM) to identify the family's vulnerability and resilience to cope with the situations. The structure, development, and family functioning are evaluated, all of which will allow the nurse to know who makes up the family, family ties, history, and interaction processes with the chronic health condition. The Genogram and Ecomap are built together with family members and are useful for delineating the internal and external structures of the family. This initial assessment helps the family to perceive itself, to evaluate and to structure behaviors and relationships, and to reorient the perceptions that they have about themselves.

Once the family's assessment is complete, the strategies for adapting to the reality and context it is going through, the probable hypotheses of suffering and the challenges in managing the conflicts triggered by the situation experienced are identified. Therefore, nurses must generate hypotheses before the meeting to explore the family's interactions, reactions, and adjustment to the situation that are created by the child's chronic condition. It is relevant that during the encounter, the nurse dialogues with the family about their concerns and its influences on their lives, confirming or refuting the nurse's initial hypothesis about the situation (Wright and Leahey 2009).

Suffering is an experience that the family of children and adolescents with a chronic health condition endure from the moment the situation is revealed to them, when their lives and interactions are altered by this context. This context generates deep suffering, which translates into a loss of meaning, sense, and hope, and marks the life of everyone in the family to the point of modifying their interactions. There are several synonyms that show the affective nature of suffering: discomfort, anguish, torment, pain, desolation, distress, and anxiety, and it encompasses several dimensions in a person's life (Marcheti 2012; Wright 2005; Ferrell and Coyle 2008). It is a response to an experience that jeopardizes their integrity and constitutes a manifestation of their dependence and vulnerability (Ferrell and Coyle 2008; Morse 2001; Rodgers and Cowles 1997; Selli 2007). It is also defined as an intense and personal experience: sufferers often feel threatened and helpless (Ferrell and Coyle 2008; Chesla 2005). Families exposed to situations of adversity caused by a chronic condition experience profound suffering that changes their lives, interfering with relationships and the family's daily life (Marcheti and Mandetta 2016).

Nurses need to understand how suffering affects the family, what changes it causes, and what meanings are attributed to it. In the family's trajectory, although there are differences in the way members experience the child's condition, they experience persistent pain that sometimes intensifies with each new situation they have to face. The intensity and duration of the family's suffering are explained by the unpredictability of the event. The condition imposes an intense burden of suffering on the family, leading them to somehow try to understand what is happening, join forces, make necessary changes, reorganize, and fight to preserve their values, beliefs, and interactions (Marcheti 2012; Marcheti and Mandetta 2016). To help nurses identify family suffering and conduct interventions with the family, we organized an illustrative figure with the hypotheses of family suffering with the experience of a child's chronic condition (Marcheti and Mandetta 2016). The family's suffering hypotheses are related to their interactions with the child's condition, with the family itself, with the health team, and with the demands and challenges they experience, and these are described in Fig. 2.

Family Suffering Hypotheses	Behavioral Responses
• Emotional and relational demands of the family in the interactions within the context of the child's chronic condition	• Difficulties accepting the chronic condition • Lack of preparation in dealing with the child's condition • Lack of knowledge about the disease and uncertainties • Submission to the unknown • Feelings of threat and powerlessness
• Demands on the family's ability to function	• Conflicts and ruptures in the family relationship • Disorganization of family life • Family overload and stressful routines • Lack of support and social support network • Difficulty making decisions • Disorientation about crisis management
• Demands and crises in the interactions with the healthcare team	• Lack of dialogue with the team • Difficulty in accessing health care and professional follow-up • Difficulty in accessing public support structures and policies • Discrimination and prejudice

Fig. 2 Hypotheses of family suffering. Source: Marcheti and Mandetta (2016)

Interventions with the Family

After identifying the hypotheses of suffering and also having validated it with the family, the nurse needs to study the possibilities of interventions that have the potential to favor changes and strengthen the family's resilience for decision-making and more successful management of the situation. It is noteworthy that in the same way that nurses identify the hypotheses that generate suffering, recognition of the strengths, and potential of the family, both individually and in the group is needed.

To conduct the intervention, the nurse considers the competencies of the family that were identified during the assessment process based upon the CFAM. Interventions should seek to alleviate suffering and identify family resources and promote empowerment through the identification of vulnerability and family resilience, according to IFCM. Identification of these elements as done during the assessment process can strengthen protective processes and enable the family to overcome the challenges they face and reinforcing their competence for future challenges. These interventions aim to develop family potential and coping strategies so that they feel empowered and can manage situations, conflicting interactions, and health care; draw out family and social resources; help the family to identify available social support networks; and promote empowerment for health care, for decision-making in relation to family care and family functioning.

Interventions offered to families follow the recommendations of the Calgary Intervention Model with Families (Wright and Leahey 2012), concerning the cognitive, affective, and behavioral domains of family functioning based on family Resilience Model from Froma Walsh (Marcheti and Mandetta 2016):

- Offer information and guidance on the child's chronic and health condition, on the management of family relationships and crises, and on resources of the community in particular about the care institutions.
- Praise the family's strengths, efforts, accomplishments, and skills in childcare.
- Offer ideas that challenge restrictive beliefs in the management of family interactions, helping the family to extract meaning from the crisis experience and the child's condition, to identify ways to reduce risk factors to their integrity, and to live with the uncertainty of the future or situations that cannot be predicted or controlled.
- Encourage the narrative of the family history, the meaning attributed to the illness, and of situations experienced in the context of the child's chronic condition, encouraging the expression of feelings and beliefs, the open sharing of thoughts and emotions that permeate the family's experience.
- Help family members to develop empathic connections among themselves.
- Encourage the acquisition of competence, trust, and connection through collaborative efforts.
- Instill hope and optimism, assuring/believing that the family is able to triumph over their adversity.
- Encourage family members to be caregivers and to organize rest and leisure.
- Mobilize family and sociocultural resources for recovery and coping with the situation, search for extra-family resources, and the development of links with available social and community networks and on resources of the community in particular about the nongovernmental organizations.
- Encourage family members to persist in their efforts, accept human limitations, and develop empathic communication strategies.
- Strengthen family relationships.
- Encourage the family to respect the individual needs of its members.
- Develop potential in the family for the care of the child with a chronic health condition.

Strategies for Intervening with the Family

These interventions are offered to the family through therapeutic conversations, intervention questions, letters, phone calls, and a family diary (Wright and Leahey 2012; Marcheti and Mandetta 2016). These strategies can be applied alone or together.

- Therapeutic conversation is an important way to establish a bond with the family. In addition, it is a communication strategy to make sure that the exchange of messages is a two-way street, so that the family is heard and recognized as having the potential for change.

- Intervention questions are aimed at informing and effecting changes in the symbolic and interactional definitions of families. An example of an intervention question is: "How do you feel when your parents dedicate time and care to your sibling with diabetes?".
- Therapeutic letters are written in a way that positively portrays the encounters and efforts of the family; they offer praise and confirm the advances and successes that the family has achieved. These are sent by mail after the first meetings with the family and as needed. A termination letter is sent after the last meeting with the family.
- Therapeutic phone calls and messages can be sent to the family during the period they have meetings via digital apps. The calls and messages are sent to encourage them in their efforts and stimulate their resilience and conversations.
- Family diary can be used by a family to document the events and history of their lived experience. It can be used as a means to demonstrate to families the strength they exhibited to face and deal with difficult situations.

The choice and conduct of interventions are influenced by the following factors: challenges experienced by the family; suffering hypothesis (Fig. 2) formulated by the nurse about the challenges and meanings that the family attribute to their experience, considering their beliefs about the lived context; respect for family beliefs, religiosity, ethnicity, and culture; connection to the strengths and potentials of the family as a unit and of its individual members; and efforts that the family have successfully made in the past and those that have been obstructed.

Based upon the aforementioned process, the intervention is proposed and planned collaboratively with the family. As a means of initiating the intervention effort, we adopted the following question: "Would you like to tell us, based on what we talked about, something that you are prepared to take on in regard to the care of _____[child's name] while _____ [partner's name] is at work?" In this manner, we always check the family's understanding of what is being proposed. In the subsequent meetings, we evaluate the responses of the family to the proposed interventions in order to identify the changes made by the family.

Finalization Process Finalization occurs collaboratively with families. The meetings finish when the families have skillfully promoted changes to overcome their situation, with renewed strength and diminished suffering. The meetings are concluded with a talk with the family and a letter of completion, highlighting the families' strengths, changes, and interactions, offering an opportunity for them to review their efforts. All consultations are registered in the Family Medical Record.

IFCM Outcomes

The evaluation of the model has been carried out through a qualitative approach, seeking to identify the family's satisfaction with the care and outcomes. The goals of care are focused on outcomes that include the family's ability to resolve their own problems and conflicts and those associated with the health system, and these include improvements in family health literacy and their participation in decision-making. Moreover, the family's ability to search for and use the community's social support network is a desired outcome of intervention services. Additionally, through the use of IFCM interventions, we expect modifications in the belief system; re-signification of the experience; and family interaction with the systems. This will be achieved through the following methods:

- Indicators of family participation: evaluation of the number of absences and rescheduling of meetings; number of families who abandon care; participation in the proposed activities (reading, films, diary)
- Student learning assessment: participation in the activities of the research group; expansion and elaboration of studies with family; construction of the family genogram and ecomap; ability to identify family strengths and identify symbolic definition; and interaction skills with families.

IFCM Project Setting It is a space dedicated to care for the family to help them deal with situations of health and illness. It is linked to the Research Group—Laboratory of Studies and Research in Family Intervention (LEPIF), and its mission is to monitor and follow up with families of children and adolescents with chronic health conditions of varying degrees of complexity. A network of other services are integrated in the Expanded Family Research and Intervention Clinic, which include outpatient clinics of the University Hospital—general pediatrics, and specialties in neuropediatrics, hematology, genetics, nephropediatrics, endocrinology, and gastro-pediatrics; Pediatric Emergency Care and Intermediate Pediatric Neonatal Care Unit at the University Hospital; Pediatric Intensive Care Unit of the University Hospital; Children's Oncology and Hematology Treatment Center; Municipal Network—Child and Adolescent Psychosocial Care Center (CAPSi) of the Municipal Health Department; and Family Health Strategy (ESF) and Rehabilitation Institutions—Pestalozzi Association of Campo Grande (APCG).

IFCM Team Members

Coordination: A Nursing Professor at Federal University of Mato Grosso do Sul, expert in Family Nursing, PhD. Leader of the Expanded Family Research and Intervention Clinic, responsible for the general coordination of the clinic, research projects and care with families. Supervisor of IFCM clinical practice.

Consultor: A Nursing Professor at Federal University of São Paulo, expert in Family Nursing, PhD. IFCM consultant participates in group meetings for mentoring and research projects.

Collaborator: A Psychologist Professor at Federal University of Mato Grosso do Sul. PhD. Responsible for psychological care and case discussion with graduate and undergraduate students.

Collaborator: A Nursing Professor at Federal University of Mato Grosso do Sul, expert in Family Nursing, PhD. Responsible for organizing the participation of undergraduate students, preparation of case discussions, and research projects.

Nurse: Responsible for the general organization of the meeting schedules at the Expanded Family Research and Intervention Clinic.

Nursing graduate students: Master or doctorate levels. They participate in clinical care under the direct supervision of the advisor. Prepare and present case discussions, follow-up worksheets, manuscripts to publication, and presentation of papers at scientific events. To participate in the IFCM, everyone must attend the preparatory course in which the content includes theoretical and practical knowledge about Family Nursing Theories; family dynamics and health and illness; therapeutic conversation skills; systems thinking skills; the use of an evidence-based approach focused on family competencies; reflections on culturally sensitive care and interpersonal relationships with the family; and nursing competencies to work with family at a general and advanced level.

Challenges and Facilitators

The facilitators that make everything possible include the openness and welcoming attitude of all the staff involved in the IFCM. Also, there is the resource of physical space offered by the University (UFMS) for the functioning of the Expanded Clinic for Research and Intervention in the Family, considering that it is near the university hospital, laboratories, and other services offered to the community. Thus, the clinical space contains the reception, waiting room, office, rooms for family group care, and children's recreation space, human resources: nurses, administrative assistant for scheduling and monitoring the premises, undergraduate and graduate students, professors of undergraduate and graduate courses in Nursing, Psychology, Nutrition and Physiotherapy, and cleaning and maintenance staff. Material resources such as forms, office supplies, hospital medical supplies, logistics, and dissemination—printed, web, radio, and TV.

Another resource is the agreement between the University (UFMS) and a nongovernmental Organization named Pestalozzi Association of Campo Grande/MS, an educational and rehabilitation institution for children and adolescents with physical, intellectual, and neuromotor disabilities. In this place, physical space is available for assistance to families, such as reception and secretary, waiting room, offices and rooms for meeting with the family, and toy library; human resources: nurses, rehabilitation, and social service professionals; material resources: telephone for contact with families, office supplies and hospital doctor, logistics, and dissemination on social networks.

The great challenge is to obtain financial autonomy for the Expanded Family Research and Intervention Clinic. However, plans and negotiations are underway for the qualification of the services provided at the clinic with the Unified Health System (SUS) to make it possible to receive the necessary amounts related to consultations and other care provided monthly.

Lessons Learned

Over the last 10 years, we have learned some lessons from the evaluation of the IFCM service by applying a qualitative approach, seeking to identify the family's satisfaction with the care received and its outcomes.

We learned that family life begins to be restored as they interact with the situations and feel strengthened by the interventions. For the families, their participation gives them a time to think and seek new ways to deal with the situations they experienced. Families have also revealed that the professional interactions that were most important for them while participating in the clinic were *being listened to*, wherein families feel they are in an environment where they can talk; be heard and share family moments; and *being encouraged* by the professional staff to enhance family strengths and abilities. The encouraging feedback enables the family to find the resources they can use to deal with challenging situations that bring about conflict and suffering. Encouragement helps to facilitate the family's competence in coping; *counseling provided by the professional staff*, wherein families receive guidance aimed at their particular experience, which helps them to manage the situation(s) that generate conflict and suffering. Families report recommendations of movies, receiving therapeutic letters, therapeutic conversations, phone calls, WhatsApp® messages, and video calls are useful; *family access to information* based upon the situational context and the family's perceived needs for guidance are viewed as helpful. This information makes it possible to reflect on the way to handle the situation that generates the family crisis. It offers elements that help the family to think of possible solutions. It gives the family the opportunity to expand their understanding of the issue that afflicts them and creates perspectives for new understandings.

Having a structured model of family care enables a better relationship between nurses and families, favoring their interaction with the health service, with other team professionals, with the community, and with students. It creates and leverages resources in the family, so that they can deal more effectively with the experience of the child's condition and recover in a stronger way, both individually and as a relational system. It stimulates the family's ability to face immediate crisis situations, increasing their competence to face future challenges, and strengthens fundamental interactional processes to encourage family coping, recovery, and resilience.

Service Adjustments Made

With the evaluation of the model carried out through a qualitative approach, we made some adjustments, such as the expansion of communication channels with families through the WhatsApp® application feature for scheduling, communication, and interaction with the family, including the provision of interventions. Therefore, there was the use of social media to disseminate the IFCM service to families with children experiencing health chronic conditions in the community.

We also made adjustments to the IFCM service, such as the organization of the flow of care in the follow-up service for newborns at the family clinic. There was also the implementation of family support groups in pediatric and neonatal inpatient units to help in the transition process of settling children with chronic conditions at home, and there was the invitation to participate in the IFCM service.

Future Implications for Clinical Practice and Research

It is time to analyze the development and evaluation of the IFCM using methodological research. It is necessary to obtain feedback from the healthcare practitioners and the families involved in its implementation.

Future plans are to implement the IFCM with other populations including adults, the elderly, and their families.

Future research is needed to evaluate family interventions in the context of the IFCM implementation. It is also important to evaluate the core competencies of undergraduate and graduate students for the implementation of the IFCM into clinical practice.

Conclusion

The application of the IFCM for families of children with chronic conditions has been carefully evaluated by the assisted families as well as by the healthcare team. The adoption of the IFCM model with an approach aimed at family interactions brings benefits that not only meet the needs and demands of the family but also promote its abilities and strengths as a system and unit of interactions. The use of the IFCM helps the nurse satisfactorily as it can contribute positively to families living in contexts of extreme adversity by offering support, having their suffering diminished, and they are thus strengthened in their experience and journey.

Useful Resources

Social media: with the aim to publicize scientific meetings, conversation circles with families who are experiencing a child's chronic illness, and opportunities for live streaming events with experts and family members.

- Instagram
  - Laboratory of Studies and Research in Family Intervention—@lepif_ufms. The focus is on healthcare professionals interested in research, researchers, master and doctoral students, and graduation students.
  - Expanded Family Research and Intervention Clinic—@clinicaampliadafamilia. The focus is to inform families interested in participating in the IFCM service.

- Facebook
  - Laboratory of Studies and Research in Family Intervention—@angelicamarchet (https://www.facebook.com/angelicamarchet)
- YouTube LEPIF—https://www.youtube.com/channel/UC4a_2AcWQ4s MrZC0gleXUyg
  - Online social media platform for scientific meetings, conversation circles with families who are experiencing a child's chronic illness; live streaming events with experts and family members; and dissemination of information on the model and approach to the family for health professionals, managers, and the community. The content is stored in the platform and can be assessed by the public interested in it.
  - A short video (6 min 12″) https://www.youtube.com/watch?v=5wMuHCxjNeA&t=87s, was posted on YouTube (2021) with the aim to provide information about the Expanded Family Research and Intervention Clinic. The location, the resources offered to families as well as the theoretical foundation of the Interactional Model of Family Care and the results obtained in the care provided are presented.

References

An M, Palisano RJ. Family-professional collaboration in pediatric rehabilitation: a practice model. Disabil Rehabil. 2014;36(5):434–40. https://doi.org/10.3109/09638288.2013.797510.

Anderson KH, Tomlinson PS. The family health system as an emerging paradigmatic view for nursing. Image J Nurs Sch. 1992;24(1):57–63. https://doi.org/10.1111/j.1547-5069.1992.tb00700.x.

Blumer H. Symbolic interactionism: perspective and methods. Upper Saddle River: Prentice-Hall; 1969.

Chesla C. Nursing science and chronic illness: articulating suffering and possibility in family life. J Fam Nurs. 2005;11(4):371–87. https://doi.org/10.1177/1074840705281781.

Clark NM. Management of chronic disease by patients. Annu Rev Public Health. 2003;24:289–313. https://doi.org/10.1146/annurev.publhealth.24.100901.141021.

Constituição da República Federativa do Brasil. Senado Federal, Brasília. 1988.

Dias BC, Marcon SS, Reis P, et al. Family dynamics and social network of families of children with special needs for complex/continuous cares. Rev Gaúcha Enferm. 2020;41:e20190178. https://doi.org/10.1590/1983-1447.2020.20190178.

Ferrell BR, Coyle N. The nature of suffering and the goals of nursing. Oncol Nurs Forum. 2008;35(2):241–7. https://doi.org/10.1188/08.ONF.241-247.

Friedman MM, Bowden VR, Jones EG. Family nursing: research, theory, and practice. 5th ed. Upper Saddle River: Prentice-Hall; 2003.

Grey M, Knafl K, McCorkle R. A framework for the study of self-and family management of chronic conditions. Nurs Outlook. 2006;54(5):278–86. https://doi.org/10.1016/j.outlook.2006.06.004.

Han KS, Yang Y, Hong YS. A structural model of family empowerment for families of children with special needs. J Clin Nurs. 2018;27(5-6):833–44. https://doi.org/10.1111/jocn.14195.

Hohashi N, Honda J. Development of the concentric sphere family environment model and companion tools for culturally congruent family assessment. J Transcult Nurs. 2011;22(4):350–61. https://doi.org/10.1177/1043659611414200.

Instituto Brasileiro de Geografia e Estatística. Censo Brasileiro de 2010. Rio de Janeiro: IBGE; 2012.

Jones PS, Winslow BW, Lee JW, et al. Development of a caregiver empowerment model to promote positive outcomes. J Fam Nurs. 2011;17(1):11–28. https://doi.org/10.1177/1074840710394854.

Knafl KA, Deatrick JA. Family management style: concept analysis and development. J Pediatr Nurs. 1990;5(1):4–14. https://doi.org/10.5555/uri:pii:088259639090047D.

Knafl KA, Deatrick JA, Knafl GJ, et al. Patterns of family management of childhood chronic conditions and their relationship to child and family functioning. J Pediatr Nurs. 2013;28(6):523–35. https://doi.org/10.1016/j.pedn.2013.03.006.

Lei No. 8.069 de 13 de julho de 1990. Dispõe sobre o Estatuto da Criança e do Adolescente e dá outras providências. Diário Oficial da União. 1990, p 13563.

Lei No. 8.080, de 19 de setembro de 1990. Dispõe sobre as condições para a promoção, proteção e recuperação da saúde, a organização e o funcionamento dos serviços correspondentes e dá outras providências. Diário Oficial da União. 1990, p 18055.

Lei No. 8.142, de 28 de dezembro de 1990. Dispõe sobre a participação da comunidade na gestão do Sistema Único de Saúde SUS e sobre as transferências intergovernamentais de recursos financeiros na área da saúde e dá outras providências. Diário Oficial da União. 1990, p 25694.

Lôpo LT, Andrade AC, Marques AC, et al. Family organization in the context of the childhood with cerebral palsy: a case study. Rev Enferm Atual Derme. 2020;94(32):e020057. http://revistaenfermagematual.com.br/index.php/revista/article/view/892. Accessed 15 Dec 2021

Marcheti MA. The family intervention program in the context of mental disability: a setting for the promotion of changes. Thesis, Universidade Federal de São Paulo. 2012.

Marcheti MA, Mandetta MA. Criança e adolescente com deficiência: programa de intervenção de enfermagem com família. Goiânia: AB Editora; 2016.

Mendes-Castillo AM, Bousso RS, Ichikawa CR, et al. The use of the family management style framework to evaluate the family management of liver transplantation in adolescence. Rev Esc Enferm USP. 2014;48(3):430–7. https://doi.org/10.1590/s0080-623420140000300007.

Minooei MS, Ghazavi Z, Abdeyazdan Z, et al. The effect of the family empowerment model on quality of life in children with chronic renal failure: children's and parents' views. Nephrourol Mon. 2016;8(4):e36854. https://doi.org/10.5812/numonthly.36854.

Mischke-Berkey K, Hanson SM. Pocket guide to family assessment and intervention. Mosby, St Louis. 1991. https://www.researchgate.net/publication/242747258_Family_Systems_Stressor-Strength_Inventory_FS_3_I. Accessed 15 Dec 2021.

Morse JM. Toward a praxis theory of suffering. Adv Nurs Sci. 2001;24(1):47–59. https://doi.org/10.1097/00012272-200109000-00007.

Nemati H, Khanouki ZM, Ghasempour M, et al. The effect of family empowerment model on quality of life in children with epilepsy in South of Iran, 2018: a randomized controlled clinical trial. Iran J Child Neurol. 2021;15(4):55–65. https://doi.org/10.22037/ijcn.v15i4.30119.

Neves ET, Cabral IE, Silveira A. Family network of children with special health needs: implications for nursing. Rev Latino-Am Enfermagem. 2013;21(2):562–70. https://doi.org/10.1590/S0104-11692013000200013.

Oliveira PP, Santos KL, Silva FL, et al. Evaluation and intervention in the family of adolescents with sickle cell disease. Rev Enferm UFPE On Line. 2017;11(4):1552–64. https://doi.org/10.5205/reuol.9763-85423-1-SM.1104201701.

Oliveira PP, Gesteira EC, Rodarte AC, et al. Avaliação de famílias de crianças com doença falciforme. Investig Enferm Imagen Desarro. 2018;20(2):1–11. https://doi.org/10.11144/Javeriana.ie20-2.afcd.

Patterson JM. Families experiencing stress: the family adjustment and adaptation response model. Fam Syst Med. 1988;6(2):202–37. https://doi.org/10.1037/h0089739.

Pettengill MA, Angelo M. Vulnerabilidade da família: desenvolvimento do conceito. Rev Latino-Am Enferm. 2005;13(6):982–28. https://doi.org/10.1590/s0104-11692005000600010.

Rodgers BL, Cowles KV. A conceptual foundation for human suffering in nursing care and research. J Adv Nurs. 1997;25(5):1048–53. https://doi.org/10.1046/j.1365-2648.1997.19970251048.x.

Selli L. Dor e sofrimento na tessitura da vida. Mundo Saúde. 2007;31(2):297–300. https://doi.org/10.15343/0104-7809.200731.2.18.

Svavarsdottir EK, Tryggvadottir GB, Sigurdardottir AO. Knowledge translation in family nursing: does a short-term therapeutic conversation intervention benefit families of children and adolescents in a hospital setting? Findings from the Landspitali University Hospital Family Nursing Implementation Project. J Fam Nurs. 2012;18(3):303–27. https://doi.org/10.1177/1074840712449202.

Tomlinson PS, Peden-McAlpine C, Sherman S. A family systems nursing intervention model for paediatric health crisis. J Adv Nurs. 2012;68(3):705–14. https://doi.org/10.1111/j.1365-2648.2011.05825.x.

Walsh F. Strengthening family resilience. 3rd ed. New York: Guilford; 2015.

Wright LM. Spirituality, suffering, and illness: ideas for healing. Philadelphia: F. A. Davis; 2005.

Wright LM, Bell JM. Beliefs and illness: a model for healing. 4th ed. Calgary: Floor Press; 2009.

Wright LM, Leahey M. Nurses and families: a guide to family assessment and intervention. Philadelphia: F. A. Davis; 1984.

Wright LM, Leahey M. Nurses and families: a guide to family assessment and intervention. 5th ed. Philadelphia: F. A. Davis; 2009.

Wright LM, Leahey M. Nurses and families: a guide to family assessment and intervention. 6th ed. Philadelphia: F. A. Davis; 2012.

From Patient Studies to a Hospital-Wide Initiative: A Mindfulness Journey

Vicki Freedenberg

Introduction

This chapter will describe the conception, development, and implementation of a comprehensive program/intervention of mindfulness and mind-body interventions at Children's National Hospital in Washington, DC. The intervention was initially developed to address the stress levels of adolescent cardiac patients using a non-pharmacological approach and ultimately became a hospital-wide program to address stress and burnout among staff, with the additional goal of the program participants using their newly developed skills to impact patients, families, and coworkers.

The program innovation, curriculum, processes employed, team/faculty-building involved, and challenges faced throughout its evolution and implementation will be described in detail. In addition, the theoretical framework used to develop the intervention will be linked to intervention outcomes.

Background

I have been an advanced practice nurse in cardiac electrophysiology for 30 years, all at the same institution, a large, academic Children's hospital in Washington, DC. Electrophysiology is the science of diagnosing and treating electrical abnormalities of the heart. Therefore, many of my young patients have implanted cardiac devices such as pacemakers (PM) and implanted cardiac defibrillators (ICD). In addition, many have inherited cardiac electrical abnormalities which increase the

V. Freedenberg (✉)
George Washington University, Children's National Hospital, Washington, DC, USA
e-mail: vfreeden@childrensnational.org

© The Author(s), under exclusive license to Springer Nature
Switzerland AG 2023
C. L. Betz (ed.), *Worldwide Successful Pediatric Nurse-Led Models of Care*,
https://doi.org/10.1007/978-3-031-22152-1_12

risk of sudden cardiac death from ventricular arrhythmias (i.e., Long QT syndrome, Brugada syndrome, and catecholaminergic polymorphic ventricular tachycardia). Some have congenital heart disease (abnormal heart structure) and have had open heart surgery with more to come in their future. They have sternotomy scars and may have decreased exercise tolerance compared to their peers. Others have structurally normal hearts with no outward appearing abnormalities but live with the fear of having a sudden life-threatening arrhythmia or receiving a shock from their ICD if they have one. Adolescents with these cardiac diagnoses face unique challenges such as cardiac device-related anxiety, school absence, physical limitations and restrictions, social isolation, peer issues, and body image changes. The social, emotional, and behavioral problems which may occur with prolonged stress can interfere with interpersonal relationships, school success, and potential to become competent adults and productive citizens (Biegel et al. 2009). Furthermore, many common medications used to treat mental health problems such as anxiety and depression can increase the risk of arrhythmias which could lead to further cardiac issues and symptoms or ICD shocks. Adolescent patients may exhibit even greater amounts of distress than adults due to fewer psychological resources (DeMaso et al. 2009). These findings suggest that adding to the unusual stresses experienced by adolescents with CHD, cardiac arrhythmias, cardiac devices, and other life-threatening cardiac illnesses may compound the long-term issues faced by this at-risk patient group.

I have witnessed these stresses firsthand with many of my patients, especially in their early adolescent and teenage years. The study of psychosocial issues in teens with cardiac devices was and is still an emerging field with little data, and I had a great desire to learn more about these issues and to find a non-pharmacological approach to help manage them. Implantable cardioverter-defibrillators (ICDs) are the treatment of choice for life-threatening ventricular arrhythmias in adult and pediatric patients (Berul et al. 2008). Pacemakers are implanted cardiac devices which are primarily used to regulate the heart rhythm due to dysfunction of the sinoatrial or atrioventricular nodes. This technology is relatively new to the pediatric population due to the decrease in size of the devices over the last decade.

In recent years, the number of studies examining psychosocial issues following ICD and pacemaker implantation has greatly increased; however, the vast majority of these studies pertain to adult patients. The results of these studies cannot be generalized to children, as adults arguably have greater intellectual, developmental, and emotional resources than their pediatric counterparts (DeMaso et al. 2009). Increased survival rates from sudden cardiac arrest in both adults and pediatric patients with ICDs have changed the focus of research from clinical outcomes to the evaluation of psychosocial factors related to the impact of living with this surgically implanted device which delivers an electrical shock to treat a life-threatening ventricular arrhythmia (Sears Jr and Conti 2006; Gradaus et al. 2004). In a study of adults with congenital heart disease (CHD), 50% of clinically interviewed patients met diagnostic criteria for at least one lifetime mood or anxiety disorder (Kovacs et al. 2009). Over 30% of these patients haven't received treatment for their mood disorders. These disorders likely started in adolescence as the incidence of anxiety disorders in adolescents with CHD is 30% compared to 7–10% in a healthy population (Kovacs et al. 2009; Wang et al. 2012; Awaad and Darahim 2015), even when the adolescent is asymptomatic from a cardiac standpoint (Wang, 2012). Social adjustment and patient-perceived health status were more predictive of depression and anxiety than medical variables. Modifiable factors such as these could be a potential focus of interventions (Kovacs et al. 2009).

Mindfulness is the cultivation of nonjudgmental awareness of our thoughts, physical sensations, and environment in the present moment, with the intent of fostering calmness and centering, and is both a practice and a way of being in the world. Mindfulness is developed by practicing a range of structured interventions such as meditation and yoga. Some popular definitions of mindfulness include:

- "Mindfulness means paying attention in a particular way; On purpose, in the present moment, and nonjudgmentally to the unfolding of experience moment by moment, as if your life depended on it" (Jon Kabat-Zinn).
- Mindfulness is a conscious, moment-to-moment awareness, cultivated by systematically paying attention on purpose in a particular way (Jon Kabat-Zinn).
- "Mindfulness is the aware, balanced acceptance of the present experience. It isn't more complicated than that. It is opening to or receiving the present moment, pleasant or unpleasant, just as it is, without either clinging to it or rejecting it" (Sylvia Boorstein).

MBSR is a structured, eight-session psychoeducational program, which was developed by Dr. Jon Kabat-Zinn at the University of Massachusetts Medical School (Kabat-Zinn 1990). This program has been in place for over four decades with multiple studies, including good quality randomized controlled trials, confirming decreased rates of anxiety and depression among many adult patient populations.

MBSR was developed in an effort to decrease stress among adults with chronic illnesses. A review of MBSR interventions in adults with cardiovascular disorders showed improvements on a range of outcomes including decreased anxiety, improved emotional regulation, less reactive coping style, decreased levels of norepinephrine, decreased blood pressure, and improved performance on exercise testing (Grossman et al. 2004). The standard MBSR program is an 8-week, 2 1/2 h per session, group psychoeducational intervention which affects positive changes in perspectives toward health and disease (Kabat-Zinn and Hanh 2009). Mindfulness interventions target emotional and cognitive self-regulation processes associated with stress (Perry-Parrish and Sibinga 2014). Mindfulness techniques taught in the MBSR program include meditation, yoga, group support, discussion of stressors, and building mindful approaches to dealing with the stressors. Positive outcomes of mindful interventions are improved coping skills, improved psychological and cognitive functioning, acceptance of experiences in the present moment, decreased autonomic arousal, and increased relaxation (Baer et al. 2012). Evidence of the benefits of the four-decade established MBSR program in adults is reported in two meta-analyses (Grossman et al. 2004; Irving et al. 2009). Benefits of the program were found across adult populations with chronic pain, fibromyalgia, cancer, anxiety disorders, and depression.

The study of mindfulness interventions in adolescents is an emerging and exciting field. Several mindfulness programs, including MBSR, have been adapted for use in adolescent populations. Program modifications include shorter sessions (90 min), fewer sessions, selecting age-appropriate mindfulness activities, and making language appropriate for youth (Biegel et al. 2009; Sibinga et al. 2011). A large published review of MBSR studies in children and adolescents includes 15 studies with sample sizes ranging from 1 to 228 and ages from 4 to 19 years (Burke 2010). Each of these studies investigated feasibility and acceptability of mindfulness-based interventions and overall conclusions, which indicate that these interventions were well-tolerated, acceptable, and safe with no adverse events reported. A study of adolescents with cancer reported increased self-confidence and a more optimistic view in coping with the illness following a MBSR intervention (Kanitz et al. 2013). As these findings reveal, teaching adolescents to think positively, cognitively restructure their thoughts, use distraction, and learn acceptance through positive interventions, may improve clinical outcomes (Compas 2006).

The small but growing research literature on MBSR interventions in adolescents shows promise of a positive effect on outcomes of anxiety, depression, and coping though this has not yet been established in adolescents with cardiac diagnoses. However, several meta-analyses have described the need for psychoeducational interventions aimed at reducing distress in adolescents with ICDs and/or CHD as well as the need for research to determine the effectiveness of such interventions (Dunbar et al. 2012; Karsdorp et al. 2007; Lane et al. 2013).

Our team completed a preliminary study to determine feasibility and acceptability of a 6-week MBSR course adapted for adolescent patients with pacemakers or ICDs ($n = 10$) (Freedenberg et al. 2015). At the time, this was the only published study investigating the MBSR intervention in adolescents with cardiac devices or any pediatric heart disease. Feasibility and acceptability were demonstrated with 100% participation with no attrition. In addition, participants' mean anxiety scores and frequency of anxiety decreased significantly from before to after the MBSR intervention. There were significant associations between coping strategies and levels of anxiety and depression after the intervention. Qualitative data showed perceived improvement in the ability to manage psychological stress and to decrease physical symptoms associated with stress with the formal and informal MBSR practices such as meditation and yoga.

Based on the outcomes of the pilot study, our group designed and implemented a 2-group randomized control trial with 46 patients who had EP diagnoses, with or without a device, and we included patients with postural orthostatic tachycardia syndrome (POTS) (Freedenberg et al. 2017).

There was an MBSR group, which met in person, and video online support group which met via Skype. Both groups met weekly for six sessions. The MBSR program was unchanged from the pilot study. The online group was purely a support group with no MBSR techniques taught, and everyone could see each other on their computer screen throughout the meeting.

We collected both quantitative data and qualitative data to examine the impact of both group interventions. Illness-related stress significantly decreased in both groups. Greater use of coping skills predicted lower levels of depression in both groups post-study completion. Higher baseline anxiety/depression scores predicted improved anxiety/depression scores in both groups. Each group reported the benefits of social support. The MBSR group further expressed benefits of learning specific techniques, strategies, and skills that they applied in real-life situations to relieve distress (Freedenberg et al. 2017).

Both the MBSR intervention and video support group were effective in reducing distress in this sample. Qualitative data elucidated the added benefits of using MBSR techniques to manage stress and symptoms. The video group format was found to be useful for teens that cannot meet in person but can benefit from group support. Both of these studies showed that adolescents with chronic illness are open to and amenable to mind-body and psychoeducational interventions such as meditation, yoga, and group support. As these published findings reveal, psychosocial interventions with stress management techniques and/or group support can reduce distress in adolescents with cardiac diagnoses (Freedenberg et al. 2017).

The positive outcomes we had in our two adolescent patient studies using a modified MBSR intervention ultimately resulted in request from cardiology and hospital leadership to develop a program for wider use in the hospital to address staff stress/burnout and make accessible to wider groups of patients. This led to the development and implementation of a staff mindfulness initiative, the *Mindful Mentors* (Freedenberg et al. 2020).

We wanted to develop and implement a program for the clinical staff in our Heart Institute to increase mindfulness with the goal of decreasing staff, patient and family stress, and making us better caregivers. Stress and burnout among medical professionals are common and costly, placing professionals, organizations, and patients at risk. Rates of physician burnout in the USA currently average around 50% with these rates increasing approximately 10% between 2011 and 2014, even as the rates of burnout among the general workforce remained steady (Shanafelt et al. 2012, 2015; McClafferty et al. 2014). Similarly concerning results have been found for nurses with burnout rates between 34 and 70% (McHugh et al. 2011; Lyndon 2016). Workplace stress is associated with decreased psychological health, quality of care, and patient satisfaction (Amutio et al. 2015). During the COVID-19 pandemic, burnout among nurses has become a critical issue. Risk factors for burnout have been identified, and the need for healthcare systems to address these factors cannot be overstated (Galanis et al. 2021).

Current organizational strategies to address well-being, stress, and burnout in healthcare providers are varied in scope (e.g., sole focus on individual mindfulness vs. broader scope of health behavior, communication, and social support, or organizational change), type of intervention (e.g., individual, group, and online), and outcome measures (Shanafelt and Noseworthy 2017; Squiers et al. 2017). Disagreement exists about which approach best serves the needs of all involved.

MBSR interventions for healthcare professionals found empirical evidence to support benefits in mental and physical health in this population (Irving et al. 2009; Krasner et al. 2009). It is traditionally taught for patients in 2.5-h blocks weekly for 8 weeks plus a 5–6-h silent retreat; programs for health professionals have been adapted to formats ranging from weekend intensives (Fortney et al. 2013) to online, asynchronous training (Kemper 2017). Various projects have attempted to develop and apply abbreviated versions of mindfulness interventions to maximize outcomes while offsetting the limitation of time with positive results (Fortney et al. 2013; Kemper 2017; Gauthier et al. 2015; Pipe et al. 2009; Bazarko et al. 2013; Foureur et al. 2013; Goodman and Schorling 2012; Romcevich et al. 2018; Kemper and Khirallah 2015).

Theoretical Model and Conceptual Framework

The model, which was used to examine the effect of a MBSR program on anxiety, depression, and coping in a patient population of adolescents with ICDs or pacemakers, was the Biopsychosocial model (BPS) (Fig. 1). The BPS was first described by psychiatrist George Engel in 1977. This is an interdisciplinary model which assumes that health and wellness outcomes and accurate diagnosis are intricately related to the patients' subjective experiences of the biological, psychological, and social dimensions of illness (Borrell-Carrió et al. 2004). The BPS model is based on general systems theory (Bertalanffy 1968) as an approach to increase holistic methods of scientific inquiry and conceptualization (Engel 1977). According to Engel (1977), variation in the clinical expression of disease, whether physical (i.e., diabetes) or psychological (i.e., schizophrenia) is related to the individual's experience of psychological, social, and cultural factors in addition to concurrent biological and biochemical factors. Engel (1977) also believed that treatment directed only at the biochemical abnormality does not necessarily restore an individual's health, even if the abnormality is amended or improved. In addition, the BPS model states that the relationship between patient and healthcare provider is a powerful influence over the therapeutic outcome, whether positive or negative, in that the psychological effects of this relationship can affect biochemical reactions and processes of the disease being treated (Engel 1977). Therefore, the healthcare provider is seen as a conduit and educator in the effort to improve the patient's peace of mind and healing powers.

The advantage of the BPS model is that physical illness, psychological illness or distress, and the social context (both individual and societal) in which the patient lives are considered equivalent and inseparable; therefore, interventions aimed at addressing all of these spheres are imperative in improving health outcomes. Figure 2 outlines the associated variables in this study and their

Fig. 1 Conceptual diagram of the bio-psycho-social model

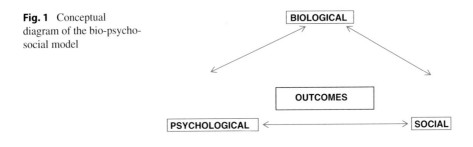

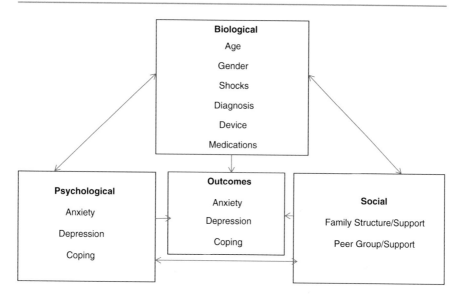

Fig. 2 Biopsychosocial model and associated variables

Biological

- Meditation
- Awareness of Breathing/Deep Breathing
- Body Scan
- Mindful eating
- Yoga\
- Guided Imagery

Psychological

- Meditation
- Awareness of Breathing/Deep Breathing
- Guided Imagery
- Pleasant/Unpleasant Events
- Negative Internal Dialogue
- Mindfulness in routine activities

Social

- Pleasant/Unpleasant Events
- Group/Paired Discussions

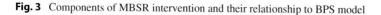

Description of the Service Model

Fig. 3 Components of MBSR intervention and their relationship to BPS model

relationship to the BPS model. In addition, the MBSR intervention which will be used in this study aims to address each component of the BPS model and fits well within this model (Fig. 3).

Organizational Components

Participants were primarily invited from the clinical staff of the Children's National Heart Institute (CNHI), as the main funding source was from an Endowed Professorship within our department, with a few clinicians from other departments who learned of the program and asked to participate. In the pilot cohort, our goal was to enlist 30 participants for the pilot cohort and we accepted 38. Participants were eligible to participate if they were a nurse, advanced practice nurse, physician, psychologist, technician, social worker, child life specialist, or chaplain. Subsequent cohorts were opened up to all hospital staff, both clinical and nonclinical. Eligible staff were sent a program description and application and invited to apply. Applications needed to be signed and approved by the participant's supervisor to ensure administrative support for attending the two all-day educational sessions (mandatory) and the monthly debrief/support sessions (whenever possible). Participants could use their administrative/educational time to attend. They did not need to use their vacation time.

Service Components

Our goal was to decrease staff stress, increase our mindful awareness as caregivers, increase calm and compassionate care, and teach simple and accessible mind-body skills (MBS) for participants to use for themselves and other staff, patients, and family members. The program invited participants to learn MBS to use as "primary prevention" tools in their daily clinical practices as well as during acute stressful moments throughout their day. As this was a pilot program, we wanted to evaluate feasibility and acceptability of a 12-month program.

We developed the 12-month longitudinal mindfulness training program (Mindful Mentors, MM) for cardiology staff at a large free-standing, academic children's hospital to answer three questions: (1) Is such a program feasible, that is, can we recruit at least 30 staff to participate and will at least 25 to complete outcome evaluations 12 months later? Will staff be able to get time off from their clinical areas to participate? (2) What quantitative outcomes (such as burnout, mindfulness, self-efficacy in providing nondrug therapies, confidence in providing compassionate care, stress, anxiety, and resilience) might be most sensitive to the intervention in a larger, controlled, and adequately powered study? (3) Does participation lead to any qualitative changes in behavior such as development and implementation of mindfulness-related projects by program participants?

We chose the critical elements of the MBSR program to pilot the Mindful Mentors program.

We wanted to reach as many staff and ultimately patients/families as possible with our program. We therefore decided to use an innovative approach using a train-the-trainer model so that we could address the personal needs of the staff, then train the staff to train other staff and coworkers, and then be able use the mindfulness techniques to help stressed and anxious patients/families once they felt comfortable.

The development of the program and its curriculum could not have occurred without administrative support for the program. Months were spent holding serial meetings with clinical unit managers to hear their feedback and input about the program in order to gain their needed support. Their belief in the program was critical in order to gain their support to allow their participating staff to use clinical work hours to be off their units to attend the trainings. In addition, hospital administrators were brought into discussions about the program for their support.

I reached out to four experts in the field of pediatric integrative medicine in the hopes of gaining their willingness to join this "mission" and help design and deliver the training. Each one of them wholeheartedly joined, and we began development of the curriculum over the next several months.

Intervention

The 12-month program consisted of an initial 16 hours of intensive, interactive education/practice over 2 days separated by 1 month, followed by 10 monthly 1-h support group/debrief sessions for participants. These monthly meetings also helped to build our "community of Mindful Mentors." The 16 h of initial training was designed by the program faculty (authors of this manuscript) who are a group of clinicians from various disciplines and institutions with vast experience in mind-body medicine. The faculty met by phone conference over several sessions to design the course in a format that would be delivered in-person to a large group of healthcare professionals. The intensive sessions include training in several mindfulness meditation techniques and brief mind-body skills (MBS) including breathing techniques and meditations, walking meditation, body scan, lovingkindness, and self-compassion meditations. Critical elements such as peer support were also used in addition to other techniques including autogenic training, gratitude meditation, guided imagery, and pediatric modifications of the techniques for use with patients. In addition, there were detailed and interactive lectures, exercises, and discussions about the science/neuroscience behind MBS, emotional boundaries, self-compassion, nonviolent, mindful and compassionate communication, misconceptions, overcoming barriers to practice, trauma-informed care, attunement and attachment practices, and mindful listening and speaking. The program taught these clinicians in a train-the-trainer format designed to prepare them to use these MBS techniques with patients, patients' families, and their own colleagues once they were comfortable in their own self-practice. Daily and weekly homework was assigned for the 4 weeks in-between the two 8-hour initial sessions. Completing the homework was encouraged, and each participant discussed their experience with it, but there was not a requirement to formally keep track of it.

The program also included monthly small group debriefing sessions to discuss how the participants were using what they learned, their perceived impact, sharing of ideas, and progress/roadblocks in their personal and professional use of the practices. In addition, each monthly session began with learning a new skill or technique. The third program component was quarterly refresher/education sessions, which were 2 hours in length and included learning new techniques and concepts such as "Compassionate Motivation" and "Clinician Mindfulness and Patient Safety." This intervention format was believed to be more feasible yet still effective for the staff to participate in that most of them "don't have time" to complete the eight-session formal MBSR program. Participants were paid their regular salary to attend the program, and they were able to use educational/administrative leave to attend. All the sessions were conducted on weekdays during normal working hours.

Team Members

The faculty who taught the 16 h of intensive training included two pediatricians who are nationally known experts in mindfulness in medicine, a doctoral prepared chaplain with extensive experience in mindfulness, communication, and trauma care; myself, a doctoral prepared RN with 27 years of experience in pediatric electrophysiology who has extensively studied the effects of a MBSR intervention in adolescents with cardiac devices and/or cardiac diagnoses; and a master's prepared MBSR expert, who teaches MBSR and develops programming in mind-body medicine for medical students. I led the monthly debriefing sessions, in which participants learned a new technique, shared techniques they had been using with themselves, other staff, and patients. Discussion also included which techniques were felt to be beneficial or not, and participants offered support, encouragement, and suggestions to each other. The quarterly education sessions were taught by two of the faculty members who were local. For the final program meeting, participants were asked to develop an individual or group project using the techniques or concepts they had learned. The final session included project presentations by each participant.

We completed our first cohort for the Mindful Mentors program—a group of 35 RNs, MDs, Social Workers, Child Life Specialists, and technicians mostly from Cardiology. Following the positive outcomes of the pilot study, we recently completed our second cohort, a group of 60 clinicians and other staff from throughout the hospital and are currently training our third cohort of 50 more clinicians, and administrative, nonclinical staff from nearly every department in the hospital.

Methods of Evaluation

For this project, feasibility was assessed using the study design and following the areas of focus described by Bowen et al. (2009) for feasibility studies.

1. Acceptability—how did the participants and their supervisors (whose commitment was needed for participation) react to the intervention?
2. Practicality—in the context of their busy clinical responsibilities, would the participants be able to participate in the "mandatory" 16-h intensive training, 2/3 quarterly education sessions, and at least 40% of the monthly debriefing sessions.

The study design of this project asked the question "Can it Work?" Our cohort design compared the quantitative outcomes and qualitative data of individuals who participated in the intervention. In this initial program, there was no randomization, though the 12-month program allowed for several outcome measurement time points.

Feasibility was assessed by recruitment and attendance at the day-long intensive sessions, the monthly sessions, and completion of the baseline, post-16-hour training, 3- and 12-month follow-up surveys.

We assessed four negative outcomes (stress, distress, burnout, and anxiety) and four positive outcomes (mindfulness, self-efficacy, compassionate care, and resilience). Quantitative data were requested to be completed at baseline (pre-16-h training), immediately post-16-h training, 3 months, and 12 months post-initial training. Qualitative program evaluation was completed after the initial 16 h of training and at 12 months, the end of the program. In addition, qualitative data were collected at the monthly debriefing sessions related to techniques that were working or not, ideas and suggestions that group members shared with each other. Comments expressed by each participant were written down and summarized by the group leader. Qualitative data were compiled and grouped by theme using the content analysis method. There was no software used to compile these data.

IRB and Ethical Approval Process

Because this was primarily a staff training initiative, the project was submitted to our IRB and approved exempt as a quality improvement initiative.

Immediately following the 16-hour intensive intervention, the variables showing the most significant improvement were self-efficacy in delivery nondrug therapies (SEND) and confidence in providing compassionate care (CCC), although anxiety and distress also improved significantly. However, after 3 months of practicing their new skills, there were significant improvements compared with baseline in every variable except resilience. These improvements were sustained at 12 months of follow-up. Furthermore, by 12 months later, there was a substantial decrease in the percentage of participants who reported missing work in the past 30 days, from 39% at baseline, 25% at 3 months, and 29% at 12 months. All participants (100%) said they would recommend the program to others and that the training met its objectives. Participants spread the word about the program to other staff, so that the following year we had twice the number of participants from throughout the hospital registering and participating in our second cohort.

Participants were asked to plan and/or implement projects in their clinical areas related to their training within 12 months after the beginning of the program. Participants generated a number of different ideas. For example, four participants jointly planned to incorporate mindfulness education in the nursing orientation curriculum on the Cardiology and Cardiac Intensive Care Units. Three participants planned to implement a weekly meditation program with staff before staff meetings and before nursing rounds. Three participants planned an innovative integrative clinical service including mindfulness meditation for parents and patients as well as acupuncture and Healing Touch for patients.

Over the 12 months of the program, the MM participants emerged as leaders and resources for their clinical units in the areas of stress reduction and MBS techniques. A noticeable culture shift also was occurring throughout the institution, as evidenced by the MM program receiving the hospital's Core Values Award, a hospital-wide competitive award which is accompanied by a grant to support program continuation and funding for research as well as projects developed by the participants. This award was developed by hospital administration to promote programs which are congruent with the hospital values of compassion, commitment, and caring, and the winner was chosen by the highest levels of administration. Over the last 2 years, well-being of staff and patients/families has become a recognized theme throughout the hospital, garnering much support throughout both clinical and nonclinical departments.

Challenges

Challenges faced in the development and implementation of this model were that it was time-consuming, there were many moving parts, and that it required support from multiple layers of people. I was very lucky to have had tremendous support from the beginning, including funding from a departmental leader who was committed to this idea from the start, and that cannot be taken for granted. In addition, I received great enthusiasm from the very beginning from the faculty that I recruited who were committed to this idea and program and have been an amazing team to work with in the development and delivery of the program. This was most definitely a team effort.

Facilitators

Other facilitators that enabled this program to be implemented were a couple of administrative support people in my department, and we're willing to add the tasks for this program to their other work, with support from their Director to do so. Funding for the program includes travel reimbursement and honorarium for recruited faculty not associated with the hospital, program supplies, and commitment from managers to count 16-h training as "work/administrative/educational hours" and not have to use vacation time. In addition, their commitment was needed to not schedule participants on the clinical units or their usual work environment for the two initial training days.

Service Adjustments Made

The pandemic hit after our second cohort finished its initial 16-h in-person training. However, our monthly debrief meetings were changed to virtual instead of in-person, which ultimately turned out to be a positive as more people could participate in these 1-hour sessions. We had to wait to recruit our third cohort until we were able to meet in-person again for the initial 16 hours of training. The initial 16 hours of training is extremely interactive, and we believed it would not have had the same impact if presented virtually. We polled the first two cohorts to get their opinion about that and all agreed.

Lessons Learned

We learned that the group size must be limited to 30–50 people to incur the benefits of group participation and interactions with each other, community building, team-building, and ideas sharing to name a few. After the initial few cohorts, some existing mentors were trained to participate in parts of the initial training (teaching techniques, group discussions). It is beneficial for them and for new participants to see where the program can take them and how they can grow as current faculty retires or is eventually unable to participate creating the need to train new faculty. Ideally, these faculty members could be recruited from our institution to lesson program costs if funding is an issue. This training strategy will also empower current mindful mentors and others in the institution who are knowledgeable and program contact and committed to the program to keep the program moving forward.

Future Implications

Future plans for this program are to continue training new cohorts, about one per year. Already some parts of the MM program are being presented in the employee orientation to all new hospital employees. This addition to the hospital new-hire orientation has been developed and led by current Mindful Mentors who are in the Human Resources and Talent Acquisition departments. We also plan to continue to collect data to track participants' outcomes and use this data to implement improvements and changes in the program. There is unlimited potential to possibly look at patient outcomes to assess differences in patient perspectives and outcomes depending on whether they had a MM for a care provider or not. The hope and goal are that clinicians who underwent the training will use techniques they learned to improve patient outcomes related to pain, stress, anxiety, etc. We also want to continue to disseminate findings and recommendations related to program implementation as this is a novel program and approach (train the trainer) to facilitate stress reduction in employees, care providers, and patients/families which could be reproduced in other systems.

Conclusion

In conclusion, our findings suggest that the MM program is feasible, can be successfully implemented and replicated with institutional support, and has the potential for beneficial effects. These benefits include meaningful outcomes of reduced healthcare provider stress and burnout, increased self-efficacy in using non-pharmacological approaches to reduce distress in patients and their families, and ongoing participant engagement. In addition, the impact of train-the-trainer approach, which is participants' teaching co-workers and other staff to use for themselves and their patients, can increase the impact of this program beyond any individual participant. The MM program has the potential to change the entire institutional culture to one which sees the value of and promotes mindfulness and mind-body approaches to improve self-care of healthcare professionals and to improve patient and family care and biopsychosocial outcomes for patients and families. Based on the successful outcomes of the pilot group, a second, larger cohort ($n = 60$) was completed and a third cohort ($n = 50$) with participants from almost every department and unit in our hospital is being trained, each in the process of developing their own innovative MM projects. Future research will include a control group and should explore the key elements of optimized implementation, as well as assessment of the impact of the program on patient care outcomes and experience.

Useful Resources

Websites specifically geared toward mindfulness for healthcare workers

https://www.mindful.org/mindfulhome-mindfulness-for-healthcare-workers-during-covid/
https://wellmd.stanford.edu/healthy/mindfulness.html
https://www.massgeneral.org/psychiatry/guide-to-mental-health-resources/mindfulness

Social media-mindfulness apps offering free memberships to healthcare providers:

https://www.calm.com/
https://insighttimer.com/
https://www.tenpercent.com/
https://www.headspace.com/covid-19

References

Amutio A, Martínez-Taboada C, Hermosilla D, Delgado LC. Enhancing relaxation states and positive emotions in physicians through a mindfulness training program: a one-year study. Psychol Health Med. 2015;20(6):720–31.

Awaad MI, Darahim KE. Depression and anxiety in adolescents with congenital heart disease. Middle East Curr Psychiatry. 2015;22(1):2–8.

Baer RA, Lykins EL, Peters JR. Mindfulness and self-compassion as predictors of psychological wellbeing in long-term meditators and matched nonmeditators. J Posit Psychol. 2012;7(3):230–8.

Bazarko D, Cate RA, Azocar F, Kreitzer MJ. The impact of an innovative mindfulness-based stress reduction program on the health and well-being of nurses employed in a corporate setting. J Work Behav Health. 2013;28(2):107–33.

Bertalanffy LV. General systems theory as integrating factor in contemporary science. Akten des XIV. Int Kongr Philos. 1968;2:335–40.

Berul CI, Van Hare GF, Kertesz NJ, Dubin AM, Cecchin F, Collins KK, Cannon BC, Alexander ME, Triedman JK, Walsh EP, Friedman RA. Results of a multicenter retrospective implantable cardioverter-defibrillator registry of pediatric and congenital heart disease patients. J Am Coll Cardiol. 2008;51(17):1685–91.

Biegel GM, Brown KW, Shapiro SL, Schubert CM. Mindfulness-based stress reduction for the treatment of adolescent psychiatric outpatients: a randomized clinical trial. J Consult Clin Psychol. 2009;77(5):855.

Borrell-Carrió F, Suchman AL, Epstein RM. The biopsychosocial model 25 years later: principles, practice, and scientific inquiry. Ann Family Med. 2004;2(6):576–82.

Bowen DJ, Kreuter M, Spring B, Cofta-Woerpel L, Linnan L, Weiner D, Bakken S, Kaplan CP, Squiers L, Fabrizio C, Fernandez M. How we design feasibility studies. Am J Prev Med. 2009;36(5):452–7.

Burke CA. Mindfulness-based approaches with children and adolescents: A preliminary review of current research in an emergent field. J Child Fam Stud. 2010;19(2):133–44.

Compas BE. Psychobiological processes of stress and coping: implications for resilience in children and adolescents—comments on the papers of Romeo & McEwen and Fisher et al. Ann N Y Acad Sci. 2006;1094(1):226–34.

DeMaso DR, Neto LB, Hirshberg J. Psychological and quality-of-life issues in the young patient with an implantable cardioverter-defibrillator. Heart Rhythm. 2009;6(1):130–2.

Dunbar SB, Dougherty CM, Sears SF, Carroll DL, Goldstein NE, Mark DB, McDaniel G, Pressler SJ, Schron E, Wang P, Zeigler VL. Educational and psychological interventions to improve outcomes for recipients of implantable cardioverter defibrillators and their families: a scientific statement from the American Heart Association. Circulation. 2012;126(17):2146–72.

Engel GL. The need for a new medical model: a challenge for biomedicine. Science. 1977;196(4286):129–36.

Fortney L, Luchterhand C, Zakletskaia L, Zgierska A, Rakel D. Abbreviated mindfulness intervention for job satisfaction, quality of life, and compassion in primary care clinicians: a pilot study. Ann Family Med. 2013;11(5):412–20.

Foureur M, Besley K, Burton G, Yu N, Crisp J. Enhancing the resilience of nurses and midwives: pilot of a mindfulness based program for increased health, sense of coherence and decreased depression, anxiety and stress. Contemp Nurse. 2013;45(1):114–25.

Freedenberg VA, Thomas SA, Friedmann E. A pilot study of a mindfulness based stress reduction program in adolescents with implantable cardioverter defibrillators or pacemakers. Pediatr Cardiol. 2015;36(4):786–95.

Freedenberg VA, Hinds PS, Friedmann E. Mindfulness-based stress reduction and group support decrease stress in adolescents with cardiac diagnoses: a randomized two-group study. Pediatr Cardiol. 2017;38(7):1415–25.

Freedenberg VA, Jiang J, Cheatham CA, Sibinga EM, Powell CA, Martin GR, Steinhorn DM, Kemper KJ. Mindful mentors: is a longitudinal mind–body skills training pilot program feasible for pediatric cardiology staff? Glob Adv Health Med. 2020;9:2164956120959272.

Galanis P, Vraka I, Fragkou D, Bilali A, Kaitelidou D. Nurses' burnout and associated risk factors during the COVID-19 pandemic: a systematic review and meta-analysis. J Adv Nurs. 2021;77(8):3286–302.

Gauthier T, Meyer RM, Grefe D, Gold JI. An on-the-job mindfulness-based intervention for pediatric ICU nurses: a pilot. J Pediatr Nurs. 2015;30(2):402–9.

Goodman MJ, Schorling JB. A mindfulness course decreases burnout and improves well-being among healthcare providers. Int J Psychiatry Med. 2012;43(2):119–28.

Gradaus R, Wollmann C, Köbe J, Hammel D, Kotthoff S, Block M, Breithardt G, Böcker D. Potential benefit from implantable cardioverter-defibrillator therapy in children and young adolescents. Heart. 2004;90(3):328–9.

Grossman P, Niemann L, Schmidt S, Walach H. Mindfulness-based stress reduction and health benefits: a meta-analysis. J Psychosom Res. 2004;57(1):35–43.

Irving JA, Dobkin PL, Park J. Cultivating mindfulness in health care professionals: a review of empirical studies of mindfulness-based stress reduction (MBSR). Complement Ther Clin Pract. 2009;15(2):61–6.

Kabat-Zinn J. Full catastrophe living: the program of the stress reduction clinic at the University of Massachusetts Medical Center. 1990.

Kabat-Zinn J, Hanh TN. Full catastrophe living: using the wisdom of your body and mind to face stress, pain, and illness. Washington: American Psychological Association; 2009.

Kanitz JL, Camus MEM, Seifert G. Keeping the balance–an overview of mind–body therapies in pediatric oncology. Complement Ther Med. 2013;21:S20–5.

Karsdorp PA, Everaerd W, Kindt M, Mulder BJ. Psychological and cognitive functioning in children and adolescents with congenital heart disease: a meta-analysis. J Pediatr Psychol. 2007;32(5):527–41.

Kemper KJ. Brief online mindfulness training: immediate impact. J Evid Based Complementary Altern Med. 2017;22(1):75–80.

Kemper KJ, Khirallah M. Acute effects of online mind–body skills training on resilience, mindfulness, and empathy. J Evid Based Complementary Altern Med. 2015;20(4):247–53.

Kovacs AH, Saidi AS, Kuhl EA, Sears SF, Silversides C, Harrison JL, Ong L, Colman J, Oechslin E, Nolan RP. Depression and anxiety in adult congenital heart disease: predictors and prevalence. Int J Cardiol. 2009;137(2):158–64.

Krasner MS, Epstein RM, Beckman H, Suchman AL, Chapman B, Mooney CJ, Quill TE. Association of an educational program in mindful communication with burnout, empathy, and attitudes among primary care physicians. JAMA. 2009;302(12):1284–93.

Lane DA, Millane TA, Lip GY. Psychological interventions for depression in adolescent and adult congenital heart disease. Cochrane Database Syst Rev. 2013;10:CD004372.

Lyndon A. Burnout among health professionals and its effect on patient safety. Agency of Healthcare Research and Quality. 2016.

McClafferty H, Brown OW, Vohra S, Bailey ML, Becker DK, Culbert TP, Sibinga EM, Zimmer M, Simon GR, Hardin AP, Meade KE. Physician health and wellness. Pediatrics. 2014;134(4):830–5.

McHugh MD, Kutney-Lee A, Cimiotti JP, Sloane DM, Aiken LH. Nurses' widespread job dissatisfaction, burnout, and frustration with health benefits signal problems for patient care. Health Aff. 2011;30(2):202–10.

Perry-Parrish CK, Sibinga E. Mindfulness meditation for children. In: Functional symptoms in pediatric disease. New York: Springer; 2014. p. 343–52.

Pipe TB, Bortz JJ, Dueck A, Pendergast D, Buchda V, Summers J. Nurse leader mindfulness meditation program for stress management: a randomized controlled trial. JONA. 2009;39(3):130–7.

Romcevich LE, Reed S, Flowers SR, Kemper KJ, Mahan JD. Mind-body skills training for resident wellness: a pilot study of a brief mindfulness intervention. J Med Educ Curric Dev. 2018;5:2382120518773061.

Sears SF Jr, Conti JB. Psychological aspects of cardiac devices and recalls in patients with implantable cardioverter defibrillators. Am J Cardiol. 2006;98(4):565–7.

Shanafelt TD, Noseworthy JH. Executive leadership and physician well-being: nine organizational strategies to promote engagement and reduce burnout. Mayo Clin Proc. 2017;92(1):129–46.

Shanafelt TD, Boone S, Tan L, Dyrbye LN, Sotile W, Satele D, West CP, Sloan J, Oreskovich MR. Burnout and satisfaction with work-life balance among US physicians relative to the general US population. Arch Intern Med. 2012;172(18):1377–85.

Shanafelt TD, Hasan O, Dyrbye LN, Sinsky C, Satele D, Sloan J, West CP. Changes in burnout and satisfaction with work-life balance in physicians and the general US working population between 2011 and 2014. Mayo Clin Proc. 2015;90(12):1600–13.

Sibinga EM, Kerrigan D, Stewart M, Johnson K, Magyari T, Ellen JM. Mindfulness-based stress reduction for urban youth. J Altern Complement Med. 2011;17(3):213–8.

Squiers JJ, Lobdell KW, Fann JI, DiMaio JM. Physician burnout: are we treating the symptoms instead of the disease? Ann Thorac Surg. 2017;104(4):1117–22.

Wang Q, Hay M, Clarke D, Menahem S. The prevalence and predictors of anxiety and depression in adolescents with heart disease. J Pediatr. 2012;161(5):943–6.

Nurse-Led Service Models: Lessons Learned Over 25 Years

Cecily L. Betz

Overview of Past and Ongoing Nurse-Led Healthcare Transition Models of Care

This chapter is designed to provide an overview of programmatic efforts that were generated over a period of 25 years pertaining to the care of adolescents and emerging adults (AEA) with a variety of long-term conditions[1] as it pertained to healthcare transition planning. In this chapter, decades of nurse-led efforts related to healthcare transition services will be memorialized with the intent of providing a chronology of programmatic efforts that were developed, implemented, and refined based upon nursing model of care that was adapted in a variety of clinical and community-based settings. The intent of this chapter is to share with the reader the evolution of model development and implementation that occurred over time in response to changing circumstances that required adaptations of the nurse-led model.

---

[1] In the United States, the terminology varies as to the designation of AEA with chronic conditions/illnesses. Authors use the following terms to denote classification of AEA that convey varied meanings: special healthcare needs, complex chronic conditions, intellectual disabilities, and developmental disabilities. For the purposes of this chapter, the terminology, long-term conditions will be used as well in addition to other commonly used designations identified in this chapter.

C. L. Betz (✉)
Center for Excellence in Developmental Disabilities, University of Southern California, Los Angeles, CA, USA
e-mail: cbetz@chla.usc.edu

© The Author(s), under exclusive license to Springer Nature Switzerland AG 2023
C. L. Betz (ed.), *Worldwide Successful Pediatric Nurse-Led Models of Care*,
https://doi.org/10.1007/978-3-031-22152-1_13

Early Beginnings

Our initial nurse-led healthcare transition programmatic efforts were influenced by our first extramural grant support from the Maternal Child Health Bureau, United States Department of Health and Human Services, entitled, *UCLA University Affiliated Program/School to Work Interagency Transition Program Southern California Transition Coalition/Healthy and Ready to Work Project* and later named *California Healthy and Ready to Work (CA-HRTW)* Project. This project was developed and implemented in collaboration with the Southern California Transition Coalition (SCTC) of the School to Work Interagency Transition Program located in West San Gabriel Valley, a suburb of Los Angeles to create an interagency transition coalition. SCTC was one of four local interagency transition coalitions that had received funding from the California School to Work Interagency Partnership (SWITP). SWITP had been established with grant support from the federal government, as a joint initiative of Departments of Education and Labor through the School-to-Work Opportunities Act of 1994 (National Transition Network 1994). The intent of this legislation was to promote "…major restructuring and significant systemic changes that facilitate the creation of a universal, high-quality, school-to-work transition system that enables all students in the United States to successfully enter the workplace" (National Transition Network 1994).

SCTC had formed an interagency coalition that worked with community-based partners from a number of organizations and agencies to improve transition services for adolescents with special healthcare needs and disabilities. Representatives from education, employment, disability-focus agencies, self-advocacy and family organizations, rehabilitation, social security and job training, transportation, community colleges, and regional occupational programs participated in SCTC. Our team joined in partnership with SCTC to introduce health issues as a component of transition planning. *CA-HRTW* facilitated the inclusion of healthcare representatives from state-funded programs for children with special healthcare needs and pediatric healthcare settings. The goals of the *CA Healthy and Ready to Work* project were to support adolescents with special healthcare needs in making the successful transition to the adult healthcare system, enrolling in an adult health insurance plan, competently managing their own special healthcare needs and obtaining the needed health-related accommodations for work, school, and living as independently as possible in the community. Programmatic efforts were also directed to providing referrals to community-based transition and adult support services for postsecondary education and training, job development and employment, and community living.

The partnership with SCTC was formative and innovative as it ushered in the opportunity to create a nurse-led model of healthcare transition that embodied an interagency approach. We recognized the importance of embracing an integrated model of care that incorporated the health, psychosocial, and developmental concerns of AEA with long-term conditions and their families as they transferred their care to the adult system of care and transition to adulthood. Given this framework of care, our approach addressed not only health-related concerns pertaining to condition self-management, their health literacy, and transfer of care issues but examined the impact of living with a long-term condition where AEA lived, worked, and played.

Based upon this holistic HCT approach, efforts were directed to developing and implementing a nurse-led transition program over 20 years ago, called *Creating Healthy Futures* (Betz and Redcay 2003). This pilot program consisted of an advanced practice nurse whose role was to assess transition-related needs for services and an interagency team who served as consultants. A diverse group of AEA with long-term conditions and their families were served; it was a pivotal opportunity to experiment with a new approach to HCT. Our team generated a number of publications based upon our *Creating Healthy Futures* program (Betz and Redcay 2002, 2005a); one of our early publications was on the role of the transition service coordinator (Betz and Redcay 2005b)

During this early period as well, the team with the input of interagency partners and interdisciplinary colleagues gathered collective input for the development of the *CA-HRTW* Transition Assessment (CA THCA) that was used in our early clinical work. This HCT assessment tool consisted of 73 items that comprehensively assessed knowledge and skills related to healthcare self-management, including those pertaining to health prevention, emergency measures/care, reproductive counseling, and safety behaviors. Other areas assessed included the use of transportation, health-related and academic accommodations at school, and understanding legal rights and protections (Betz et al. 2003). At the time, this pilot program was not sustainable beyond the grant funding project period, which was disappointing. However, the knowledge gained from this pilot program was later applied to our subsequent clinical, educational, and research efforts.

Movin' On Up

An opportunity arose in 2011 to replicate the original *Creating Healthy Futures* model into an outpatient clinical setting at Children's Hospital Los Angeles for youth and young adults with spina bifida. Replication of this model required modifications given the clinical setting wherein this model was implemented. Our model required changes in the service delivery model in order to adapt to the clinical services arrangements, needs of the youth and families, and reimbursement options for services. This nurse-led model of healthcare transition services has been sustainable for over 10 years.

Initially, it was envisioned to schedule the HCT clinic separately from the usual clinic schedule. This arrangement was found to be not feasible for several mitigating factors. The staffing needed to support a stand-alone clinic was not feasible fiscally and logistically. Administrative staffing was not available, and availability of conference rooms was limited. However, of primary consideration was the burden that would be imposed on families for coming to another clinic on another day of the week. The reality of that arrangement meant that families with limited resources would be required to spend additional funds for travel. Hosting the clinic at another time would cause considerable inconvenience for families who would have to get their child and other siblings ready to come to the hospital or make other arrangements for childcare. Another significant issue that deterred the proposed scheduling was the youth would be missing part or all of a school day, which was not in their best interests.

Given the aforementioned constraints, it was decided that HCT services would be integrated within the flow of the usual spina bifida clinic services. A revised plan for the implementation of the HCT was devised that accommodated the clinic logistics, staffing availability, and be responsive to the needs of youth and families. It was determined that the most feasible approach would be to have weekly team conferences that could be reimbursed according to the payer's code and provide direct HCT services that would be integrated into the clinic weekly schedule. Both of these service components were integrated components of the *Movin' On Up* HCT service program (Betz et al. 2015).

Movin' On Up weekly conferences consist of interdisciplinary team members who provide discipline-specific input regarding the HCT progress of youth and their families. Typically, the team conferences involve the HCT service coordinator who organizes the conference meetings and reviews current HCT status as it pertains to condition self-management, coordination for service referrals, needs for durable medical equipment, supplies, braces, and assistive devices. Other issues reviewed are the needs for scheduling/updating annual and, as needed, specialty service evaluations (i.e., urology, physical therapy), current status and needs for academic and health-related accommodations, as well as engagement in social and recreational activities. Our team also reviews future planning needs as it pertains to postsecondary education and training, living arrangements, and employment.

Team meeting members include the spina bifida nurse care manager, social worker, physical therapist, and pediatrician/spina bifida specialist. Other members of the spina bifida clinic team are accessed on an as needed consultative basis. Team conferences enable review, monitoring, and revision of healthcare transition planning goals. At the conclusion of each team conference meeting, the revised set of goals are generated until the next conference team meeting. Generally speaking, conferencing on youth occur approximately twice a year. For youth whose needs are of pressing concern (i.e., postoperative needs for in-home schooling, social challenges) and for those who are approaching age 21 and the termination of pediatric care, they may require additional conferences.

Direct HCT nursing consultation services are provided during the weekly half-day morning spina bifida clinics. During these clinics, the HCT specialist meets with youth and their families to review the current status of issues pertaining to healthcare transition planning. Issues addressed during direct consultation encounters are highly dependent upon the current needs the youth and/or families identified. It is not unusual that issues previously identified as pressing are no longer an issue as it has been resolved or another priority is now identified by the youth and family. Examples of issues that are discussed include the status of CIC self-management, school bullying, obtaining academic and health-related accommodations needed at school, review of job training options, and accessing community-based recreational programs. It is also an opportunity to meet with new patients who meet eligibility criteria for HCT services, which are provided to all youth who are 10 years and older regardless of insurance status.

Involvement in the *Movin' On Up* program has enabled our team to explore issues relevant to healthcare transition planning that are not often explored in the literature. The theoretical framework of our transition program is based upon a comprehensive healthcare transition planning approach that addresses health-related concerns that are not only relegated to chronic care management and illness concerns. Having a chronic condition impacts every aspect of an individual's life. For children and youth, their chronic condition can affect their school performance, peer relationships, and involvement in sports and recreational activities and their aspirations for the future. Therefore, we have been and continue to be interested in learning more about the lived experiences of transition-aged youth with the ultimate aim of improving their quality of life and lived experiences.

To that end, we conducted several studies pertaining to the student's school experiences. Our team investigated youth's understanding of their individualized education plan (IEP), which is an academic plan of instruction support and services for students who qualify for special education services (Betz et al. 2019). An IEP is an individualized plan based upon the needs of each student to assist him/her to achieve academic goals for the school year. Our team was interested in obtaining empirical data to better understand the extent to which students enrolled in our study understood what an IEP is and how an IEP can be helpful to them academically. Findings revealed that students had limited understanding of the purpose of an IEP and its relevance to their own academic activities.

We conducted another study to explore the types of academic and health-related accommodations students with spina bifida received in the school settings (Betz et al. 2022a). Our interest in exploring this phenomenon in the school setting was not only to gather empirical data but to raise this issue as a relevant to the provision of comprehensive healthcare transition services. Our findings revealed that the most frequently identified educational accommodation was enrollment in special education and the most frequently identified health-related accommodations students with spina bifida received was assistance with clean intermittent catheterization. Other academic accommodations that were most often reported were adaptive physical education, tutoring, and home schooling.

These studies illustrate that there are relevant and important areas of assessment and intervention that need to be considered with the provision of healthcare transition planning services. In order to support the AEAs transfer of care to adult healthcare services and transition to adulthood, assisting the AEA to learn to manage their chronic care needs in a variety of settings wherein they work, live, and play is essential. Learning to self-manage their needs in diverse settings is necessary to promote optimal health and quality-of-life outcomes and the AEA aspirations for adulthood.

Future Development in Intellectual Disabilities and Developmental Disabilities

More recently in 2021, our team was awarded a grant *Community-Based Transition Pilot Program* by the Administration on Community Living to generate a pilot plan for the transition program for individuals with intellectual disabilities and developmental disabilities (ID/DD). This project has enabled our team to undertake new efforts to develop and implement programmatic efforts for individuals with intellectual disabilities and developmental disabilities (ID/DD). These efforts include hosting Transition Summits for professionals and family members, production of white papers that address policy-related topics relevant to transition for ID/DD, and constructing a blueprint for a transition pilot program for youth and young adults with ID/DD.

As well, our team is involved with program development efforts in designing a pilot HCT program for transition-aged youth with ID/DD and co-occurring mental health conditions as this is an underserved group of AEA with ID/DD. Our goal is to obtain extramural support for this pilot program. To that end, our team conducted a survey of three major groups of stakeholders (i.e., providers, community-based organization/resource representatives, and disabilities advocates) to elicit their perceptions about the need for HCT services for this group of AEA with ID/DD with co-occurring mental health conditions. This data will be used in our grant proposal to demonstrate the need for this model of care. As well, our team is currently working on generating publications based upon the survey data that we collected from 277 respondents (Betz et al. 2022b).

As has been recounted with our team efforts in providing nurse-led healthcare transition services, there have been varied opportunities that presented themselves to enable our service model to be implemented and be sustainable. We have discovered over the years that sustainability of nurse-led service models can be a challenge. However, having administrative and institutional support for programmatic efforts are foremost factors to ensure sustainability. Our team has been fortunate to have continued support for our *Movin' On Up* nurse-led HCT program. It is our fervent hope and desire that our program continues in the spina bifida clinic in the years to come and that we are able to leverage our efforts into other programs for AEA with ID/DD and those with ID/DD and co-occurring mental health conditions.

Based upon our decades of clinical efforts, our team has acquired insights and understandings with the development and implementation of nurse-led programs. Nurse-led service models involve considerable time, effort, resources, creativity, and institutional support. Nurse-led service models are not developed and implemented in a vacuum; these service programs require the collaboration of a network of support. The following portion of this chapter provides readers with the "lessons learned" with nurse-led service model development.

Lessons Learned

In this chapter section, lessons our team learned with the development and implementation of nurse-led healthcare transition model of care are presented. Many of the "lessons learned" as described below are applicable to nurse-led efforts undertaken by nurse innovators whose practice involved different age groups of children with a variety of needs and is embedded within traditional healthcare settings or conducted in settings with full practice authority (American Nurses Association 2020; Bosse et al. 2017; Stucky et al. 2020). As ANA asserts, Full Practice Authority refers to the "…APRN's ability to utilize knowledge, skills and judgment to practice to the full extent of his or her training." The "lessons learned" that are presented include timing is pivotal, partnerships are essential, measuring outcomes are needed, infrastructure support, HCT services need to be individualized, flexibility not rigidity is needed, referral support is needed, and dissemination is important.

Timing Is Pivotal The timing of a nurse-led service model is a key factor in its development and implementation. In the early 1990s, our team had received extramural funding to create a nurse-led community-based primary care clinic for individuals with intellectual and developmental disabilities. A nurse-practitioner staffed this early project. This project encountered a number of challenges in terms of staffing issues, outreach and recruitment of individuals for care, logistical support, and a clearly defined plan of operation. This innovation was created long before other similar programs were established. Although the model was not sustainable beyond the project period, it did provide the impetus for the development of other programs similar to this original model. Nevertheless, this early model of care served as a precursor to the development of our later nurse-led models of care.

Partnerships Are Essential Throughout the span of more than 25 years of service development, research, and policy-making, partnerships have been essential to supporting and influencing our collective efforts. With our early efforts, partnerships and collaborative efforts helped to shape the development of our model of care that was unique and innovative at a time wherein the focus of state of practice and research was primarily focused on the transfer of care. As we described previously, our partnership with SCTC was hugely influential with the conceptual development of our nurse-led healthcare transition service model. As reflective of our comprehensive nursing approach with the provision of healthcare transition services, our publications have reflected our involvement and interest with AEA lived HCT experience such as exploring issues associated with school-related services and accessing community resources (Betz et al. 2019; Betz and Redcay 2005a). Over the past many years, our team has been involved with a HCT network, the International and Interdisciplinary Health Care Transition Research Consortium (HCTRC) (Ferris et al. 2011). Through collaboration with HCTRC, we have shared HCT knowledge and clinical acumen that have enhanced our own programmatic efforts. These collaborations have led to other projects that have resulted in joint publications, projects, and hosting of monthly HCTRC zoom meetings and the Annual HCTRC Research Symposiums (Betz et al. 2014; Fair et al. 2015). Currently, members of the *Community-Based Transition Pilot Program* Partnership Advisory Team are advising our team with pilot HCT planning efforts. Their recommendations and assistance with these program development efforts have been invaluable in moving forward with the development of this nurse-led service model.

Measuring Outcomes Is Needed The effectiveness of services can only be verified with measurement of outcomes. The primary focus of measuring outcomes has been on the transfer of care. That is, researchers have engaged in limited tracking of AEA following their transfer of care to adult providers. Generally, in the current literature, indicators of a successful HCT outcome have been the first appointment with the adult provider and care coordination between pediatric and adult providers (Suris and Akre 2015). A significant challenge with tracking pediatric patients into another system of care is the lack of resources available to continue monitoring. Longitudinal studies require allocation of resources for staffing support to conduct the follow-up. Staffing for a project of this type likely extends beyond the resources available within the program needed for a longitudinal study that include staff with statistical, research, and database development expertise. Another widespread challenge for longitudinal research is that lack of connectivity/linkages among service systems in some countries. In the United States, there are few states that designate an identifier to the user across systems of care. Most often, when a pediatric patient exits pediatric care, the identifier within the insurance plan is discarded and replaced with a new identifier for the new service system, thereby making tracking a challenge.

Some issues have been raised as to what HCT outcomes should be considered for measurement (Coyne et al. 2017). In a recent review of transition outcomes, authors noted that standardization of transition outcomes are needed as currently there is lack of uniformity in the conceptual meaning and measurement of transition outcomes (Coyne et al. 2017). Several Delphi studies were conducted that resulted in a list of indicators that should be considered for outcomes measurement (Fair et al. 2015; Suris and Akre 2015). More recently, discussions have been raised that it is timely to revisit this topic given the advances and developments in HCT research and practice.

Infrastructure Support Key to the development of any nurse-led model is infrastructure support. This form of support is invaluable and contributes greatly to the sustainability of the project. Infrastructure support comes in the form of intramural or extramural support. The types of intramural support our project team has encountered over the years have not always been quantifiable as financial support. Our team has been fortunate to create collaborations and partnerships with other transition and adult-related agencies that served as referral sources and informational resources that enabled our team to be more informed and adept HCT service providers to the AEA and families we served which we have described previously in the section on Partnerships Are Essential.

As well, our collaborations and partnerships created new opportunities for joint programming and projects. For example, in one of our transition projects, our Partnership Advisory Team was instrumental in supporting our efforts to host two Transition Summit meetings, one for professionals and another for families and self-advocates. Our advisory members were key to the success of our Transition Summits as they volunteered as speakers or provided introductions to other speakers with the subject matter expertise. Our team would not have been able to host these Transition Summits if not for their support and involvement with this effort.

We have learned over the years that extramural support is certainly an ideal opportunity to create and pilot a program, but it is not sustainable. Other sources of financial support are needed and essential for programmatic sustainability. In our own experience, seeking extramural programmatic support can be challenging, particularly as the field of healthcare transition expands and grows. Therefore, other avenues of sustainable support need to be explored. Fortunately, for our program, we were able to access one of the financial advisors to assist the team in accessing funding support through a government program to enable sustainable funding. This individual was a pivotal resource in enabling the continuation of services.

More recently, we have discovered through a collaboration with one of our advisory board members that we may be able to create a training program that heretofore would not have been possible without this collaborative effort. As well, we have been advised by colleagues over the years of smaller and larger pockets of funding support for ancillary projects that contribute to the overall mission of our HCT efforts.

HCT Services Need to Be Individualized We discovered in our programs that the life course of AEA does not follow predictable patterns. During a HCT planning encounter, the adolescent may identify a self-management priority such as working on developing competence with a daily condition-related management task such as weight management. That priority may not be as evident with a subsequent encounter as other factors intervened such as undergoing major surgery based on medical necessity resulting in decreased physical activity level. Other developmentally related events such as changing schools, access to after-school activities, and friendships can affect HCT planning. Individualization of care is the bedrock of providing services that are based on an adolescent-centered and family-centered framework of care. That is, services are predicated on the AEA and family's interests, needs, and preferences.

Flexibility not Rigidity Is Needed Being adaptable is essential to any long-term programmatic effort, particularly those that are nurse-led. Having an attitude that is open to recommendations and opportunities that present themselves enables new pathways to programmatic development. A new opportunity for service development may initially seem undesirable; however, upon further reflection and consideration with the team, this new venue can and very often lead to growth of not only the program itself but contributes to the professional development of the team members as well.

Importantly, in the burgeoning field of healthcare transition, innovations are being introduced that impact service development, policymaking and research. For example, in the early days when the concept of healthcare transition was first introduced, the age range suggested for initiating transition service was in late adolescence and more narrowly focused. The early literature and to a certain extent even today, HCT planning tends to be focused on the transfer of care (Chu et al. 2015; Hart et al. 2019). More recently published articles describe models of care that are more comprehensive in approach that include other components of services such as an emphasis on learning self-management and navigation skills, service referrals to transition, and adult services and coordination of care (Betz and Coyne 2020).

Nursing models of HCT have become more evident in the literature and in service settings. Evidence of the influential role of nurses in the field of HCT is to peruse the literature for examples of nursing HCT models and scholarly papers (Betz and Coyne 2020; Grady et al. 2021). In 2020, the National Institute of Nursing Research in conjunction with the National Association of Pediatric Nurse Practitioners sponsored a 2-day meeting at NINR, National Institutes of Health: Research Roundtable: Care Transitions from Pediatric to Adult Care: Planning and Interventions for Adolescents and Young Adults with Chronic Illness (Betz 2021; Grady et al. 2021). Later that same year, Lost in Transition Workshop was hosted by National Institute of Child Health and Human Development and National Institute of Health, signifying the recognition of this important area for research development.

Referral Support Is Needed   Our team has learned that providing referral information is not always a sufficient strategy, particularly for AEA. A foremost consideration is the extent to which AEA have had previous experience in making a "cold call" to a transition-related or adult service agency. We have observed that this can be a very intimidating experience, especially when the AEA has not previously called an agency independently. Our team discovered that several strategies can be used to assist AEA in reaching out to an agency for assistance.

We begin with role playing and coaching the script and actions needed to make the call. This is a necessary precursor step before the AEA actually makes the call. Following that preliminary step, the AEA makes the call, while we are in the room preferably on speaker phone so that we can provide assistance with the conversation/request being made. These strategies have been found to be more effective in supporting AEA to make the call with staff assistance.

There are relevant sources for consideration to be made when providing referrals. Many of the agencies have phone trees that can be challenging to navigate.

Assisting an AEA through the phone tree can be very helpful. In today's world, technology reigns supreme for younger generations as evidenced with characterizations of Generations X, Y, Z and the Alpha Generation. Integrating technology into providing referrals is effective and efficient. During the appointment, accessing the websites of referral agencies enables having a screenshot to be taken. This is a more lasting and convenient method for obtaining and retrieving information when needed.

Dissemination Is Important The field of HCT will only advance with the sharing of ideas, evidence, model development, and research. Our team realized early on the importance of sharing our work in practice, service, scholarship, and policy-making as a means of contributing to the literature that provides understanding and knowledge of the science and practice. Colleagues will only learn of others work through dissemination opportunities whether it be at conferences, involvement in practice, and research networks as has been mentioned previously, engagement in institutionally led efforts for HCT activities, participation in professional associations' HCT policy-making, and through publishing efforts ranging from newsletters to peer-reviewed publications.

Our team published several clinically oriented articles that were generated from our work with our first grant funded by the Maternal Child Health Bureau, United States Department of Health and Human Services. These early papers focused on introducing the concept of healthcare transition to pediatric nurses (Betz 1998a, b). As well, we published papers on our nurse-led HCT program, the role of the transition service coordinator, and our interagency approach to HCT that have been referred to in this chapter. As mentioned previously, our team has published several research studies including a randomized control trial (Betz et al. 2010) and systematic reviews. Through these publishing efforts, we have been able to communicate with colleagues our findings and experiences as well as contribute to the expanding HCT literature.

Conclusion

This chapter has provided the reader with an overview of collective experience with the development and implementation of nurse-led healthcare transition models of care. As has been discussed in this chapter, over the period of many years, nurse-led models originally developed can and do evolve in response to changing situations, emergence of new evidence to shape HCT practice, and scope of nursing practice developments such as authorization of Full Practice Authority for nurse practitioners in states across the United States. Based upon our experience, a selection of "lessons learned" gained with the development and implementation of nurse-led models of care is offered.

References

American Nurses Association. ANA's principles for advanced practice registered nurse (APRN): full practice authority. 2020. Accessed November 12, 2020. https://www.nursingworld.org/~49f695/globalassets/docs/ana/ethics/principles-aprnfullpracticeauthority.pdf.

Betz CL. Adolescent transitions: a nursing concern. Pediatr Nurs. 1998a;24(1):23–8.

Betz CL. Facilitating the transition of adolescents with chronic conditions from pediatric to adult health care and community settings. Issues Compr Pediatr Nurs. 1998b;21(2):97–115.

Betz CL. Nursing's influence on the evolution of the field of health care transition and future implications. J Pediatr Health Care. 2021;35(4):408–13. https://doi.org/10.1016/j.pedhc.2021.01.001. Epub 2021 May 28. PMID: 34053794.

Betz CL, Coyne I. Transition from pediatric to adult healthcare services for young adults with long-term conditions: an international perspective on nurses roles and interventions. Cham: Springer; 2020.

Betz CL, Redcay G. Lessons learned from providing transition services to adolescents with special health care needs. Issues Compr Pediatr Nurs. 2002;25(1):33–61.

Betz CL, Redcay G. Creating healthy futures: an innovative nurse-managed transition clinic for adolescents and young adults with special health care needs. Pediatr Nurs. 2003;29(1):25–30.

Betz CL, Redcay G. An exploratory study of future plans and extracurricular activities of transition age youth and young adults. Issues Compr Pediatr Nurs. 2005a;28:33–51.

Betz CL, Redcay G. Dimensions of the transition service coordinator role. J Spec Pediatr Nurs. 2005b;10(2):49–59.

Betz CL, Redcay G, Tan S. Self-reported health care self care needs of transition-aged youth: a pilot study. Issues Compr Pediatr Nurs. 2003;26(3):158–81.

Betz CL, Smith KN, Macias K. Testing the transition preparation training program: a randomized controlled trial. Int J Child Adolesc Health. 2010;3:595–608.

Betz CL, Ferris ME, Woodward JF, Okumura MJ, Jan S, Wood DL. The health care transition research consortium health care transition model: a framework for research and practice. J Pediatr Rehabil Med. 2014;7(1):3–15. https://doi.org/10.3233/PRM-140277. PMID: 24919934.

Betz CL, Smith KA, Van Speybroeck A, Hernandez FV, Jacobs RA. Movin' on up: an innovative nurse-led interdisciplinary health care transition program. J Pediatr Health Care. 2015;30(4):323–38.

Betz CL, Hudson S, Lee J, Smith KN, Van Speybroeck A. Adolescents and emerging adults with spina bifida knowledge of their individual education program: implications for health care transition planning. J Pediatr Rehabil Med. 2019;12:393–403. https://doi.org/10.3233/PRM-180578.

Betz CL, Hudson S, Skura A, Rajeev N, Smith KN, Van Speybroeck A. Academic and health-related accommodations used by students with spina bifida in school settings. J Pediatric Rehab. 2022a. https://doi.org/10.3233/PRM-210116.

Betz, CL, Mirzaian, CB, Deavenport-Saman A, Hudson SM. Health care transition for adolescents with intellectual and developmental disabilities (IDD) and those with IDD and co-occurring mental health conditions: stakeholder perspectives. J Ment Health Res Intellect Disabil. 2022b. https://doi.org/10.3233/PRM-210116.

Bosse J, Simmonds K, Hanson C, Pulcini J, Dunphy L, Vanhook P, Poghosyan L. Position statement: full practice authority for advanced practice registered nurses is necessary to transform primary care. Nurs Outlook. 2017;65(6):761–5. https://doi.org/10.1016/j.outlook.2017.10.002.

Chu PY, Maslow GR, von Isenburg M, Chung RJ. Systematic review of the impact of transition interventions for adolescents with chronic illness on transfer from pediatric to adult healthcare. J Pediatr Nurs. 2015;30(5):19–27. https://doi.org/10.1016/j.pedn.2015.05.022. Epub 2015 Jul 22. PMID: 26209872; PMCID: PMC4567416.

Coyne B, Hallowell SC, Thompson M. Measurable outcomes after transfer from pediatric to adult providers in youth with chronic illness. J Adolesc Health. 2017;60(1):3–16. https://doi.org/10.1016/j.jadohealth.2016.07.006. Epub 2016 Sep 7. PMID: 27614592.

Fair C, Cuttance J, Sharma N, Maslow G, Wiener L, Betz C, Porter J, McLaughlin S, Gilleland-Marchak J, Renwick A, Naranjo D, Jan S, Javalkar K, Ferris M. International and interdisciplinary identification of health care transition outcomes. JAMA Pediatrics. 2015. https://doi.org/10.1001/jamapediatrics.2016.3168.

Ferris ME, Wood D, Ferris MT, Sim P, Kelly B, Saidi A, Bhagat S, Bickford K, Jurczyk I. Toward evidence-based health care transition: the health care transition research consortium. Int J Child Adolesc Health. 2011;3(6):479–86.

Grady KL, Rehm R, Betz CL. Understanding the phenomenon of health care transition: theoretical underpinnings, exemplars of nursing contributions, and research implications. J Pediatr Health Care. 2021;35(3):310–6. https://doi.org/10.1016/j.pedhc.2020.12.003.

Hart LC, Patel-Nguyen SV, Merkley MG, Jonas DE. An evidence map for interventions addressing transition from pediatric to adult care: a systematic review of systematic reviews. J Pediatr Nurs. 2019;48:18–34. https://doi.org/10.1016/j.pedn.2019.05.015.

National Transition Network. Youth with disabilities and the school-to-work opportunities act of 1994. 1994. Accessed March 14, 2022. https://mn.gov/mnddc/parallels2/pdf/90s/94/94-POU-YWD.pdf.

Stucky CH, Brown WJ, Stucky MG. COVID 19: an unprecedented opportunity for nurse practitioners to reform healthcare and advocate for permanent full practice authority. Nurs Forum. 2020;2020:1–6. https://doi.org/10.1111/nuf.12515.

Suris JC, Akre C. Key elements for, and indicators of, a successful transition: an international Delphi study. J Adolesc Health. 2015;56(6):612–8. https://doi.org/10.1016/j.jadohealth.2015.02.007. PMID: 26003575.

A Paediatric Eczema Shared Care Model

Jemma Weidinger, Richard Loh, Roland Brand,
Sandra Salter, Sandra Vale, Maria Said,
and Stephanie Weston

Introduction

In this chapter, we provide an overview of the eczema shared care model which was piloted in Western Australia (WA) in 2018–2021 and share our lessons learned. The National Allergy Strategy describes a shared care model as a patient-centred approach to care that uses the skills and knowledge of a range of healthcare professionals who share joint responsibility with the patient, ensuring the patient receives the right care, at the right time, from the right health professional(s), in the right place (National Allergy Strategy 2019).

Eczema is also commonly referred to as atopic dermatitis or atopic eczema. For the purpose of this chapter, the term eczema will be used.

With eczema and food allergy increasing in Australia and eczema being the leading cause of the global burden from skin disease (Langan et al. 2020) coupled with long specialist waiting times, there was a pressing need to address timely access to care for children with eczema.

Recent research shows the altered skin barrier in people with eczema has a key role in the development of food allergy (Sugita and Akdis 2020) and suggests sensitisation to allergenic foods may occur through this impaired skin barrier (Lack

J. Weidinger (✉) · R. Loh · R. Brand · S. Weston
Perth Children's Hospital, Nedlands, WA, Australia
e-mail: Jemma.Weidinger@health.wa.gov.au

S. Salter
The University of Western Australia, Perth, WA, Australia

S. Vale
National Allergy Strategy, Guildford, WA, Australia

M. Said
Allergy and Anaphylaxis Australia, Sydney, NSW, Australia

C. L. Betz (ed.), *Worldwide Successful Pediatric Nurse-Led Models of Care*,
https://doi.org/10.1007/978-3-031-22152-1_14

2011). Current research also suggests introduction of common food allergens in the first year of life (including high-risk infants with moderate to severe eczema) may reduce the risk of developing food allergy (Fleischer et al. 2021). Therefore, an urgency exists to effectively manage paediatric eczema to reduce the risk of food allergy development in this population.

Previously, patients referred to dermatology for eczema were seen solely by consultants or dermatology registrars, doctors in a dermatology specialist training program (with consultants supervising) at Perth Children's Hospital (PCH) who had limited time to explain the management of eczema to patients and parents, and, therefore, typically had poorer compliance with treatment. After identifying this as an issue, funding from PCH Foundation was sought and subsequently obtained to develop a new paediatric eczema shared care model (Eczema Model). The intention was to better link the expertise of dermatology and other specialties including allergy and immunology, general practice and pharmacy with others involved in the process of eczema management including patient support organisations. The pharmacy model of care will be described later in the chapter.

Through this, our goal was to optimise eczema management in children and provide more timely access to care. With the allocated funding, a nurse practitioner (NP) position was created, and a NP-led paediatric eczema service was established at PCH to address waiting times and improve access to care. A combined multidisciplinary eczema and allergy clinic for infants and young children with eczema and food allergy or food allergy concerns was also established to optimise eczema management and promote timely introduction of common food allergens where clinically appropriate. This multidisciplinary clinic involves a consultant immunologist, advanced immunology trainee, eczema nurse practitioner, allergy nurse and paediatric accredited practising dietitian. Eczema resource development for community and health professionals was undertaken in collaboration with national partner organisations—the National Allergy Strategy (NAS) and Allergy & Anaphylaxis Australia (A&AA), a national consumer organisation. The NAS shared care model (National Allergy Strategy 2019) for allergic disease was adopted as a framework for the Eczema Model. A collaborative pharmacy eczema model of care (CPEM) was also developed in partnership with the School of Allied Health/Discipline of Pharmacy at The University of Western Australia. Overarching themes and guiding principles identified by pharmacists and consumers informed the CPEM and will be discussed in detail later in this chapter.

Engagement with young people who have eczema and parents/carers of children with eczema was undertaken. Additionally, engagement with a range of health professionals including general practitioners (GPs), community and hospital pharmacists, paediatricians and dietitians was also undertaken. Efforts included enhanced resource development and patient and health professional education to optimise paediatric eczema care state-wide.

Background

Overview of the Need for an Eczema Model/Target Population/Setting

Eczema is a common chronic inflammatory skin disorder characterised by dry skin, recurrent eczematous lesions which flare and settle and intense itch (Langan et al. 2020). Eczema affects people of all ages and ethnicities. The worldwide prevalence of eczema ranges from 0.2% to 24.6% with the highest prevalence of childhood eczema in Africa and Latin America (Sugita and Akdis 2020). Eczema begins in infancy for 60% of children (Sugita and Akdis 2020) and can persist into adulthood. While not life-threatening, eczema can have a significant psychosocial impact on the affected child and their family and can adversely affect growth and development, school performance, mental health, social life and general quality of life (Barbarot et al. 2022, Carvalho et al. 2020; Lewis-Jones 2006). Eczema is the leading cause of the global burden from skin disease (Langan et al. 2020) and is associated with increased risk of other atopic diseases such as food allergy, asthma, allergic rhinitis, as well as mental health disorders (Langan et al. 2020; Martin et al. 2013). The pathophysiology is complex and involves genetic and environmental factors, epidermal dysfunction and T-cell-driven inflammation (Langan et al. 2020).

Age, race and ethnicity add to the complex immune response in patients with eczema (Leung 2015). Evidence suggests darker skin pigment can be challenging to assess and eczema severity is often under-recognised, leading to more severe and persistent symptoms, more sleep disturbance and poorer overall health (Leung 2015; Torjesen 2019). Previous studies have shown racial and ethnic differences in the epidemiology of atopic eczema, with non-white children having higher incidence and prevalence compared with white children (Poladian et al. 2019; Kim et al. 2019). A significant proportion of people with eczema are vulnerable children from culturally and linguistically diverse families (Wan et al. 2019; Kaufman et al. 2018; Fischer et al. 2017). We have found a disproportionate number of these children in our eczema and allergy clinics. A recent retrospective audit found more than a third of children with refractory eczema who presented to the PCH dermatology outpatient clinic on multiple occasions for their eczema were of Asian ethnicity and two thirds had a history of skin infection.

Food allergy occurs in around 10% of infants, 4–8% of children and about 2–4% of adults in Australia (Sugita and Akdis 2020). Recent research suggests the altered skin barrier in people with eczema has a key role in the development of food allergy (Sugita and Akdis 2020). Evidence suggests that sensitisation to allergenic foods may occur through topical application of food protein (in food-containing skin products) as a result of the impaired skin barrier, while regular consumption of these foods at an early age may actually result in tolerance (Sweeny et al. 2021). This has been termed the dual-allergen-exposure hypothesis (Sweeney et al. 2021; Lack 2011). Therefore, an urgency to effectively manage eczema to prevent food allergy development also exists. Early evidence-based treatment is essential in treating the skin disease of eczema and potentially additional atopic diseases (Sugita and Akdis 2020; Langan et al. 2020). When developing a shared care model for paediatric eczema (including a NP-led paediatric eczema service), the above key factors were all taken into consideration.

Impetus for Development of the Eczema Model

The population prevalence of eczema in Australia is estimated to be 20.3% in infants (Martin et al. 2013). Each year in WA, 6000 infants will develop eczema resulting in a large number of dermatology referrals and ever-increasing waitlists. In WA, there is only one paediatric tertiary hospital for a population of approximately 600,000 (Australian Bureau of Statistics 2022). Given the increasing and urgent need for more paediatric eczema services, our three paediatric general dermatology clinics a week at PCH, staffed by a dermatologist, dermatology registrars and a clinical nurse specialist, is insufficient for the population, and novel systems are needed to optimise patient care and outcomes.

A model of care is broadly defined as the way health care and services are delivered for a person or population group as they progress through stages of a condition, injury or event (New South Wales Agency for Clinical Innovation 2013). The overall objective of a model of care is to ensure people get the right care, at the right time, by the right team and in the right place (New South Wales Agency for Clinical Innovation 2013; Networks WH 2014).

An Eczema Model was proposed by the Department of Dermatology, Immunology and Allergy at PCH and involved a multidisciplinary team (listed later in this chapter). This model was developed to achieve timely access to evidence-based, best-practice advice and management, together with effectively coordinated health care and support, as close as possible to where the person and their family live. That is, "the right care, at the right time, from the right health professional(s), in the right place" (National Allergy Strategy 2019, p. 1).

The Process Undertaken to Develop and Implement the Eczema Model

Developing and implementing the Eczema Model involved a number of steps: laying the groundwork for the Eczema Model including staffing, sourcing funding, establishing a collaboration to support Eczema Model planning and training, and resource development.

Laying the Groundwork for the Eczema Model

Initially, funding was sought from the PCH Foundation for the Eczema Model to reduce the 3-year dermatology wait list at PCH. This Eczema Model proposal included funding for an eczema nurse practitioner, additional sessions for paediatric dermatologists and development of education resources for health professionals and patients. Only part of the proposal was funded as the PCH Foundation believed funding for health professional positions was not in their remise. However, they were keen to progress with a model of care to improve knowledge of health professionals and initially agreed to fund a NP to develop eczema resources including for GPs and other health professionals involved in eczema care. With further negotiation, that funding was allocated to an eczema NP position of 1.0 full-time equivalent (FTE), comprising 50% allocated to providing a clinical service to reduce hospital waiting times for children with eczema and 50% for eczema resource development. In-kind support from medical, nursing and dietetic staff from the Department of Dermatology, Immunology and Allergy at PCH was also obtained.

Acknowledging the integral role of GPs in eczema management in primary care, the decision was made to split the funding to 0.8 FTE for NP duties and 0.2 FTE for a GP dedicated to resource development for GPs. That transpired but the GP employed was unable to continue and consequently an alternative arrangement was made with pharmacists—the Collaborative Pharmacy Eczema Model of Care (CPEM).

All project key performance indicators in relation to wait time reduction, improved referral processes, education and resource development were achieved. However, as funding was limited and specifically aimed at resource development, the project was restricted in what it could achieve for a multidisciplinary paediatric eczema service, particularly for potential broader service offerings such as tele-dermatology and a complex dermatology clinic.

Collaboration Efforts Involved with Eczema Model Planning

The allocated funding for a NP position of 0.8FTE over a 3-year period provided the human resource to establish a new Eczema Model including a NP-led paediatric eczema service. The Eczema Model sought to reduce waiting times and improve access to care and eczema support, deliver a combined multidisciplinary eczema/allergy clinic for infants and young children and undertake eczema resource development.

In addition, collaboration, consultation and engagement with key partners in the Eczema Model were undertaken. This involved children with eczema and their parents/caregivers including those from culturally and linguistically diverse backgrounds, stakeholders from the PCH Department of Dermatology, Immunology and Allergy, nurses, dieticians, GPs, paediatricians, pharmacists, the NAS and A&AA.

The NAS, a unique partnership between the Australasian Society of Clinical Immunology and Allergy (ASCIA) and A&AA, was developed in 2015 in consultation with 57 stakeholder groups and organisations, representing consumers, health professionals, government and industry. The NAS identifies gaps with existing allergy care in Australia and provides a coordinated plan to guide future actions that will improve the health and quality of life for Australians with allergic disease and minimise the burden on individuals, their caregivers, healthcare services and the community (National Allergy Strategy 2015). In 2018, the NAS undertook a national shared care model for allergy scoping project; hence, the NAS was a key stakeholder to engage in developing the Eczema Model.

Feedback from children with eczema and their parents/caregivers was sought in a number of ways including focus groups and patient/parent satisfaction surveys, which helped inform the Eczema Model. The consultation process also provided insight into required educational resources and underpinned resource development for children with eczema, parents, carers and health professionals.

Collaboration, Training and Resource Development

Collaboration, training and resource efforts are described in this section. These efforts as presented below include eczema resources for health professionals and consumers, community webinars and seminars, an eczema school kit, a primary care decision-making algorithm and a GP management plan.

Eczema Resources for Health Professionals and Consumers

In collaboration with the NAS and ASCIA, a paediatric eczema e-training course for health professionals was developed. This resource was reviewed by experts in dermatology, allergy and immunology and is hosted on the publicly accessible ASCIA e-training platform. Other eczema resources developed for the Eczema Model included videos and infographics for all stakeholders—infants, children and young people with eczema, parents/caregivers and health professionals. These resources were created by a NAS Working Group comprising individuals with high-level eczema expertise. Although the project was WA focused, it was considered important to create nationally consistent education and information for health professionals and consumers, which engagement with the NAS was able to provide.

Community Webinars and Seminars

Knowledge of eczema management and patient care in the community has also been enhanced through webinars and seminars with maternal and child health, school health and primary care nurses, GPs, paediatricians, pharmacists and dietitians in metropolitan, outer metropolitan and rural and regional areas across WA. Eczema webinars in collaboration with A&AA were also developed for consumers.

Eczema School Kit

In relation to further resource development as part of the Eczema Model, A&AA received funding from the PCH Foundation to share the Eczema Support Australia's Eczema School Kit with schools and parents of children with eczema in WA. Schools and parents have free access to the Eczema Support Australia's Eczema School Kit. The School Kit comprises a booklet for the parent, a booklet for school staff and useful templates. Schools and parents in WA can receive a hard copy or be sent a link to the School Kit to help improve the health and well-being of children with eczema while at school.

Primary Care Decision-Making Algorithm and GP Management Plan

As previously mentioned, a GP was recruited to work on our Eczema Model to provide guidance in relation to development of eczema resources and enhanced education in primary care. Improved education and resources were developed and made available to support GPs in making clinical and referral decisions, including a decision-making algorithm and GP management plan (see Appendices 1 and 2). The PCH GP Liaison was instrumental in working with us and with WA Primary Health Alliance to promote these resources. The Eczema Model was piloted in WA, and we worked in collaboration with the NAS and A&AA to prepare national roll out of this model.

Finally, part of our funding was also allocated to develop a Collaborative Pharmacy Eczema Model of Care (CPEM), described in detail below. It was recognised pharmacists are easily accessible members of the healthcare team and are able to support patients and their families through disease, treatment education and non-pharmacological measures (Wong et al. 2017). However, there are few systems in place to guide pharmacists in caring for eczema patients.

Theoretical Framework

Multidisciplinary approaches to eczema management have previously been developed in appreciation of the complex range of factors that affect disease control (LeBovidge et al. 2016). The NAS, including ASCIA, A&AA and other key stakeholder organisations, developed a proposed shared care model for allergic conditions in 2018 (Fig. 1). This model is a patient-centred approach to care which involves a range of health professionals including GPs, specialists and pharmacists across different levels of health services and is proposed to improve access to care.

When establishing the Eczema Model, the NAS model for allergic conditions was adopted (National Allergy Strategy 2019) with the aim of ensuring the patient receives the right care, at the right time, from the right health professional(s), in the right place. This framework was based on the *Framework on Integrated People-Centred Health Services* from the World Health Organization (WHO), which stipulates equity in access for everyone, everywhere to access the quality health services they need, when and where they need them (World Health Organization 2016).

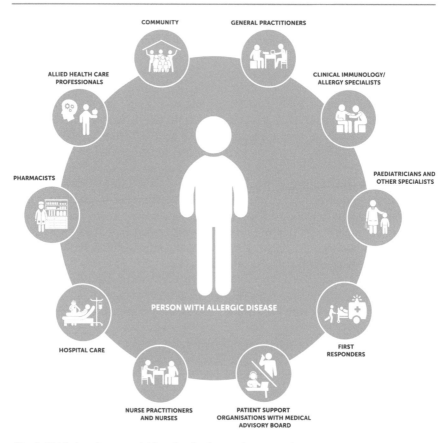

Fig. 1 NAS shared care model for allergic disease. Source: National Allergy Strategy (2022)

Components of the Shared Care Model for Allergic Diseases

Shared care models in Australia usually involve primary health care as it is the first point of contact people have with the health system (National Allergy Strategy 2019, p. 4). Primary health care plays an important role in the prevention, management and appropriate referral of patients with allergic conditions (National Allergy Strategy 2019, p. 4). However, the very principle of a shared care model is that all healthcare providers work together to provide optimal, coordinated care. In addition, our shared care model sought novel ways to improve patient access to optimal care. The CPEM and nurse-led eczema model are examples of this, and we will be referring to the CPEM and nurse-led eczema model in more detail. These discipline-specific components of care demonstrate the necessity of interdisciplinary approaches to care. There are also other shared management components such as the role of allied healthcare professionals and first responders such as community pharmacists in addressing the needs of children with eczema.

Collaborative Pharmacy Eczema Model of Care

As part of the Eczema Model, a CPEM for children with eczema in WA is being developed, overseen by a multidisciplinary expert advisory group (see Appendix 3).

Guidance resources for the CPEM were identified from the New South Wales (NSW) Agency for Clinical Innovation (ACI) and the WA Health Networks. Both resources were used to define a model of care and understand the development process for the CPEM (New South Wales Agency for Clinical Innovation 2013; Networks WH 2014).

The CPEM expert advisory group considered a comprehensive set of pharmacy and health guidance documents and resources. These included the Professional Practice Standards for Pharmacists (version 5, Pharmaceutical Society of Australia) (Pharmaceutical Society of Australia 2017). These standards give pharmacists direction for providing therapeutic goods (such as prescription items and over the counter moisture management products) and providing health information to patients with eczema and their families. In particular, the following standards were considered:

- Pharmacy practice principles, including education, counselling and referral, to achieve quality use of medicines and promote patient-centred health and well-being
- The role of the pharmacist as a key contributor to patient-centred care, collaborating as a member of the healthcare team
- Practices for medication supply that reflect prescriber intentions, therapeutic need, and are consistent with quality use of medicines and the patient's health goals and values
- Provision of healthcare information that is tailored to the individual patient
- Overarching principles underpinning disease state management services to assist patients in managing their own chronic disease

The CPEM Expert Advisory Group has also been guided by national plans, strategies and policies, including Australia's Long Term National Health Plan 2019, Australia's Primary Health Care 10 Year Plan 2022–2032, the National Medicines Policy 2000, and the report, Pharmacists in 2023 (Pharmaceutical Society of Australia, 2019): For patients, for our profession, for Australia's health system.

The CPEM project objectives include the following:

1. Conduct a literature review and environmental scan to identify and examine resources and guiding documents, such as existing models of care, educational materials and other pharmacy-specific documents relevant to paediatric eczema.
2. Conduct consumer consultation to understand the consumer experience with paediatric eczema care, particularly in terms of pharmacy interactions, and obtain perspective on a collaborative pharmacy eczema model of care.
3. Conduct pharmacist consultation to understand pharmacist perspectives of their role in paediatric eczema management and on a CPEM.

4. Triangulate results of objectives 1–3 to identify elements for a proposed CPEM.
5. Use Delphi methodology to achieve consensus and prioritise proposed CPEM elements and to identify components of each element.
6. Integrate elements to develop the proposed CPEM.
7. Develop an implementation plan for the proposed CPEM.

Data from objectives 1–3 were triangulated to identify CPEM *elements* and CPEM element *enablers*. CPEM *elements* refer to the components identified through objectives 1–3 as necessary for the proposed CPEM. The way in which the CPEM elements will be actioned in the proposed CPEM is referred to as CPEM *enablers* (Schneider et al. 2021). Gaining input and consensus from stakeholders on both the CPEM elements and enablers will form the basis of the Delphi study. The resulting agreed CPEM elements and their associated enablers will form the basis for the design of the proposed CPEM, the final output of this project.

The proposed CPEM will define the role of WA pharmacists as part of the patient's eczema management team, and the tools and resources they require to provide the right care, at the right time for children with eczema in the community. The model will also provide guidance on management steps and referral pathways. The patient group of interest for the CPEM project is WA children from birth to 6 years of age. As community pharmacists see eczema patients across all stages of disease, eczema severity considered in this project may range from mild to severe and include patients who have not yet been diagnosed but are suspected to have eczema, as well as those with inactive disease. This project aims to develop a proposed CPEM for the pharmacist component of the NAS shared care model for allergic conditions (Fig. 1).

The adapted NSW ACI project process chart as applied to the first three stages of CPEM development is shown in Fig. 2 (New South Wales Agency for Clinical Innovation 2013).

Guiding principles of the model of care included (New South Wales Agency for Clinical Innovation 2013):

- Patient centric
- Localised flexibility and consider equity of access
- Supports integrated care
- Supports efficient utilisation of resources
- Supports safe, quality care for patients
- Has a robust and standardised set of outcome measures and evaluation process
- Is innovative and considers new ways of organising and delivering care
- Sets the vision for services in the future

In the CPEM project, consumers with lived experience of caring for a child with eczema aged 0–6 years were invited to share their perspectives on paediatric eczema care, particularly in terms of pharmacy interactions, and on how they envisaged a CPEM to operate. Data were collected using a community conversation format. A community conversation is an event that adapts the internationally recognised World

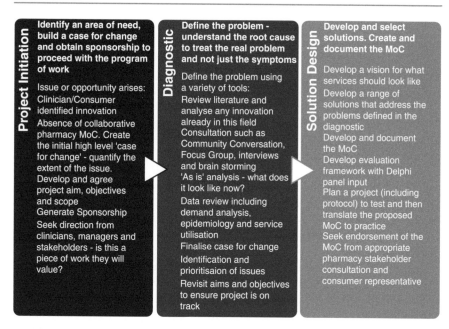

Project Initiation

Identify an area of need, build a case for change and obtain sponsorship to proceed with the program of work

Issue or opportunity arises: Clinician/Consumer identified innovation
Absence of collaborative pharmacy MoC. Create the initial high level 'case for change' - quantify the extent of the issue.
Develop and agree project aim, objectives and scope
Generate Sponsorship
Seek direction from clinicians, managers and stakeholders - is this a piece of work they will value?

Diagnostic

Define the problem - understand the root cause to treat the real problem and not just the symptoms

Define the problem using a variety of tools:
Review literature and analyse any innovation already in this field
Consultation such as Community Conversation, Focus Group, interviews and brain storming
'As is' analysis - what does it look like now?
Data review including demand analysis, epidemiology and service utilisation
Finalise case for change
Identification and prioritisaion of issues
Revisit aims and objectives to ensure project is on track

Solution Design

Develop and select solutions. Create and document the MoC

Develop a vision for what services should look like
Develop a range of solutions that address the problems defined in the diagnostic
Develop and document the MoC
Develop evaluation framework with Delphi panel input
Plan a project (including protocol) to test and then translate the proposed MoC to practice
Seek endorsement of the MoC from appropriate pharmacy stakeholder consultation and consumer representative

Fig. 2 The National Allergy Strategy describes a shared care model as a patient-centred approach to care that uses the skills and knowledge of a range of healthcare professionals who share joint responsibility with the patient, ensuring the patient receives the right care, at the right time, from the right health professionals(s), in the right place

Café method, designed for open conversations with a group of people around a specific topic (Consumer and Community Involvement Program 2020). In our work, the World Café method allowed parents of children with eczema to explore broad ideas in an informal, friendly setting. Parents were grouped based on the age of their child and across three rounds discussed who they see for help with their child's eczema, how they manage their child's eczema and how pharmacists could help with their child's eczema.

Separately, four focus groups were conducted with pharmacists in rural and metropolitan areas within WA to gain insight into their perspectives and experience in paediatric eczema management, and how they saw a CPEM operating, particularly from a practical viewpoint. Results from the consumer and pharmacist consultation and the environmental and literature scan were then triangulated to identify elements for the proposed CPEM and themed to provide an overarching purpose for the model.

Three overarching themes were identified that the proposed CPEM needs to address:

- Access to timely care, resources and support
- Consistency of care across all healthcare professionals in collaborative eczema care team (via evidence-based education, model of care)

- Collaboration between healthcare professionals, the eczema patient/parent/carer and all other members of the eczema patient's care team in order to provide personalised care

Ongoing development of the proposed CPEM is underway with expert review of the CPEM elements and enablers set to inform the final document. Once complete, the CPEM will be piloted in pharmacies in WA in an integrated approach linking patients with eczema, nursing, hospital, clinic, immunology, allergy and consumer organisations with pharmacy.

Description of the Nurse-Led Model

Organisational Components

As part of this Eczema Model, a NP-led paediatric eczema service was established within the dermatology department at PCH. Perth Children's Hospital is the specialist paediatric hospital and trauma centre in WA, providing medical care to children and adolescents 15 years of age or under. The hospital provides treatment for emergency presentations as well as for patients requiring inpatient, outpatient and daystay care. The hospital is located in Nedlands, Perth, WA, and has 298 beds. The hospital forms part of the Child and Adolescent Health Service which includes neonatology, community health and the child and adolescent mental health services.

Components of the Service Model

When developing the Eczema Model, we recognised the importance of involving a multidisciplinary expert advisory group (see Appendix 3). This group comprised of clinical immunology/allergy specialists, dermatologists, general practitioners, eczema nurse practitioner, pharmacist, National Allergy Strategy Manager, Allergy & Anaphylaxis Australia CEO (consumer representative) and the project lead for the CPEM project.

The eczema NP supports the dermatology team by independently managing lower risk and lower complexity referrals to optimise topical therapy thereby reducing the need for systemic therapy, allowing specialist dermatology registrars and consultants to manage complex cases. The NP works autonomously and in collaboration with other members from the multidisciplinary team including dermatologists, immunologists, nurses, dieticians, pharmacists, GPs and psychologists.

The majority of eczema referrals at PCH are triaged to the eczema NP who sees and treats infants, children and adolescents 15 years of age or under with varying degrees of eczema severity. In the NP-led paediatric eczema outpatient clinic at PCH, the patient attends in person, via telehealth or telephone depending on the nature of the eczema concern, whether it is a new referral or follow-up and where the patient lives. When required, the NP orders pathology and diagnostic tests, prescription of necessary medications, initiates referrals to relevant healthcare providers and discharges suitable patients.

The combined dermatology allergy clinic, a rapid eczema allergy support service, is a newly established multidisciplinary hospital outpatient-based clinic at PCH, developed as part of this new eczema shared care model for young children with eczema and food allergy or food allergy concerns. The clinic is staffed by a clinical immunologist, immunology advanced trainee, eczema NP and allergy nurse to perform skin prick testing where clinically appropriate. The purpose of this clinic is to optimise eczema management early for those children with moderate-to-severe eczema and promote introduction of common allergenic foods in the first year of life to help reduce the risk of developing a food allergy.

This combined dermatology allergy clinic is also a teaching clinic for paediatric trainees which fosters an understanding of the link between dermatological and allergic conditions, the roles of the eczema NP and allergy nurse and how a multidisciplinary team can provide a greater service together in one clinic. The provision of multidisciplinary care facilitates coordination of care during a single visit rather than having a patient seeing these healthcare providers on different days at potentially different locations resulting in multiple hospital clinic visits for the patient and their family.

Position Requirements of Those Involved with the NP-Led Model

The NP is registered with the Australian Health Practitioner Regulation Agency (AHPRA) and endorsed by the Nursing and Midwifery Board of Australia. AHPRA is the national organisation responsible for implementing the National Registration and Accreditation Scheme across Australia. The NP must also be credentialed and have a documented defined scope of practice in accordance with the Child and Adolescent Health Service Nurse Practitioner Credentialing and Scope of Practice Policy (CAHS 2022).

Methods of Evaluation

Data from the NP-led eczema clinics were collected in relation to patient/parent satisfaction as well as patient-reported outcome measures. Several tools were used to measure outcomes associated with care provided, which included atopic eczema symptoms and severity as well as quality of life. We demonstrated improved clinical outcomes using the patient-oriented eczema measure (POEM) scoring system. We also evaluated quality-of-life outcomes using Infants' Dermatitis Quality of Life Index (IDQOL) and Children's Dermatology Life Quality Index (CDLQI). Eczema severity scores including Scoring Atopic Dermatitis Index (SCORAD), a scoring index combining extent, severity and subjective symptoms and Eczema Area and Severity Index (EASI) were also used to measure clinical outcome.

Evaluation tools used to measure clinical outcomes	
Evaluation tools	Clinical outcomes measured
Patient oriented eczema measure (POEM)	Monitoring atopic eczema severity Focus on the illness experienced
Infants' dermatitis quality of life index (IDQOL)	Administer to infants/toddlers ages 0–3 years, 11 months Examines the extent to which dermatitis affects the child's life
Children's dermatology life quality index (CDLQI)	Administer to children ages 4–16 years; although given the cartoon figures up to 11/12 years of age may be most developmentally appropriate Examines extent to which skin problem affects the child's life
Scoring atopic dermatitis index (SCORAD)	Used to determine the body area and severity of eczema Uses rule of 9 to calculate body area affected Intensity is measured using Likert scale from 0 (none) to 3 (severe) to measure the intensity of the following signs: redness, swelling, oozing/crusting, scratch marks, skin thickening and dryness
Eczema area and severity index (EASI)	Used to measure the body area and severity of atopic eczema Area of body affected is scored ranging from 0 to 100% Signs scored on Likert scale 0 (none) to 3 (severe) based on following signs: redness, skin thickness, scratching and lichenification

We demonstrated significant reduction in waiting times from over 3 years to within 3 months improving hospital key performance indicators for children with eczema. Cost-effectiveness was also demonstrated which will be discussed in the following section. Feedback from patients and parents/carers through survey and community conversation was obtained. Staff feedback was also considered.

Challenges and Facilitators

Challenges

Like any new model or concepts, development of this model required time to discuss with nursing, medical and allied health colleagues with regard to the merits of the model to gain support with implementation.

Not having a dedicated project officer or sufficient clerical support allocated to development of the shared care model was challenging at times, however utilising that funding for GP and pharmacist involvement was invaluable. Due to personal circumstances, our GP left the project early on and was not replaced. Although GP resources were developed, it would have been beneficial to have GP support when implementing these new resources into general practice. We utilised the Hospital Liaison GP who was most helpful in liaising with WA Primary Health Alliance to promote the revised and newly developed resources in primary care. The combined multidisciplinary dermatology allergy clinic relied on the goodwill of the dietitian, nursing and medical staff from the immunology department, and clinician leave was not consistently covered.

Facilitators

Early engagement and support from Medical Co-Leads and Head of Department for Dermatology and Immunology was instrumental in the success of this model of care. Mentorship from colleagues throughout Australia was also a significant facilitating factor.

Address Financing/Reimbursement

To ensure sustainability of service provision and to maintain resource development once the pilot phase of the model was complete, we worked with our hospital business manager and demonstrated cost-effectiveness of the NP-led service. In relation to activity-based funding, we were able to demonstrate a financially viable service.

Service Adjustments Made

To better support our GPs in primary care, we developed an eczema algorithm and an eczema pre-referral guideline. The aim was to encourage more evidence-based management to effectively treat eczema thereby improving patient outcomes and improving quality of eczema referrals. This has also reduced some of the topical corticosteroid fears among parents and clinicians and has streamlined patient referrals for those GPs who have adopted it. Information provided in the algorithm was also emphasised in the GP webinars we delivered.

Since establishing the Eczema Model, parents of children with eczema have received more education through the NP-led clinic as well as the existing dermatology clinical nurse specialist clinic which has improved compliance with treatment and complemented the overall service provided. Previously, patients with eczema were seen solely by Dermatology Registrars (with Consultants supervising) who had limited time to explain the treatment and therefore typically had poorer compliance with treatment.

Lessons Learned

Nursing and medical mentors as well as support from nursing, medical and allied health colleagues were greatly beneficial. Early engagement with national partner organisations was also very helpful to ensure we had a shared vision for the Eczema Model.

Some of the eczema myths which parents have believed in the past have prevented adequate treatment of their child's eczema. This was also compounded by the lack of knowledge and confidence in prescribing appropriate quantity and correct type of topical corticosteroids in primary care. Reported parent comments from some clinicians regarding topical corticosteroid dangers also resulted in 'corticophobia' (fear of topical corticosteroid use) and suboptimal eczema management seen in our patient cohort. A general lack of knowledge regarding type of moisturiser use and general skin care measures was also evident in the community. A shared care approach was helpful in addressing these issues across the various disciplines.

Confusion exists in the general community among parents and some healthcare providers regarding the association of eczema with food allergy. In the past, many parents believed that eczema was caused by food allergies, which resulted in them seeking a cure by elimination diets. These myths have been clarified and explained during education sessions for parents and also during GP webinars and nursing education sessions. Having an aspect of the shared care model particularly focusing on eczema and food allergy/food allergy concerns enabled rapid access to eczema support and allergy specialist review to address parental concerns and promote the timely introduction and regular consumption of common allergenic foods where appropriate.

Overall, the most important lesson learned is that we need to spend more time with patients and parents to explain eczema and its management and to dispel any myths, which in turn improves treatment compliance and more optimal patient outcomes. Consumers and pharmacists overwhelmingly cited adequate time for discussion, education and explanation of eczema and its management as having a positive impact on eczema outcomes for patients. On the other hand, time constraints contributed to frustration, isolation and delay in obtaining appropriate treatment. Balancing time and resources are critical components of the model, and the shared (or collaborative) approach seeks to enable time across the health professions by better sharing the load within a framework that maintains the right treatment messages for the patient at the right time in the right place.

Future Implications for Clinical Practice and Research

Our dermatology team is pursuing options for expansion to community outreach services to provide more timely access to care closer to home. Further exploration and development of appropriate resources for children with eczema from culturally and linguistically diverse families are currently being undertaken. The need for psychologist support for children with refractory eczema requiring multiple outpatient clinic visits for their allergic disease is also being addressed. As a paediatric dermatology tertiary service, we are also keen to be more involved in eczema research and new eczema treatments for children with eczema.

Conclusion

We used a robust, multi-phase process informed by evidence, theoretical frameworks, existing guidance documents and professional and consumer engagement to create an eczema model of care (Eczema Model) and a CPEM.

Our Eczema Model was piloted in WA in 2018–2021 and has highlighted the many benefits of having consumers and a multidisciplinary group of experts working together towards a common goal: that of improved paediatric eczema management and better service provision. Importantly, consumer involvement from the beginning has been integral to the process of developing our shared care model, paediatric eczema service and educational resources.

Our CPEM will be completed in 2022 and is planned to be implemented in the community via a pilot in 2023. We recognise that the ACI implementation phase of development requires the support of the health system to execute the changes needed. Endorsement and sponsorship of the CPEM business case, building the capability of the workers involved and developing a communication plan are some of the steps that may be required during this phase. Ongoing monitoring and evaluation of standardised outcome measures, with adjustments to practices where necessary, are included in the sustainability phase to optimise the model of care and its impact.

From a health system perspective, there are no specific federal initiatives in place for paediatric eczema as it is not currently a national health priority area. This may impact implementation of our Eczema Model that would span across all health services. However, Australia's Primary Health Care 10 Year Plan shares a vision for enhanced access to primary healthcare services for all Australians to support health and well-being in the community. The value of our Eczema Model in providing prioritised care with limited resources is evident from early feedback from users of the system. For the CPEM, future Community Pharmacy Agreements promise funding for more professional services, and the National Digital Health Strategy will enable better communication and information exchange between healthcare providers, facilitating a truly patient-centred, collaborative approach.

Useful Resources

- Nip Allergies in the Bub website (preventallergies.org.au)
- 250K for teens and young adults (250K - A hub for young people living with severe allergies)
- ASCIA (Australasian Society of Clinical Immunology and Allergy (ASCIA)

- Allergy & Anaphylaxis Australia (Allergy & Anaphylaxis Australia (allergy-facts.org.au)
- Eczema Support Australia Eczema School Kit—https://www.eczemasupport.org.au/school-kit/
- Patient Oriented Eczema Measure (POEM)—https://www.nottingham.ac.uk/research/groups/cebd/resources/poem.aspx
- Infants' Dermatitis Quality of Life Index (IDQOL) https://www.cardiff.ac.uk/medicine/resources/quality-of-life-questionnaires/infants-dermatitis-quality-of-life-index
- Children's Dermatology Life Quality Index (CDLQI) https://www.cardiff.ac.uk/medicine/resources/quality-of-life-questionnaires/childrens-dermatology-life-quality-index

Appendix 1: Eczema Decision-Making Algorithm

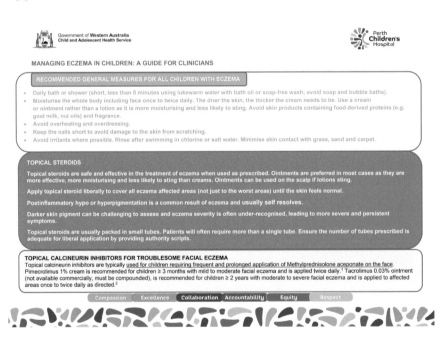

Government of **Western Australia**
Child and Adolescent Health Service

Perth
Children's
Hospital

MANAGING ECZEMA IN CHILDREN: A GUIDE FOR CLINICIANS

RECOMMENDED GENERAL MEASURES FOR ALL CHILDREN WITH ECZEMA

- Daily bath or shower (short, less than 5 minutes using lukewarm water with bath oil or soap-free wash; avoid soap and bubble baths).
- Moisturise the whole body including face once to twice daily. The drier the skin, the thicker the cream needs to be. Use a cream or ointment rather than a lotion as it is more moisturising and less likely to sting. Avoid skin products containing food derived proteins (e.g. goat milk, nut oils) and fragrance.
- Avoid overheating and overdressing.
- Keep the nails short to avoid damage to the skin from scratching.
- Avoid irritants where possible. Rinse after swimming in chlorine or salt water. Minimise skin contact with grass, sand and carpet.

TOPICAL STEROIDS

Topical steroids are safe and effective in the treatment of eczema when used as prescribed. Ointments are preferred in most cases as they are more effective, more moisturising and less likely to sting than creams. Ointments can be used on the scalp if lotions sting.

Apply topical steroid liberally to cover all eczema affected areas (not just to the worst areas) until the skin feels normal.

Postinflammatory hypo or hyperpigmentation is a common result of eczema and usually self resolves.

Darker skin pigment can be challenging to assess and eczema severity is often under-recognised, leading to more severe and persistent symptoms.

Topical steroids are usually packed in small tubes. Patients will often require more than a single tube. Ensure the number of tubes prescribed is adequate for liberal application by providing authority scripts.

TOPICAL CALCINEURIN INHIBITORS FOR TROUBLESOME FACIAL ECZEMA
Topical calcineurin inhibitors are typically used for children requiring frequent and prolonged application of Methylprednisolone aceponate on the face. Pimecrolimus 1% cream is recommended for children ≥ 3 months with mild to moderate facial eczema and is applied twice daily.[1] Tacrolimus 0.03% ointment (not available commercially, must be compounded), is recommended for children ≥ 2 years with moderate to severe facial eczema and is applied to affected areas once to twice daily as directed.[2]

Compassion | Excellence | Collaboration | Accountability | Equity | Respect

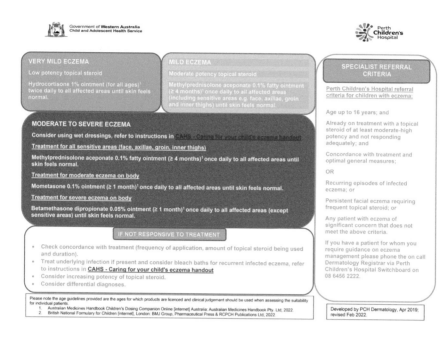

Developed by PCH Dermatology, Apr 2019; revised Feb 2022.

Appendix 2: GP Management Plan

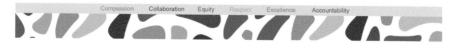

		2. Ensure adequate amounts of topical steroid are prescribed. 3. Wet dressings are helpful if the child is waking at night with itch and for stubborn eczema areas. See attached Caring for your child's eczema health facts.	
	Control and minimise infections	1. Good hand hygiene (wash hands) before and after applying skin care products. 2. Don't 'double dip' into tubs or containers storing skin care products. 3. Consider bleach baths if there is infected eczema or recurring skin infections (discuss with GP). 4. Antibiotics when required (uncommon).	Parents/Guardian GP
		Provide PCH Eczema Treatment Plan (see attached).	

I, _____ agree to the preparation of the above treatment plan for _____

Signed: _____

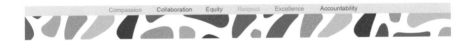

Compassion   Collaboration   Equity   Respect   Excellence   Accountability

Appendix 3: Advisory Group Members

Collaborative Pharmacy Eczema Model of Care Expert Advisory Group (Alphabetical by Surname)

- Dr Melinda Boss, Senior Research Fellow, Pharmacy, The University of Western Australia
- Dr Roland Brand, Dermatologist, Perth Children's Hospital
- Dr Kenneth Lee, Senior Lecturer, Pharmacy, The University of Western Australia
- A/Prof Richard Loh, Paediatric Clinical Immunology/Allergy Specialist, Perth Children's Hospital
- Dr Michael O'Sullivan, Consultant Clinical Immunologist, Perth Children's Hospital
- Dr Natalia Popowicz, Senior Lecturer, Pharmacy, The University of Western Australia
- Maria Said, Chief Executive Officer, Allergy and Anaphylaxis Australia
- Dr Sandra Salter, Project Lead, Senior Lecturer, Pharmacy, The University of Western Australia
- Jessica Schneider, Research Officer, Pharmacy, The University of Western Australia
- Dr Liza Seubert, Head, Discipline of Pharmacy and Deputy Dean—School of Allied Health, The University of Western Australia
- Sandra Vale, Manager, National Allergy Strategy

- Jemma Weidinger, Eczema Nurse Practitioner, Perth Children's Hospital

Multidisciplinary Expert Advisory Group (Alphabetical by Surname)

- Dr Roland Brand, Consultant Dermatologist and previous Head of Department, Perth Children's Hospital during which time the eczema shared care model was established and piloted
- Dr Maree Creighton, Perth Children's Hospital, Liaison General Practitioner
- A/Prof Richard Loh, Clinical Immunology/Allergy specialist, Perth Children's Hospital
- Dr Cory Lei, General Practitioner
- Dr Michael O'Sullivan, Consultant Clinical Immunologist, Perth Children's Hospital
- Maria Said, Chief Executive Officer, Allergy & Anaphylaxis Australia
- Dr Sandra Salter, Senior Lecturer, Pharmacy, The University of Western Australia and Project Lead, Collaborative Pharmacy Eczema Model of Care
- Sandra Vale, Manager, National Allergy Strategy
- Jemma Weidinger, Eczema Nurse Practitioner, Perth Children's Hospital
- Dr Stephanie Weston, Consultant Dermatologist and current Head of Dermatology Department, Perth Children's Hospital

References

Australian Bureau of Statistics. Births, by year and month of occurrence, by state. 2022. https://explore.data.abs.gov.au/vis?tm=births&pg=0&df[ds]=ABS_ABS_TOPICS&df[id]=BIRTHS_MONTH_OCCURRENCE&df[ag]=ABS&df[vs]=1.0.0&hc[Measure]=Births&pd=2000%2C&dq=1..5.A&ly[cl]=TIME_PERIOD.

Barbarot S, Silverberg J, Gadakari A et al. The family impact of atopic dermatitis in the pediatric population: results from an International cross-sectional study. J Pediatr. 2022;246:220–26 e5.

Carvalho D, Aguiar P, Mendes-Bastos P, Palma-Carlos A, Freitas J, Ferrinho P. Quality of life and characterisation of patients with atopic dermatitis in Portugal: The QUADEP Study. J Invest Allergol Clin Immunol. 2020;30(6):430–38.

Child and Adolescent Health Service. Nurse practitioner credentialing and scope of practice policy. 2022. https://healthpoint.hdwa.health.wa.gov.au/policies/Policies/CAHS/CAHS.PM.NursePractitionerCredentialingAndScopeOfPractice.pdfreference.

Consumer and Community Involvement Program. Types of consumer and community involvement. 2020. https://cciprogram.org/researcherservices/types-of-community-involvement/.

Fischer A, Shin DB, Margolis DJ, Takeshita J. Racial and ethnic differences in healthcare utilization for childhood eczema: an analysis of the 2001-2013 medical expenditure panel surveys. J Am Acad Dermatol. 2017;77(6):1060–7. https://doi.org/10.1016/j.jaad.2017.08.035.

Fleischer DM, Chan ES, Venter C, et al. A consensus approach to the primary prevention of food allergy through nutrition: guidance from the American Academy of Allergy, Asthma, and Immunology; American College of Allergy, Asthma, and Immunology; and the Canadian Society for Allergy and Clinical Immunology. J Allergy Clin Immunol. 2021;9(1):22–43. https://doi.org/10.1016/j.jaip.2020.11.002.

Kaufman BP, Guttman-Yassky E, Alexis AF. Atopic dermatitis in diverse racial and ethnic groups—Variations in epidemiology, genetics, clinical presentation and treatment. Exp Dermatol. 2018;27(4):340–57. https://doi.org/10.1111/exd.13514.

Kim A, et al. Racial/ethnic differences in incidence and persistence of childhood atopic dermatitis. J Invest Dermatol. 2019;139(4):827–34.

Lack G. Early exposure hypothesis: where are we now? Clin Transl Allergy. 2011;1(1):71. https://doi.org/10.1186/2045-7022-1-S1-S71.

Langan SM, Irvine AD, Weidinger S. Atopic dermatitis. Lancet. 2020;396(10247):345–60. https://doi.org/10.1016/S0140-6736(20)31286-1. Erratum in: Lancet. 2020;396(10253):758. PMID: 32738956.

LeBovidge J, Elverson W, Timmons W, et al. Multidisciplinary interventions in the management of atopic dermatitis. J Allergy Clin Immunol. 2016;138(2):325–34. https://doi.org/10.1016/j.jaci.2016.04.003.

Leung D. Atopic dermatitis: age and race do matter! J Allergy Clin Immunol. 2015;136:1265–7. https://doi.org/10.1016/j.jaci.2015.09.011.

Lewis-Jones S. Quality of life and childhood atopic dermatitis: the misery of living with childhood eczema. Int J Clin Pract. 2006;60(8):984–92.

Martin PE, Koplin JJ, Eckert JK, et al. The prevalence and socio-demographic risk factors of clinical eczema in infancy: a population-based observational study. Clin Exp Allergy. 2013;43(6):642–51. https://doi.org/10.1111/cea.12092.

National Allergy Strategy. National allergy strategy: improving the health and quality of life of Australians with allergic disease. 2015. https://www.nationalallergystrategy.org.au/download.

National Allergy Strategy. Scoping a shared care model for allergic conditions: background information paper. 2019. https://www.nationalallergystrategy.org.au/images/doc/Background_document_Shared_Care_March_2019.pdf.

National Allergy Strategy. Shared care model for allergic diseases infographic. 2022. https://www.nationalallergystrategy.org.au/projects/shared-care-model-for-allergy.

Networks WH. Model of care overview and guidelines. Government of Western Australia Department of Health, 2014.

New South Wales Agency for Clinical Innovation. Understanding the process to develop a model of care: an ACI framework. 2013. https://www.aci.health.nsw.gov.au/__data/assets/pdf_file/0009/181935/HS13-034_Framework-DevelopMoC_D7.pdf.

Pharmaceutical Society of Australia. Professional practice standards. 2017. https://my.psa.org.au/servlet/fileField?entityId=ka1Oo0000001DYHAA2&field=PDF_File_Member_Content__Body__s.

Pharmaceutical Society of Australia. Pharmacists in 2023: for patients, for our profession, for Australia's health system. 2019. https://www.psa.org.au/wp-content/uploads/2019/02/Pharmacists-In-2023-digital.pdf.

Poladian K, et al. Atopic dermatitis in adolescents with skin of color. Cutis. 2019;104(3):164–8.

Schneider J, Salter SM, Boss M, Weidinger J, Vale S, Loh R, et al. Collaborative pharmacy model of care - interim report. Crawley: The University of Western Australia; 2021. p. 28.

Sugita K, Akdis CA. Recent developments and advances in atopic dermatitis and food allergy. Allergol Int. 2020;69(2):204–14. https://doi.org/10.1016/j.alit.2019.08.013.

Sweeney A, et al. Early intervention of atopic dermatitis as a preventive strategy for progression of food allergy. Allergy Asthma Clin Immunol. 2021;17(1):30.

Torjesen I. Atopic dermatitis in teens with skin of colour. Dermatology Times. 2019. https://www.dermatologytimes.com/view/atopic-dermatitis-teens-skin-color.

Wan J, Oganisian A, Spieker AJ, et al. Racial/ethnic variation in use of ambulatory and emergency care for atopic dermatitis among US Children. J Invest Dermatol. 2019;139(9):1906–13. https://doi.org/10.1016/j.jid.2019.02.024.

Western Australian Health Networks. Model of care overview and guidelines. Western Australia: Government of Western Australia Department of Health. 2014. http://cedd.org.au/wordpress/wp-content/uploads/2014/04/Model-of-Care-Overviewand-Guidelines-WA-Health-Networks.pdf.

Wong I, Tsuyuki R, Cresswell-Melville A, et al. Guidelines for the management of atopic dermatitis (eczema) for pharmacists. Can Pharm J. 2017;150(5):285–97. https://doi.org/10.1177/1715163517710958.

World Health Organization. Sixty-Ninth world health assembly. Framework on integrated, people-centred health services. 2016. https://apps.who.int/gb/ebwha/pdf_files/WHA69-REC1/A69_2016_REC1-en.pdf.

Breatheasy: A Nurse-Led 'Care Through Family' Service Model

Natasha North and Minette Coetzee

Introduction

This chapter describes an expert paediatric nurse practitioner-led service model that has ensured that children with tracheostomies no longer spend extended periods of time in the hospital but at home with their families. This service model formed the basis for developing a conceptual model called *Care Through Family*, which is presented together with a brief description of its development.

This chapter begins with a summary of the key literature relating to worldwide increases in the number of children surviving critical illness, injury and prematurity and associated support needs for children and families living with chronic and complex health conditions. We describe important aspects of African societal and professional cultures which inform distinctive local practices related to the active involvement of mothers/primary caregivers in caring for their hospitalised children. A contrast is made with the resource-intensive response to caring for technology-dependent children in higher-income health systems.

Against this background, we present an account of one highly innovative nurse-led programme supporting families and children with tracheostomies and on home ventilation. Key elements of the impetus for establishing the service model, which became known as the *Breatheasy programme*, are described. These drivers included an urgent need to find alternatives to institutional care for a growing population of children living with tracheostomies and/or requiring home ventilation in a large metropole in South Africa, including a significant proportion of families living in informal settlements on the urban periphery. The practical realities of this are explored further below (see *The contextual lens* below). Specific challenges that the

N. North (✉) · M. Coetzee
The Harry Crossley Children's Nursing Development Unit, University of Cape Town,
Cape Town, South Africa
e-mail: natasha.north@uct.ac.za

© The Author(s), under exclusive license to Springer Nature
Switzerland AG 2023
C. L. Betz (ed.), *Worldwide Successful Pediatric Nurse-Led Models of Care*,
https://doi.org/10.1007/978-3-031-22152-1_15

programme sought to respond to included enabling mothers in a variety of living situations to provide care at home by managing airway patency and led to the design of a new approach to tube changes and cleaning.

Background Information

In this section, we provide the background and context of the Breatheasy programme. It places tracheostomy and home ventilation programmes in the context of global shifts in childhood mortality and morbidity. We describe the context for an innovative nurse-led service model, led by an expert paediatric nurse practitioner (PNP) which has ensured that more than 1000 children with tracheostomies and on home ventilation have gone home to their families since its inception in 1989. Finally, we introduce the conceptual model of *Care Through Family*.

Infant and Child Mortality and Morbidity Shifts

Improved technologies and treatment options are leading to more children surviving illness and injury (Cohen et al. 2011). As survivorship increases, so does the likelihood that some children will live with long-term functional and health resource-use consequences including technology reliance and/or complex polypharmaceutical needs (Cohen et al. 2011). These conditions involve an increased risk of frequent and prolonged hospitalisations. While inpatient care in hospitals meets complex treatment needs, this care cannot adequately encompass the social, emotional, developmental, intellectual or spiritual needs essential to long-term well-being. This trend towards increased survival is also being seen in lower-resourced and more fragile health systems. This includes the *sub-Saharan African region* (*defined by the United Nations* as the 54 African nations situated south of the Sahara desert) where more children are also surviving communicable, maternal, neonatal and nutritional diseases as a result of improvements in access to care and better treatments (Westwood and Stemming 2019; Bigna and Noubiap 2019). These children often require more frequent prolonged hospital stays, which are harder to accommodate in sub-Saharan Africa's healthcare systems. Paediatric services are largely concentrated in central urban areas and with limited bed capacity for this population. Institutional facilities for children with complex care needs are few. The shortages of appropriately skilled health professionals in many sub-Saharan countries pose additional challenges in meeting the short- and longer-term care needs of children who are technology-dependent.

Children with a Tracheostomy

The need for a tracheostomy to manage an obstructed airway and long-term invasive ventilation is one of the outcomes of surviving congenital and early childhood illness or injury. Medical historians have dated the first tracheostomies to ancient Egyptian times, pre-dating the first paediatric intensive care unit (PICU) by more than 5000 years (Dunbar and Andropoulos 2012). Today, however, health professionals have become accustomed to a service model in which children with a tracheostomy in situ receive a prolonged period of close medical supervision in hospital, and an acceptance that safe discharge home should include home-based nursing care by professionals, with ready access to technological support (Baker et al. 2016; Hartnick et al. 2017; McKeon et al. 2019). Such models of service provision are not widely available in the lower-resourced health systems of many sub-Saharan African countries (Groenendijk et al. 2016). Hospital-based care for a child with a tracheostomy is designed to mitigate the risks associated with an artificial airway. The two major risks that must be managed are the need to maintain patency of the tube by avoiding blockage, typically from secretions, and the need to avoid the tube becoming dislodged. Care involves stabilising and securing the tube, ensuring that inspired air is humidified, managing excess secretions through suctioning and changing the tube. The stoma requires cleaning, protection and in the early stages dressing. Care of the hospitalised child is usually organised around care regimes of constant monitoring, bathing, clothing and feeding.

These regimes cannot fully meet the child's social, emotional, developmental, intellectual or spiritual needs. As for all children, these needs are best met in the context of capable and engaged families. But care regimens also are often too complex to simply send children home, and the challenges of coordinating this intricate care outside of hospital are considerable. While tracheostomy and ventilation home care programmes do exist in high-resourced countries, the complexity of the child's needs mean that there are many children in high-, middle- and low-income countries who spend extended periods of time in hospitals and care facilities, away from home and their families.

Care in Lower-Resourced Settings

Clinicians caring for children with tracheostomies in lower-resourced health systems in Africa must either resign themselves to prolonged hospital stays or reframe these children's care to utilise available resources. 'Resourceful' is a descriptor we often hear in the context of African healthcare innovation. The service model described in this chapter is an excellent example of looking differently at resources. An expert paediatric nurse reframed what she had and harnessed her clinical expertise with the determination of her own experience of being a mother to consider the possibilities of a different model of care for children with tracheostomies and their families. Caring for a child with a tracheostomy requires three essential resources: a competent team of caregivers, a safe place and access to necessary equipment and supplies. We propose two important lenses that enable a reframing of the way that these resources are secured. One is the contextual lens—the societal context in which care occurs. The second is a lens that focuses on what we have and what we can work with, rather than what we do not have. This is a lens similar to abundance thinking (Covey 1989), one that lends itself well to the solution-focused approach so characteristic of the Breatheasy Programme.

The Contextual Lens

The service model presented in this chapter is situated in Cape Town, South Africa, a low-middle income country with a child population of 19.7 million, equivalent to just over one-third of the country's total population (Hall 2020). Cape Town is a busy metropole, the legislative capital of South Africa that has experienced rapid urbanization, and significant poverty and hardship are a reality of many residents. In 2018, over half of South Africa's children (59%) lived below the 'upper bound' poverty line, and 30% lived in households where no adults were employed. In these households, social assistance grants are an important source of income for caregivers to meet children's basic needs (Hall 2020). Between 10% and 25% of households in large urban areas may live in informal settlements (UN-HABITAT 2021; StatsSA 2016). These settlements feature many dwellings (shacks) that have been constructed on municipal land that is not demarcated for habitation. Such areas have little or no infrastructure such as roads and are not serviced with water, sanitation or electricity (DHS 2009). Access to basic amenities in informal settlements is improving: just over half (55%) of households in informal settlements have access to a safe electricity connection, and 71% of children have access to a piped water connection providing safe water either inside the dwelling or on the immediate site (Children's Institute 2019). Access to amenities can be much lower in highly rural areas.

While the statistics tell an important part of the story, a full understanding of the context of care for children requires that we look with a different lens at the context of healthcare delivery. South African and wider African societal cultures understand that personhood lies in community or Ubuntu. In isiXhosa, one of the three languages of the region, Ubuntu is defined as '*Umntu ngumntu ngabantu*': a person is a person through other persons. This is an expression of an African ethos based in communalism rather than individualism (Senghor 1965): so a child is a child through his or her family, and the family is family through the child. As identity is in belonging, the mother is a mother through her child and her community. This means she does not require permission to care or to mother. Her personhood is integrated with her caring and her mothering. Loss of this role means loss of this personhood, and for the child often the loss of a capable mother. When a child is hospitalised, this ethos extends to assuming that mothers are competent to fully engage in the child's required treatment regime while also nurturing a mother's inherent ability to care (Haegert 2000). Rooted in this relational ethic, extended families in African settings often take on additional caring responsibility for children, who are very rarely placed in institutional care, even when an onlooker viewing with a different lens may consider families available resources as insufficient.

A Solution-Focused Lens

The second contextual lens is about the focus on what we have to work with rather than what we do not have. Healthcare professionals are well trained in identifying what is wrong. Numerous differential diagnoses should lead an astute clinician to a definitive diagnosis of the problem or deficit. While this is an approach that serves us well in assessing illness, it lets us down when assessing the capacity and resources of children and their families. Clinicians identify problems and set expectations by comparing children and families to what is a relatively ill-defined 'normal'. As a result, the resources embedded in the social and cultural norms of the communities that nurses and families come from are easily missed.

As we will see, the Breatheasy service model reframes care for children by utilising both these lenses: a contextual lens which recognises the capacity of mothers and families and a solution-focused lens focused on what we have and what we can work with, rather than what we do not have. This reframing extends to the three essential resources. A competent team of caregivers must include mothers, extended family members and the wider community. A safe place is maintained within the circle of the mother–child dyad, wherever they are, recognising that a safe environment is not defined by brick walls. Access to necessary supplies can be ensured without a complex distribution chain when families take responsibility, and the type of equipment used is appropriate to the situation. Initially this included durable, foot-operated suction pumps that have more recently been replaced with handheld suction equipment.

Researching Clinical Practice

As a team of nurse scholars, our awareness of this successful service innovation, together with other promising African nursing practices in partnering with mothers to care for their hospitalised children, informed the design of a research study (North et al. 2019). The research settings where nursing practices were observed were all in South Africa, but the types of facilities and the nature of the geographical settings were diverse, including a nurse-led programme for technology-dependent children at a tertiary paediatric hospital in the Cape Town metropolis (the *Breatheasy* programme); an Intensive Care Unit (ICU) in a regional hospital in the largely rural Overberg region; a neonatal unit at a secondary health facility in an area of Cape Town which experiences significant localised poverty and deprivation; a general paediatric ward in a tertiary hospital in the Cape Town metropole; and a paediatric ward in a district hospital in a deep rural area of KwaZulu-Natal (North et al. 2020). We used a qualitative observational case study design, working with five teams of nurses to develop detailed descriptions of how nurses at each setting partnered with mothers in the care of their hospitalised child. We spent around a week with each team observing care and interviewing nurses and families to develop detailed descriptions of practice. We used visual research methods including graphic facilitation, sociograms and photographic elicitation to construct a detailed picture of routines, activities and environments.

Comprehensive accounts of 'real' nursing practices were constructed through 1:1 and group interviews, exploring the underlying rationales and values. Comprehensive case study reports were produced for each setting (see, e.g. North et al. 2020) and reviewed by key nurse participants. We found evidence of distinctive values and culturally specific caring practices, including 'standing with mothers', 'promoting a healthy whole' (by minimising separation of the mother and child) and 'letting the mother be the nurse'. After analysis of the data, researchers and key nurse participants worked together to develop statements reflecting the model of care. The end product was a description of nursing practice in the form of a conceptual model of nursing care ordered around six thematic domains. We called this model 'Care Through Family'. Each domain has a guiding principle, in the form of an illustrative statement reflecting the philosophies of care in the five sites. Having introduced the six domains of the Care Through Family conceptual model of nursing care, we will use the model as an organising framework to present a detailed account of the nurse-led *Breatheasy* service model in the next section.

Description of the Breatheasy Programme

In this section, we provide a detailed description of the organizational and service components of one service model, the *Breatheasy Programme*. Core information regarding programme design, team roles and responsibilities, and a brief description of the services provided are presented. An in-depth description of the practices involved in implementing the nurse-led model is presented in relation to the six components of the *Care Through Family* model, with specific examples of observed practice and quotations illustrating the beliefs and actions of nurses and mothers involved in the programme.

The Service Model

Breatheasy is a service which aims to empower and enable families to provide safe, competent home care to children reliant on a tracheostomy or artificial ventilation. Caregiver participation is key. Established in 1989, around 1000 children with tracheostomies have successfully been discharged home and managed in the community. The majority of children no longer need a tracheostomy by the time they reach school age, thanks to physiological maturation or successful surgical interventions. In this tracheostomy and ventilation home care service, an expert paediatric nurse practitioner (PNP) supports the child's journey from the clinical decision to create a tracheostomy, through insertion of tracheostomy, intensive care unit then high care and, in the majority of cases, home. It follows a primary healthcare approach, being centred on the child rather than the place of care, and therefore care delivery spans primary, secondary and tertiary care settings. The multi-site nature of the programme includes children at home, in the wards and in the Paediatric Intensive Care Unit at the Red Cross War Memorial Children's Hospital. The number of children enrolled in the programme at any one time varies considerably but is often around 150. This includes the children that are at home and those managed as in-patients in the ten beds available for admissions on a specialist paediatric ward. Over time, the service has extended to an advisory service for hospitals elsewhere in the Western Cape, other areas of the country and neighbouring countries.

The majority of children on the programme are high risk but medically stable and are cared for at home by their primary caregiver (usually their mother, grandmother or aunt). These children are seen by the PNP at a monthly follow-up clinic, if they live within travelling distance. Children who live out of area are followed up by local doctors, who consult with the PNP and team as needed. The most intensive period of engagement with a child and family is when the child first receives the tracheostomy, and during the period leading up to discharge home. Although the most intensive phase of interaction occurs while the child is an inpatient and the mother is undergoing training, the *Breatheasy* programme continues when the child goes home. There are a number of ways through which ongoing support is provided. The 'red card' ensures priority treatment and readmission so that the child is assured of rapid access to care by the specialist team if needed. Mothers are also given a mobile phone number to call for advice, and calls are answered by 24/7. Families are able to return to the ward to collect supplies at any time and at no cost to the family. These measures ensure that families remain in direct contact with the PNP and the ward team. This needs to be understood in the context of a lower-resourced healthcare system, where specialist community services do not exist.

Staffing

The *Breatheasy* programme was developed by Sister Jane Booth, an expert paediatric nurse practitioner (PNP) now with more than 40 years' experience of paediatrics, specialising in paediatric tracheostomy care at the Red Cross War Memorial Children's Hospital, Cape Town. Two paediatric nurses were appointed as additional nurse coordinators, anticipating Sister Booth's retirement in 2020. Other staff include ward nurses, doctors, allied health professions and ward housekeeper, and cleaners are essential to its in-hospital operation.

The *Breatheasy* team and the ward staff are a stable team overall, with many long-standing staff members particularly at consultant and senior nursing level. New nurses are inducted 'like new mothers', with no strong distinction made between what nurses need to know and what mothers need to know to care safely for a child.

Individuals are clear about what their role is and what they are responsible for within the multidisciplinary team. Ward nurses' roles are understood as being concerned with the daily planning and provision of nursing care. Overall care coordination and integration of social and psychological factors alongside physical care are the remit of the PNP and nurse co-ordinators, who orchestrate the contributions of the wider multidisciplinary team.

Inter- and Multidisciplinary Teamwork

The PNP convenes and leads a weekly multidisciplinary ward round of approximately 2 hours duration. The focus is on acute and long-term clinical decision-making regarding management of children on the programme. This meeting is the channel for all long-term decision-making pertaining to discharge and management, consultants, registrars and medical officers of various specialties, including ENT, pulmonology and intensivists. Allied professionals—speech and language therapist, social worker, physiotherapist and dietician, also attend and sometimes one of the ward nurses. The consultant's report on the medical aspects of the child's care and the PNP leads the discussion about social and family issues and readiness for discharge.

> The key to the multidisciplinary ward round is ensuring that everyone is clear what their contribution is. A lot of thought has gone into designing the format so that the presentations and dialogue flows, the quality of contributions is high, and everyone feels they have a contribution to make and knows what it is. (PNP)

> There are so many doctors on the various teams, they need to do their own thing really. It's impossible to have them interfering in the home discharge programme... I don't report to them. The multidisciplinary ward round is about them reporting to me, on the clinical aspects, and me and everyone else communicating about social and family issues and readiness for discharge. (PNP)

Preserving the Mother–Child Pair

The *Breatheasy Programme* strongly embodies a fundamental concept of the *Care Through Family* approach, which is that the family are the child's normal carers and the normal place of care for the child is the home. It is part of the *Breatheasy Programme* design that mothers or a family member who will have a significant role in caring for the child outside hospital should be present in hospital at all times as training is ongoing. Ultimately, the mother and family *are* the 'safe place' in which the child will be cared for.

If a mother is not the child's usual carer, the team may encourage the main carer to be the person who stays with the child in hospital so that they experience the intensive training and care required by the child. Some families alternate between either the mother or father or grandmother being present to accommodate other family needs and provide opportunities for better quality rest. For simplicity, and following the custom of the programme, we refer to the caregiver accompanying the child as their 'mother'.

A second way in which the *Breatheasy Programme* aligns with the *Care Through Family* model is the emphasis placed on ensuring that the mother's usual role in caring for the child continues with as little interruption as possible—including in the days immediately after surgical formation of the child's stoma. Mothers that we interviewed for our research did not describe having their role in caring for their child interrupted while they are in hospital, other than during short periods of critical illness or during surgical procedures. The PNP conceptualises this as nurses taking responsibility for the technical environment of treatment surrounding the child rather than taking responsibility for the child.

> I think it's a positive [involving families]. The more people who can care for the patient when he goes home, the better… because at the end of the day it stays "her" child. It's never going to be my child. (Ward nurse)

Mothers therefore perceive their role in providing hands-on care for their child as continuous. Nurses also provide direct care, but mothers experience the nurses' interventions as assisting and unobtrusive and delivered in a way that does not detract from the mothers' role as primary caregiver.

Enabling Continuous Presence

Since preservation of the mother–child pair is essential for the well-being of their children and the effective running of the programme, this must be practically enabled both in hospital and at home. Policies and amenities in the hospital ward are organised to support the continuous presence of mothers. During their stay in hospital, 'kangaroo chairs' (upright chairs that convert into sleeping couches) are provided for mothers, next to their child's bed. Nurses on the ward support normal home practices regarding sleeping as far as possible.

Parents have access to The Friends of the Children's Hospital parents' resource centre when their child is in the hospital. The mothers' room contains showers and laundry facilities, and space for parents to relax and socialise. There are toilets available for mothers to use on the ward, and meals for parents are served here three times daily by the friends. This level of assistance is not always available at other hospitals in South Africa. The PNP emphasises that the mothers are being prepared to take their child home and that they need to be able to care for the child there, rather than in hospital, so the hospital environment is made as home—like as possible:

> We are teaching all the time by example. So if I am making a bed with a mum, I will be looking for nice blankets, and making a little nest [to support the child in an optimal position], and making it look lovely. But all the time we are trying to make it look like it will at home, and thinking of how they are going to do it. (PNP)

At the beginning of the training period, mothers are provided with a 'trachy bag' made by volunteers. The bag is the right size to carry suction equipment and supplies for the tracheostomy, wherever the mother and child go. Inside is a small pocket with a Velcro zip in which a spare tracheostomy tube and a pair of scissors are kept for an emergency trachy change. This bag immediately becomes the mothers' property, and she is responsible for keeping it stocked and ensuring it is with her at all times. Towards the end of the training process, the mother is encouraged to take the child off the ward by themselves, spending gradually longer periods of time with the child, away from the ward. Increasingly the mother becomes familiar with this new role without a safety net of health professionals when the child is at home.

Once again, the mother and family *are* the 'safe place' in which the child will be cared for—wherever they go—and the innovation of the trachy bag helps ensure access to necessary supplies.

Belief and Trust

It is a clear expectation of the programme that on completion of the initial inpatient training period, mothers will be able to care for their child independently, without direct assistance from healthcare professionals. The *Breatheasy* team expect it to take between 2 weeks and 1 month of supportive training for a mother to feel confident to take a child home from hospital. The child is discharged when the mother indicates her readiness and is competent, and the child is clinically stable, regardless of the length of time spent in hospital. It is quite usual for children to go home within a month of the creation of the stoma. Tasks that mothers must become competent in include adapted feeding (including breastfeeding and often tube feeding), administration of prescribed medication and daily tracheostomy tube changes. The *Breatheasy* programme practice is to change the tracheostomy tube daily. A second clean tube is at the ready for insertion, while the previous day's tube is cleaned with soap and water, and a pipe cleaner and toothbrush are used to remove the biofilm plaque build-up inside of the tube. Mothers are also helped to recognise the signs and symptoms that their child needs to be suctioned, how to recognise if a tube is becoming blocked and what to do in emergency situations. It is clear that mothers carry a very significant level of responsibility for their child's welfare. At home, a mother cannot shout for help or rely on other people to know what to do. In our research, mothers talked to us about needing to be able to rely on their own training and ability. Mothers also talked about being able to deal with emergency situations:

> That first day at home I was very nervous, very shaky. But I did it [removed and cleaned the tube] myself. (Mother)

> One day she turned blue and I had to help her. (Mother)

Frequently, the comments mothers made demonstrated personal empowerment as well as pride in the knowledge and skills they have developed and the progress they have made:

> I had to learn a lot with him. I am [like] a home-based nurse, I know everything now, why they put the trachy in, how to clean a trachy, how to take it in and how to put it back in and how to suction. (Mother)

While nurses understand the emotional impact, on very young mothers in particular, they consistently express belief and confidence in mothers' ability to overcome their initial shock and fear:

> They are scared at first but as time goes by they just embrace it. (Nurse Coordinator)

Psychological Support and Empathy

For the *Breatheasy Programme* to achieve its goals, it is not enough for mothers simply to be physically present. Mothers are an essential resource as part of the 'competent team' caring for the child, so they must be psychologically present and able to provide engaged care for their child. Nurses express a high level of awareness of the emotional strain that mothers are under, informed by professional insight and, for many, the ability to empathise with mothers as mothers themselves. Nurses' awareness of the mother's life experience extends to life beyond the hospital ward, indicating an appreciation of the fact that the home and community rather than the hospital ward are the child's usual place of care. Nurses are also sensitive to the living circumstances in which families must manage children with complex care needs. This awareness extends to the child's home environment:

> I don't stay in a house, I stay in [an informal dwelling or shack], and so at night when it's cold, it's very cold. (Mother)

> Sister Booth has organised housing for people, even electricity. We write letters to the council motivating for things. You get involved… I do home visits [for children on ventilation] and it helps a lot to be able to know where a child will sleep, where they will do their exercises, where they will keep their medicines. (Physio)

The approach to visiting a family home illustrates this psychological support and empathy well. While the PNP describes taking all mothers and children home in the initial years, she soon realised that having spent the time in the ward meant that mothers knew well what they would need to care for a child with a tracheostomy home. She describes how proud mothers often are to show her around their home. Rather than point out what they do not have she is able to assist a mom with repositioning a shelf or safely adding an extension cord to reach a socket. Preparing a home with a family who are preparing for home ventilation is more complex and happens ahead of the discharge. In these settings the PNP often enrols wider community support from the local council, non-profits or volunteer organisations. Once again however, the mother and family lead the visit and preparation of the space.

While the emotional burden of managing a child with a tracheostomy is considerable, it varies over time. The family of a newly tracheostomised child is likely to experience considerable anxiety, and there will inevitably be times at later stages when the child is sick or encounters problems. Healthcare providers working in a hospital setting are likely to encounter a disproportionate number of families who are anxious or in difficulty. But this does not represent the whole situation. Many children on the programme become stable, and there can be long periods which are relatively untroubled. Others outgrow the need for a tracheostomy, are decannulated or no longer require ventilation. Parents at this stage are likely to have a very different perspective than they did at the outset. Even where children are receiving palliative care, the tracheostomy or ventilation supports a better quality of life overall than would otherwise have been the case. The emotional burden that families face is not downplayed by the programme but consistently seen in the context. An assessment of quality of life in children and families in the *Breatheasy* programme found that children and their families are empowered to live independently of the hospital system and appear to be thriving (Din et al. 2020).

Mothers as a Capable Resource

As described, it is quite usual in many African healthcare settings for mothers to be seen as an essential part of the team caring for the child on the ward. The *Breatheasy* programme is no exception, and mothers regard themselves and are regarded by nurses, as capable resources for their children both in hospital and at home. Asides from meeting their child's basic care needs and learning how to manage their tracheostomy, mothers in the programme also help to care for one another. 'New' mothers on the ward receive intensive input from nurses but are also expected to progress a rapid rate:

> … but then we get admissions and the new mum becomes the old mum and I help, but she has to do it on her own. [Next] I let the mum do it [remove and clean the tube]… [and soon] it's their turn, because they relax faster if they get involved early on. It depends on the mums. (Nurse)

'Old' mothers (of all ages!) are seen as trustworthy sources of information and emotional and practical support for 'new' mothers entering the programme and are asked to orientate new mothers to the ward environment and to aspects of basic care. Nurses exhibit confidence in the quality of the knowledge that is transmitted in this way. This is a further example of the way that the programme harnesses all available resources. There is a support group for mothers which meets weekly, which inpatient and outpatient mothers attend voluntarily, often travelling some distance to attend. These practices are typical of the resourceful mindset that the *Breatheasy* service model cultivates. Even the earliest nursing assessment by the PNP seeks to map and articulate a family's resources from the first encounter. Genograms, a visual 'family tree' which usually depict inheritance of illness, look very different in the *Breatheasy* patient folders. Instead of being solely a map of a family's medical history and patterns of hereditary conditions, in this programme, the 'family tree' often includes a neighbour with a vehicle and an 'aunty' who provides childcare for a sibling. These people are important family resources in caring for the child at home.

Sharing Knowledge

The continuous presence of mothers shapes the nature of the learning experience, providing a richness and intensity to the exchange of knowledge and information, and accelerating the rate at which mothers learn, both from team members and from one another. The continuous presence of mothers also enables normalisation, supporting mothers to adjust to their child's altered care needs very rapidly:

They [mothers] embrace it into their lives. It is new, but it just needs to become a part of their routine. (PNP)

Sister Booth told me how to wash him, she kept telling me he is a normal baby, and there is nothing wrong with him. I was shocked, what happens if the water goes into his trachy, or runs down his neck, but she said he is normal, and that is what I keep in the back of my mind, he is not a different baby. (Mother)

The staff are happy to include the extended family in training, and nurses are aware that many mothers train the rest of the family over time. Nurses feel mothers have peace of mind if a second family member also has some knowledge of the tracheostomy and recognise that mothers need a backup to help facilitate normal life, e.g. shopping.

Yes, but what the mothers do when they are at home… they are so smart, they train the rest of the family. (Ward Nurse)

The approach to training recognises the wide variations in literacy and educational background, and in particular the fact that many mothers in this setting may be unable to read English, or any complex written information. Mothers are given a training manual with clear photographic information (Booth n.d.) There is also a strong emphasis on practical demonstration and coaching, and most learning on the programme occurs by 'being with' rather than 'being taught'. Oversight of the training in tracheostomy care and provision of initial instruction, demonstrations and supervising first procedures by mothers are the responsibility of the PNP or specialist nurse coordinators. As we have seen, the first learning encounter is usually between the mother and one of the specialist nurse coordinators and is centred on the ordinary daily activity of washing the baby/child. The rapid rate at which mothers are expected to learn and the fact that they are involved in hands-on care almost immediately are a key part of the approach.

… that strong message that the quicker you learn, the quicker you can go home. (specialist Nurse Coordinator)

The ward nurses reinforce training at the bedside, ensuring consistency. Ward nurses typically work alongside mothers, demonstrating, explaining and progressively involving mothers in care to the point where mothers undertake procedures under supervision and then independently. Nurses use their knowledge to help mothers anticipate and plan interventions and care, helping mothers to know what to expect. Nurses are so good at providing this unobtrusive and highly responsive input that some mothers feel confident to take the lead in hands-on care in as little as 2 days. Nurses will reinforce a mother's growing sense of confidence in her abilities, although mothers are still observed and supported.

[The specialist Nurse Coordinator] changed the trachy on the Thursday and showed me what to do and I just watched. On the weekend I changed it myself. On the Monday Sister Booth watched and said I could go home. (Mother)

While the length of the training process may vary, it is clear that it is remarkably rapid, with a minimum of 2 weeks and a mean of 23–30 days (Groenendijk et al. 2016).

Factors That Support Care Through Family

In this section, we describe a range of supportive factors and innovations that support the successful operation of the *Breatheasy* service model. Firstly, we describe a clinical practice innovation (daily cleaning and changing of the tracheostomy tube) which is seen as central to improving outcomes for children. Secondly, we revisit the essential resources and inputs required to successfully implement the *Breatheasy* programme, aligned with the *Care Through Family* conceptual model. We briefly discuss these supportive factors and innovations in the light of evidence from the wider scientific knowledge base as well as published outcome evaluations of the *Breatheasy* programme.

Daily Changing of the Tracheostomy Tube

One highly innovative aspect of the *Breatheasy* programme is the daily practice of changing the tracheostomy tube. All nurses, mothers and children in the *Breatheasy* programme gain mastery of this daily routine. In the paediatric population, the respiratory tract (and therefore the lumen of the tracheostomy tube) is small, and the most common tracheostomy-related cause of death is tube obstruction (Ng 2021). The PNP noticed that children's tubes often obstructed despite having just been suctioned to remove secretions. Having examined numerous tubes, she was convinced that the biofilm that built up in these narrow tubes became dislodged by suctioning and then occluded the tube. While the presence of biofilm is well recognised in the oral cavity and tubing used in various treatments (Solomon et al. 2009), there seems to be more research interest in their microbiology than in the possibility of the dislodged film occluding narrow artificial airways. While there is no global consensus regarding how frequently tracheostomy tubes should be changed (Ng et al. 2022), the science behind this intuition has been carefully considered (Benner & Tanner, 1987) and outcome measurement appears to support the practice in the context of the *Breatheasy* programme, with survival outcomes for the *Breatheasy* programme comparable with that of high-income countries (Van der Poel et al. 2017). This practice of mastering the daily changing of the tracheostomy tube and securing it with clean tape may be the mainstay of early discharge home, and further research is needed to fully understand its contribution.

Resources and Inputs

Earlier in this chapter, we highlighted three essential resources and inputs required to successfully implement the *Breatheasy* service: a competent team of caregivers, a safe place and access to necessary supplies. These resources and inputs include inter- and multidisciplinary team working arrangements, as well as ways in which resources are mobilised to meet the costs of implementation, medical technology and devices. The 'solution-focused' approach to overcoming challenges such as a lack of electricity or water supply at home will be explained. Practical considerations regarding the physical accommodation of mothers have already been described above (see *Enabling continuous presence*). We also proposed two important lenses that enable a reframing of the way that these resources are secured. The first lens focuses on the societal context in which care occurs. The second lens is focused on what we have and what we can work with rather than what we do not have.

A Competent Team of Caregivers

From what has been described above, it should be clear that mothers, extended family members and the wider community are an integral part of the team caring for the child. Yet while the service model that this chapter describes may initially be seen or categorised as a family centred-care model by those unfamiliar with African society, it is different in fundamental ways. The main difference is in how families are recognised. Much 'family-centred' practice holds that 'that the perspectives and information provided by families, children, and young adults are important in clinical decision making' during periods of care by professionals (American Academy of Pediatrics 2012). It follows that the mother and family are important supports of children and—since their relationship has been disrupted by a medical event—ways must be found to allow them more access, invite them into more conversations with professionals and instil in them a new set of knowledge, attitudes and skills.

In contrast, the ethos of the *Care Through Family* conceptual model (which the *Breatheasy* programme exhibits so clearly) is to be fully supportive of the mother and family in the role that they never lost. If they never lost the responsibility of mothering and care, if they never lost their personhood as mother, they do not need to be allowed or helped to come back. They never left. In higher-resourced health systems, poor socio-economic circumstances are often assumed to be reasons not to discharge a child with a tracheostomy. Three published evaluations of the *Breatheasy* programme confirm that tracheostomy care at home is feasible under difficult socio-economic circumstances provided that a structured tracheostomy education and a caregiver training programme are in place (Din et al. 2020; Groenendijk et al. 2016, Van der Poel et al. 2017). With adequate enrolment and training of family caregivers, home-care nursing is not necessary. Readmissions or other negative outcomes do not appear to be associated with the carer's education level, socio-economic status or informal housing (Din et al. 2020).

A Safe Place

As we have seen, ultimately, the mother and family are the 'safe place' in which the child will be cared for. The goal in ensuring a safe environment in this lower-resourced setting is not to establish a 'hospital at home' or a 'special school'. The innovation of the 'trachy bag', given to mothers at the start of training, exemplifies this mindset: the child will have what they need, wherever they go. An independent nonprofit organisation (The Children's Hospital Trust) raises funds for the programme. These funds meet the costs of equipment needed to send children home with suction machines, ventilators, humidifiers, oximeters and so forth. The hospital is gradually incorporating these costs into the hospital budget. A hospital voluntary organisation also provides additional items when needed. The solution-focused lens recognises the capacity in lower-resourced families and communities and ensures these are utilised to best effect. The 'solution-focused' approach driven by the expert nurse extends to overcoming challenges such as a lack of electricity or water supply at home, through negotiating with the municipal authorities to provide amenities. More than once, this has resulted in a whole street being connected to the electricity supply.

Challenges and Service Adjustments Made

Challenges

The major challenges involved in establishing and running the Breatheasy programme are quite apparent in the description above. The significant hardship experienced by many of the families participating in the programme and the absence of a safety net of community-based health professionals available to provide direct assistance to families at home might in other circumstances have been seen as insurmountable barriers. Yet the achievements of the Breatheasy programme demonstrate just how successfully these obstacles were overcome.

The account of the Breatheasy Programme presented above draws on a 20-year process of development and refinement. Numerous adjustments and modifications have been made over the years to improve the service model and its operation. In this section, we highlight two main areas, not addressed above, where the design of the programme required innovations in relation to professional accountability and employment arrangements.

Service Adjustments

It remains highly unusual in South Africa's health system for a specialist service such as *Breatheasy* to be nurse-led. Because of the level of training and high level of autonomous expert practice on the part of the PNP, it was agreed with facility management that the expert paediatric nurse practitioner would have a dual reporting line. This involved a line management relationship with the nursing manager for the facility, who was responsible for annual performance reviews and other contractual matters, as well as a 'dotted reported line' to the clinical leadership of the Pulmonology and ENT teams at the hospital, which was designed to ensure clinical and professional accountability appropriate to the PNP's scope of practice.

Further adjustments were required following the extension of the service beyond the Red Cross War Memorial Children's Hospital. As word of the programme's success spread, the PNP responded to requests to provide the service to children at a leading private specialist hospital (Netcare Christiaan Barnard Memorial Hospital) and to the pulmonology services at other hospitals in South Africa's Western Cape. Children receiving care from the service have been discharged home to other South African provinces, neighbouring countries and remote island locations. This type of multi-centre service provision, spanning both public and private sectors, was not anticipated by South Africa's nursing employment framework. After negotiation, it was agreed that the PNP would provide the service to these other facilities in addition to her full-time work at Red Cross War Memorial Children's Hospital, with remuneration under the RWOPS policy (Remuneration for Work Outside the Public Service). Both these adjustments are to some extent a 'workaround' solution in the continuing and regrettable absence of Advanced Nurse Practitioner or Nurse Consultant roles within the national employment framework for nurses in South Africa. While Sister Booth holds advanced diplomas in paediatric nursing and advanced paediatric nursing which qualified her for entry on the South African Nursing Council register as an Advanced Paediatric and Neonatal Nurse Practitioner, she was developing a responsive service model for which she had the training and clinical expertise before the employment framework for Advanced Nurse Practitioners was established.

Lessons Learned

The nursing practices and organisational policies embodied in the *Breatheasy Programme* and presented in the *Care Through Family* model represent distinctive nursing practice innovations. The knowledge embedded in them is a completely appropriate African response to an African situation and may also have something to offer to other settings. The deliberate practices and lenses related to the role of mothers and families in the *Breatheasy* programme contrast with models of care provision originating in higher-resourced settings including Europe and America, such as family-centred care, and contrast with informal practices in local African settings still aligned with European service models designed a century ago (Davies 2010) which simply tolerate the presence of mothers, as well as local institutional policies which limit mothers' presence to varying extents.

The Care Through Family Self-Assessment Tool

Based on the research study described above (see *Researching clinical practice*), we have developed a *Care Through Family* self-assessment tool to guide nursing teams through a facilitated process of reflection and further practice development. The approach and questions were informed by established best practices in self-assessment related to practice improvement (South et al. 2005; Measure Evaluation for United States Agency for International Development and the Health Data Collaborative 2019). The self-assessment process involves gathering objective examples of practice, reflecting on the subjective beliefs and attitudes embodied in these practices, and thinking critically about any gaps between what nurses 'know' and what nurses 'do'. Nurses then record their self-assessment on a user-friendly spreadsheet which automatically calculates scores. Self-scoring is presented visually as a spider chart, and nurses are prompted to use the information to plan improvements in their practice and subsequently to review progress (Fig. 1).

The *Care Through Family* model simply formalises the concepts that we have observed in excellent African nursing practice. In the final section of this chapter, we discuss why this matters.

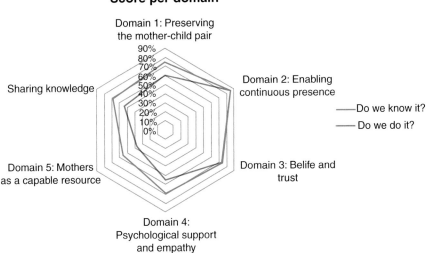

Fig. 1 A Care Through Family practice assessment

Future Implications for Clinical Practice and Research

The best of nursing care in South Africa, such as that embodied in *Breatheasy*, is shaped by cultural and societal values, as well as resourcefulness, resilience and professional expertise. But nursing practices are also shaped by the professional and organisational cultures of health systems that, through the legacy of colonisation, are not often aligned with cultural or societal values. There remains an enormous gap between the way that many nurses are prepared through their training, and the reality and scope of practice that they face. As part of a growing community of children's nursing educators across the African continent, we endeavour to incorporate this awareness into our teaching and learning. However, the absence of more formally articulated models of authentic and excellent African nursing practice is a hindrance (Nyondo-Mipando et al., 2020).

There is considerable scope for further work to conceptualise Afrocentric models of nursing practice in relation to involving families in the care of hospitalized children. As more descriptions of children's nursing practice in Africa are published (see, e.g. Phiri et al. 2017), there will be more important global conversations about the ways that nurses work with families in a wider variety of societies and contexts.

The focus of our ongoing research activity at the Children's Nursing Development Unit is on observing, documenting understanding and articulating the reality of children's nursing practice in Africa, with a particular focus on family involvement, which is such an invisible mainstay of nursing practice in many African settings. Our goal is to move family involvement from being an implicit practice to one that is formally articulated and valued. In doing so, we stand to generate knowledge that will enrich nursing in Africa as well as colleagues working in higher-resourced settings, in a way that respects the authentic contribution of Africa's nurses. This is an essential part of the process of decolonialising nursing knowledge. There is currently work underway in two areas that pertain to clinical practice and research:

- Training a new generation of Advanced Practice Nurses in paediatrics, equipped to lead practice change, through a professional master's programme at the University of Cape Town—with a curriculum that equips nurses to recognise and explicitly embrace the essential role that families play in caring for children in hospital and at home.
- Support and expert facilitation for children's nurse leaders and their teams to implement nurse-led *Care Through Family* practices in African paediatric settings.

Conclusion

> The Breatheasy programme is life changing. There is no hope of a normal life for these children and it gives them hope. It gives them quality of life. (Operational Manager)

This chapter has presented a successful nurse-led service innovation—the *Breatheasy programme*—which has informed an Afrocentric conceptual nursing care model—*Care Through Family*. In addition to providing a real alternative to extended hospitalisation for children with tracheostomies and/or requiring ventilation, the model of care described provides inspiration and encouragement for nurses in a variety of other settings to reflect on the extent to which elegantly simple, solution-focused approaches, an abundance mindset and the capacity of mothers and families can contribute to establishing new nurse-led models of care in their own clinical and community-based settings.

Useful Resources

For more information about the *Breatheasy* programme visit www.breatheasyprogramme.org.za

The *Care Through Family Conceptual Model of Children's Nursing Care* and the *Care Through Family Practice Assessment Tool* by Natasha North, Angela Leonard, Candice Bonaconsa and Minette Coetzee can be downloaded at https://open.uct.ac.za/handle/11427/38442 and are licensed under Creative Commons CC BY-NC 4.0. The terms of the license lets others remix, adapt, and build upon this work non-commercially. New works must acknowledge this source.

Follow The Harry Crossley Children's Nursing Development Unit on Twitter @ HCCDU or visit the website at http://www.childrensnursingunit.uct.ac.za/

Acknowledgements Sister Jane Booth is a visionary advanced nurse practitioner in paediatrics who conceived and ran the *Breatheasy* Programme until her retirement in 2020. We thank Jane and colleagues on the nursing and wider team involved in the *Breatheasy* programme for making it possible for us to spend time with you.

We acknowledge with gratitude the nursing leadership and teams at all the hospitals that participated in the Care Through Family study, for their willingness to engage so actively in making their practices visible and reflecting on the nature of their nursing practice. We recognise your commitment to providing the best possible care to the children and families who depend on you.

The Care Through Family study was assisted by researchers at CNDU: Stephanie Sieberhagen, Angela Leonard and Candice Bonaconsa.

Appendix

Preserving the mother–child pair	*Guiding principles*: The goal is to ensure that the mother's role in caring for the child continues with as little interruption as possible, with the nurse partnering with the mother to meet additional aspects of care required by the child's condition. The normal place of care for the child is the home, and the family are their normal carers
	Attributes • Preserving the mother–child dyad is of paramount importance, and active steps are taken to prevent or minimise disruption and separation (preserving the mother's role as the child's main care provider) • Mothers continue to provide practical care (bathing, nappy changes, feeding etc.) as they would at home to the maximum extent that the child's condition allows • The home is recognised as the child's normal place of care, with nurses and mothers working together openly towards the child's return home as soon as they are able • The specific developmental needs of infants, babies, children, adolescents and the needs of their parents are recognised and incorporated • Where possible, home routines are continued in hospital, or new routines are designed with returning home in mind • Arrangements are made for mothers to have access to ongoing support and relief, for example, through visits by the extended family and faith communities
Enabling continuous presence	*Guiding principles*: Policies and amenities are directed towards enabling the presence of mothers. Accommodation, space and amenities are organised to enable mothers' continuous presence
	Attributes • Mothers are present with their child at all times, spending most of the day and night with their child • Policy in this setting recognises that the continuous presence of mothers is essential for children • The setting includes space for mothers to rest and sleep (e.g. a bed or a chair) • Mothers have ready access to the equipment, materials and supplies they need to care for their child and themselves
Belief and trust	*Guiding principles*: Nurses and mothers have innate confidence in mothers' abilities to learn and to cope, and high expectations about the speed at which they will become competent in new activities
	Attributes • The continuous presence of mothers in this setting contributes to improved psychological outcomes for the child • Most mothers are competent to provide care (with training, if required). Exceptions are rare • Nurses and mothers have innate confidence in mothers' abilities to learn and to cope, and high expectations about the speed at which they will become competent in new activities • Mothers have responsibilities in this setting

Psychological support and empathy	Guiding principles: Enabling mothers to be physically and psychologically present and equipped to care involves empathetic practical and psychological support and the integration of social and psychological factors alongside physical care
	Attributes • Mothers are supported to be psychologically present, as well as physically present, in order to provide engaged care for their child • Nurses are alert to signs that mothers are struggling to engage and work to draw the mother into being fully present • Authentic personal relationships between nurses, mothers and children help to minimise emotional disengagement in difficult situations • Nurses look after both the mother and child and show empathetic awareness of the psychological and physical strains that the mother faces
Mothers as a capable resource	*Guiding principles*: Mothers are regarded as a resource within the healthcare system for their children in hospitals and at home by both nurses and mothers
	Attributes • There is a place where mothers can socialise and interact • Mothers are encouraged to form a mutually supportive community • The transmission of knowledge and support between mothers is a valued activity • The support that mothers can give to one another, drawing on their experiences, is valued by nurses
Sharing knowledge	*Guiding principles*: The transmission of knowledge between nurses and mothers happens through 'being with' and 'being taught'. The process through which mothers become competent to manage the child's needs outside of hospital is dynamic and responsive to the mother's individual situation and progress.
	Attributes • The continuous presence of the mother is central to the learning process • Starting from admission, nurses actively encourage mothers to learn about and provide additional aspects of care, as required by the child's condition • Nurses make use of both formal training sessions and informal, responsive teaching and learning opportunities at the bedside to equip mothers with the knowledge they need • Nurses work alongside the mother–child pair, demonstrating, explaining and progressively involving mothers in care to the point where mothers undertake new caring activities under supervision and then independently • Normalisation of the mother's role in meeting the child's altered care needs is achieved through a combination of both planned and opportunistic inputs • Information and knowledge, including professional nursing knowledge, is shared freely with mothers, rather than guarded protectively • Nurses invite mothers to share information about changes in the child's condition and are responsive to what mothers say • Nurses come alongside mothers to provide information and feedback in a way that upholds the mother's position as the child's main carer

References

Baker CD, Martin S, Thrasher J, Moore HM, Baker J, Abman SH, Gien J. A standardized discharge process decreases length of stay for ventilator -dependent children. Pediatrics. 2016;137(4):e20150637. https://doi.org/10.1542/peds.2015-0637.

Benner P, Tanner C. How expert nurses use intuition. Am J Nurs. 1987;87(1):23–34.

Bigna JJ, Noubiap JJ. The rising burden of non-communicable diseases in sub-Saharan Africa. Lancet Glob Health. 2019;7(10):e1295–6. https://doi.org/10.1016/S2214-109X(19)30370-5.

Booth J. The breatheasy training manual. How to look after your child with a tracheostomy. n.d. ISBN: 978-0-620-54265-4. Available from: http://breatheasyprogramme.org/uploads/6ba5c6 7c361fb06ba9c67c3f/1442588335920/Home-Care-Book-final-email.pdf.

Children's Institute, University of Cape Town. Children count: statistics on children in South Africa. 2019. Available from: http://childrencount.uct.ac.za/indicator.php?domain=3&indicator=41. Accessed 10 Dec 2021

Cohen E, Kuo DZ, Agrawal R, Berry JG, Bhagat SK, Simon TD, Srivastava R. Children with medical complexity: an emerging population for clinical and research initiatives. Pediatrics. 2011;127(3):529–38. https://doi.org/10.1542/peds.2010-0910.

Committee on Hospital Care and Institute for Patient-and Family-Centered Care (2012). Patient- and family-centered care and the pediatrician's role. Pediatrics, 129(2), 394–404. https://secure-web.cisco.com/1AEEUhdF0vWKnCY_ QBZTwcsTJU7TG3O34S7HakqoYWd1EmMHv4RTrrYQx_wFhrUvCcSR1gXqh5ZDvVw- mDALjVDlkOsZCJgi8hsJLuumAhv3y91eMG_WquisQk5SRqIXeNV5frSIlRwmd0Y8vD_ bOjO15GecXZ42sfhNok4LM-MJca4lCXR7Ny2nftJzGTpxfslOL-RMaelnoMkphmbwYSZ- BL86AUFfd-bOMVLxxIFVXsNoOTv_eF6H0d3ogYEz7CR0ynury0vVwyeOB- fRRT5cNLygO68bb5iH1TLDdNQK3PtAsU9yMsBgxbW0AlZQyuKj63JULD8_TPiRL_ WHI4KvvvGSrcQpsne-q3NRgDwPzwSz5WuIPn00jfjYFz3aLb7imsCFJ5t8mXAI7D3brBO 62LcOc9LUXhekqnDvez3DGmBs5WeVvBQbOoqiaGtDvERlGS9y_12ylRXTJEggRfDapw/ https%3A%2F%2Fdoi.org%2F10.1542%2Fpeds.2011-3084.

Covey SR. The 7 habits of highly effective people, vol. 1. New York: Simon & Schuster; 1989.

Davies R. Marking the 50th anniversary of the Platt report: from exclusion, to toleration and parental participation in the care of the hospitalized child. J Child Health Care. 2010;14(1):6–23. https://doi.org/10.1177/1367493509347058.

Department of Human Settlements (DHS). 'Upgrading of Informal Settlement programme', Part 3, Volume 4 of the National Housing Code; 2009. p. 16.

Din TF, McGuire J, Booth J, Lytwynchuk A, Fagan JJ, Peer S. The assessment of quality of life in children with tracheostomies and their families in a low to middle income country (LMIC). Int J Pediatr Otorhinolaryngol. 2020;138:110319. https://doi.org/10.1016/j.ijporl.2020.110319.

Dunbar BS, Andropoulos DB. History of pediatric anesthesia. Gregory's Pediatr Anesth. 2012:15–26. https://doi.org/10.1016/B978-0-323-06612-9.00041-9.

Groenendijk I, Booth J, van Dijk M, Argent A, Zampoli M. Paediatric tracheostomy and ventilation home care with challenging socio-economic circumstances in South Africa. Int J Pediatr Otorhinolaryngol. 2016;84:161–5. https://doi.org/10.1016/j.ijporl.2016.03.013.

Haegert S. An African ethic for nursing? Nurs Ethics. 2000;7(6):492–502.

Hall K. Demography of South Africa's children. In: May J, Witten C, Lake L, editors. South African child gauge 2020. Cape Town: Children's Institute, University of Cape Town; 2020. http://www.ci.uct.ac.za/cg-2020-food-and-nutrition-security.

Hartnick C, Diercks G, De Guzman V, Hartnick E, Van Cleave J, Callans K. A quality study of family-centered care coordination to improve care for children undergoing tracheostomy and the quality of life for their caregivers. Int J Pediatr Otorhinolaryngol. 2017;99:107–10. https:// doi.org/10.1016/j.ijporl.2017.05.025.

McKeon M, Kohn J, Munhall D, Wells S, Blanchette S, Santiago R, Graham R, Nuss R, Rahbar R, Volk M, Watters K. Association of a multidisciplinary care approach with the quality of care after pediatric tracheostomy. JAMA Otolaryngol Head Neck Surg. 2019;145(11):1035–42. https://doi.org/10.1001/jamaoto.2019.2500. PMID: 31536099; PMCID: PMC6753653.

Measure Evaluation for United States Agency for International Development and the Health Data Collaborative. Health information systems interoperability maturity toolkit: users' guide. Version 1.0. Updated Jan 2019. Available from https://www.measureevaluation.org/resources/publications/tl-17-03a. Accessed 12 Apr 2020.

Ng J, Hamrang-Yousefi S, Agarwal A. Tracheostomy Tube Change. [Updated 2021 Jul 31]. In: StatPearls [Internet]. Treasure Island (FL): StatPearls Publishing; 2021 Jan. Available from: https://secure-web.cisco.com/1B8WlJWMOCtKZb6ieckK8Z1-8niseX5QwSCIH-HXj0KtMRUqFFULYWkZNpQ6Oiz_ZmXSayAlL3SHojhbOUFAL_2Rj2OdRLwd-aL_u4VaRaf92tSdQRY4qLfeFFByWcBvezmhvBmg11YKjWS50cSDc1guY-w3W7TsRy-TgUTAHNnAaFGe3czpLYyfpwDExQ8GliZl6e7GjEXpB9Vb5YJ3Ek7O_giZdtVwqhOMeBzVW_KynkHK5sZn-gxW7SrLJ-hWXJwNIekZBOZ44CyLLFNzzaJ1VIjqmRR4uEF8sLHfYBmpdt09oRbt3_dzkeaFAr9i1ac4sjE8zZRZbhbjVKz-d9QqJES0srWFLPwVs8FAvQTJXi5HDfL1-LW4o4EOXWZtK5fosi00evYor2VsZFR0h_INECdurK3bcd0sxDyK3TMED8ICaZ3KG1dRB8DlTltDNIkpu7eoD6zC2_oWDXUN-s1WbEw/https%3A%2F%2Fwww.ncbi.nlm.nih.gov%2Fbooks%2FNBK555919%2F.

Ng J, Hamrang-Yousefi S, Agarwal A. Tracheostomy tube change [Updated 2022 July 25]. In: StatPearls [Internet]. Treasure Island, FL: StatPearls Publishing; 2022. Available from: https://www.ncbi.nlm.nih.gov/books/NBK555919/.

North N, Sieberhagen S, Bonaconsa C, Leonard A, Coetzee M. Making children's nursing practices visible: using visual and participatory techniques to describe family involvement in the care of hospitalised children in southern African settings. Int J Qual Res Method. 2019;18:160940691984932. https://doi.org/10.1177/1609406919849324.

North N, Leonard A, Bonaconsa C, Duma T, Coetzee M. Distinctive nursing practices in working with mothers to care for hospitalised children at a district hospital in KwaZulu-Natal, South Africa: a descriptive observational study. BMC Nurs. 2020;19(1):1–12.

Nyondo-Mipando AL, Woo Kinshella ML, Bohne C, Suwedi-Kapesa LC, Salimu S, Banda M, Newberry L, Njirammadzi J, Hiwa T, Chiwaya B, Chikoti F, Vidler M, Dube Q, Molyneux E, Mfutso-Bengo J, Goldfarb DM, Kawaza K, Mijovic H. Barriers and enablers of implementing bubble Continuous Positive Airway Pressure (CPAP): perspectives of health professionals in Malawi. PLoS One. 2020;15(2):e0228915. https://doi.org/10.1371/journal.pone.0228915.

Phiri PG, Kafulafula U, Chorwe-Sungani G. Registered nurses' experiences pertaining to family involvement in the care of hospitalised children at a tertiary government hospital in Malawi. Africa J Nurs Midwifery. 2017;19(1):131–43. https://hdl.handle.net/10520/EJC-898b3e858.

Senghor I. On African socialism. Stanford, CA: Stanford University, 1965. Cited in: Haegert S (2000) An African ethic for nursing? Nurs Ethics 7(6).

Shung-King M, Lake L, Sanders D & Hendricks M (eds) (2019) South African Child Gauge 2019. Cape Town: Children's Institute, University of Cape Town. https://secure-web.cisco.com/182BkJlbwqezewgJpq1DDYl8j9AWlq9IVarylcwF4NeiAastH--7urm-UhCDKrK2Wot-seAUw4xm7cAeS2OOSddtirr1nGz6rVMJuiclUsN2mmRTSsn3Y7N2zVLkTB-RHgp6qG63guw6329ldaue0JBI7AT1encyOPIJajiyGNX7tgrRuWS65Oi11X9tdMYYS3YVUVz-pg3T_RgOTQmyll7Gye5nwDK0gQ7fbUsHGF6xvpnxwqRlsYy2CVIUyFqJ006i4hkyPkvDU99SEuXeuWY8pRKIqAd_v9_uxcK6IaleiF_wQD2092sjyMF-O9NdZGBIvkFQy8qROufee-kWwMOCyo57Z2_tvu1dYlywsbJzt6EnLCJPO7uG854jlYWhEA5-p65T-AAvgRxaR3ylJn-tazd2atCNOSwUeP4sF0Tdh66u-WrBEBrS2hbiTX01V3fOh5WPBgdODoGmqTtTn-fq5umQ/http%3A%2F%2Fwww.ci.uct.ac.za%2Fcg-2019-child-and-adolescent-health.

Solomon DH, Wobb J, Buttaro BA, Truant A, Soliman AM. Characterization of bacterial biofilms on tracheostomy tubes. Laryngoscope. 2009;119(8):1633–8.

South J, Fairfax P, Green E. Developing an assessment tool for evaluating community involvement. Health Expect. 2005;8(1):64–73.

StatsSA. GHS series volume VII: housing from a human settlement perspective. 2016. Available at: http://www.statssa.gov.za/?p=6429. Accessed 10 Dec 2021.

United Nations Human Settlements Programme (UN-HABITAT) Population living in slums (% of urban population) - South Africa. Available at: https://data.worldbank.org/indicator/EN.POP.SLUM.UR.ZS. Accessed 10 Dec 2021.

Van der Poel LA, Booth J, Argent A, van Dijk M, Zampoli M. Home ventilation in South African children: do socioeconomic factors matter? Pediatr Allergy Immunol Pulmonol. 2017;30(3):163–70. https://doi.org/10.1089/ped.2016.0727.

Westwood A, Stemming W. Long term health conditions in children: towards comprehensive care. Part Two, Child and adolescent health – leave no one behind South African Child Gauge 2019 CG2019- (5) Long term health conditions in children.pdf. 2019.

Leading a Nurse Practitioner-Designed Newborn Circumcision Clinic

Vivian W. Williams, Laura J. Wood, and Debra Lajoie

Introduction

Boston Children's Nurse Practitioner (NP)-Led Newborn Circumcision Clinic (NCC) is operationalized within the hospital's Department of Urology. The program offers newborn circumcision to infants not previously circumcised in the immediate newborn period. The model enables NPs to practice to the full extent of their education, expertise, and scope of practice. In the NCC, NPs assess, implement, and evaluate procedure-related care needs for infants and families. The creation of this novel NP-led clinic included the following components: (a) validation of unmet community and parent needs; (b) alignment with both state- and institutional-level credentialing and privileging requirements; (c) capture and integration of qualitative needs assessment data obtained through parent interviews; (d) internal value realization planning to understand the financial, operational, and patient-family experience impacts (Kibby et al. 2015); and (e) ongoing quality, safety, and experience assessments administered in surveys to patient families related to this model. At the time this NP-led, family-focused circumcision model was first conceptualized, there was also a growth in the design, adoption, and dissemination of innovative nurse-led models of care nationally as recognized by the AAN (Mason et al. 2015). Within Boston Children's pediatric healthcare delivery system, the organization had previously implemented and disseminated findings related to the impact of nurse practitioner-led clinics (Buxton et al. 2017). The NP NCC model further aligns with the organization's commitment to improving the

V. W. Williams (✉)
Department of Urology, Boston Children's Hospital, Boston, MA, USA
e-mail: Vivian.Williams@childrens.harvard.edu

L. J. Wood · D. Lajoie
Boston Children's Hospital, Boston, MA, USA

health of the community through equity, diversity, and inclusivity practices. Expanding access to care and the growth of advanced practice registered nurse (APRN) care models such as the NP NCC is consistent with this commitment.

Background Information

NCC Needs Assessment

Prior to the creation of the organization's Newborn Circumcision Clinic (NCC), the Department of Urology offered male newborn circumcision at age 1 year in the operating room, with a brief general anesthetic. Infants who had prolonged neonatal intensive care unit (NICU) stays, other minor medical issues at birth, and those who had penile anatomy identified at birth were considered to be inappropriate for clamp style circumcision and often left without an option for newborn circumcision unless treatment was deferred until the child was old enough to safely undergo a general anesthetic. The design of the NCC is similar to the Flinter and Bamrick (2017) model described as having been informed by the creation of innovative professional practice driven by a need to create a sustainable, affordable, and patient-family centric model that further served to advance professional practice.

The creation of this NP-led clinic was guided by the following goals: (a) to create a safe option for infants undergoing circumcision in the newborn period by eliminating the associated risks, costs, and child/family stressors associated with a surgical procedure coupled with a general anesthetic; (b) to develop a sustainable and replicable care delivery model, available to spread and scale regionally, nationally, and internationally; and (c) to further align this care delivery model with the quadruple aim to improve the patient experience of care—including quality and satisfaction, population health, and the per capita cost of health care (Feeley 2017). These drivers shaped the development of this model at a time when there were few similar programs available to reference.

Once we defined the populations we intended to serve, the next step focused on stakeholder identification and engagement. It was critical to identify parent, community, and interprofessional stakeholders to validate the proposed model. Key stakeholders included the following:

- Senior surgeon leaders from the Department of Urology.
- Senior nurse leaders spanning inpatient and ambulatory services.
- Marketing and communications colleagues to guide the development of clear and consistent internal and external messaging.
- Operations and facility experts were identified to define space, resource, and equipment requirements aligned through a detailed process mapping approach (see Fig. 1).
- Family members reflecting a wide range of socioeconomic backgrounds to ensure the clinic was developed to improve access for all the populations that we serve.

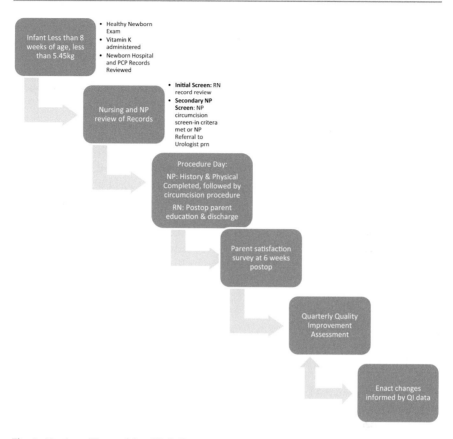

Fig. 1 Newborn Circumcision Clinic Processes

Both curriculum design experts and surgical faculty supported nurse practitioner skill development, working together to create a plan to assess and validate competencies and to develop policies, procedures, and family education materials. Information technology experts were enlisted to guide the development of standardized documentation templates used in the electronic health record. Quality improvement experts contributed to the creation of an outcome measurement plan. Additionally, finance colleagues collaborated to model projects costs, revenue, and reimbursement and to consider value realization more broadly.

A measurement plan was developed to obtain data from multiple sources including the following:

- Parent perspectives related to their experience, satisfaction, and recommendations.
- NP skill and competency validation.
- Quantitative measures to confirm quality and safety-focused outcomes.

When the program was initially designed, there was little guidance available describing nurse practitioner transition to practice in relationship to this NP-led care model. The American Academy of Pediatrics (AAP) Taskforce on

Circumcision (2012) recommended circumcision be performed by trained and competent practitioners. The AAP taskforce reinforced the importance of appropriate patient selection including ensuring infants are otherwise healthy and in a stable healthy state—all while acknowledging that significant acute complications are rare. Furthermore, the taskforce underscored the importance of patient and family education materials to assist parents with decision-making and treatment considerations (AAP Taskforce on Circumcision 2012).

Evidence reviewed provided direction to support the development of this care delivery model. Horowitz and Gershbein (2001) reviewed newborn circumcisions performed during a 2-year period and found that Gomco clamp circumcision beyond 3 months of age had substantial morbidity. A retrospective review of males undergoing newborn circumcision over a 2-year period found that infants weighing more than 5.1 kg identified a potential higher risk for bleeding and long-term complications from circumcision (Kim et al. 2019). Additionally, Gerber et al. (2019) reviewed circumcisions performed by an advanced practice provider (NP or Physician Assistant) versus circumcisions performed by a pediatric urologist, finding no difference in clinical outcomes for children either over or under 4.5 kg. The study recommended further evaluation of age and weight parameters. The study authors also noted a significant difference in the need for circumcision revision in older versus younger children, with children greater than 30 days of age requiring revision more often, supporting the potential benefit of access to clinics such as the NCC in the first month of life.

Incomplete neonatal circumcision is a common problem often requiring circumcision revision under a general anesthetic when the child is 1 year or older (Task Force on Circumcision 2012). Boston Children's Department of Urology performs approximately 500 circumcision revisions annually for children referred regionally, highlighting the scope and burden of this problem. Kokorowski et al. (2013) found the incidence of circumcision revision to be increasing by 119% at free standing children's hospitals between 2004 and 2009. This work was used to guide the selection of a target population of newborns who could safely have circumcisions performed in the NP clinic setting instead of the operating room with general anesthesia.

Based upon our expertise performing circumcision in the newborn period, we anticipated an opportunity to improve the outcomes of newborn circumcision through a reduction in circumcision revision rates both within our organization and well beyond. Within our healthcare delivery organization and nationally, we learned from colleagues that NP-led clinics were successfully and safely providing care in a wide range of practice settings. Together with a decade of national findings based upon acute, critical care, primary care service delivery further substantiated the value of advanced practice providers in patient care management, care continuity, satisfaction, and safe, high-quality care delivery (Kleinpell et al. 2019; Liu et al. 2020).

Target Population and Setting

Boston Children's Hospital, Boston, Massachusetts, is a quaternary care center and teaching hospital with 454 licensed inpatient beds, 4 satellite campuses, and 264 specialized clinical programs. Boston Children's Department of Urology is currently ranked as the number one pediatric urology department by US News and World Report (2021). Regionally distributed satellite settings and a community health center enable improved access to care in support of a broad range of families and communities. Initially, the NCC was housed in the Boston main campus and has since moved to the satellite facility in Waltham, MA, accessible via public transportation. The clinic takes place within a procedural suite that is part of the Department of Urology ambulatory clinic.

Care was taken to assure the proper selection of patients who could safely benefit from the NP-led care model. The NCC is designed for otherwise healthy newborns less than 8 weeks of age and less than 12 lb (5.5 kg). Exclusion criteria for the NCC include the following:

- Medically unstable or ill infants, with evidence of infection or skin rashes.
- A family history of bleeding anomalies.
- The presence of congenital anomalies of the penis.

In a retrospective cohort study of 234 patients in the NCC, Williams et al. (2020) found that the majority of patients served were white ($n = 60$; 25.6%) and 15.4% ($n = 36$) were Hispanic/Latino ethnicity. Patients requesting care in the NCC have not had a circumcision in the newborn period. The most common reason for referral to the NCC was concern for anatomical anomaly of the penis (53.8%), parental preference (15.4%), or other comorbidities (14.5%) (Williams et al. 2020). Not all infants who presented to the NCC met the screening criteria to be treated in this setting.

Designing and Implementing the NCC

When the NP-led NCC was initially conceptualized, Massachusetts' state Nurse Practitioner practice regulations did not allow independent prescribing authority and required physician supervision within a collaborative agreement (KFF 2015). The NCC was initially designed to reflect this model of NP care delivery. As policy advocacy continued, Massachusetts NPs were granted Full Practice Authority on January 1, 2021, as recommended by *The Future of Nursing: Leading Change, Advancing Health* (Institute of Medicine 2011). Effective September 3, 2021, Certified Nurse Practitioners (CNPs) as well as Certified Registered Nurse Anesthetists (CRNA) with a minimum of 2 years of supervised practice may engage in prescriptive practice without supervision upon submission of an attestation to the Board of Registration in Nursing of completion of a minimum of 2 years of supervised practice by a Qualified Healthcare Professional (244 CMR 4.0: Advanced Practice Registered Nursing).

Initially, our model was a nurse practitioner-led, physician supervised clinic, aligning with regulatory guidelines; however, this model evolved to a NP-led, physician supported clinic, consistent with the organization's team-based care practices supporting interprofessional collaboration and professional practice while maintaining fidelity to each team member's privileges. This philosophy was reflected by our early initial development of the physician-supported care model which we then transformed to a collaborative, co-managed model, now beginning to emerge in the literature (Norful et al. 2019). In January 2021, Massachusetts expanded the NP's scope of practice to improve timely patient access to high-quality care when *An Act promoting a resilient health care system that puts patients first* ((MA Bill S.2984, 191st (2019-2020)) was signed into law.

A multidisciplinary committee was formed comprised of senior nursing and hospital leaders, Department of Urology leaders, NPs, RNs, and an operations team spanning finance and facilities. We conducted a literature review regarding existing NP-led procedural clinics and found a paucity of literature. That said, the literature supported the fact that newborn clamp style circumcision is well tolerated by infants and a relatively low-risk procedure with few major complications (Task Force on Circumcision 2012). We reached out to hospitals nationally and identified one existing NP-led circumcision clinic at another nationally ranked children's hospital. Our team completed a site visit to observe their practice and better understand the processes developed by their team. Early key stakeholder investment was noted as critical to the success of developing both clinical and reimbursement models. We recognized the important influence of stakeholders with significant institutional power and influence would have in the creation and success of innovative practice. It was critical to have these stakeholders involved with the planning process. Stakeholder alignment requires clear delineation of the mission, program drivers, current practice landscape, and program structure (Flinter and Bamrick 2017).

Through proactive planning, including a comprehensive literature review, specific criteria were established to identify program inclusion criteria. Next, a training program was jointly developed by urologists, anesthesiologists, and NPs to establish key competencies required for the NP to be privileged to administer a local penile block and to perform circumcision. Procedural guidelines were collaboratively established.

Theoretical Framework

Two theoretical frameworks guided the initial development of the Boston Children's NCC, the Institute for Healthcare Improvement (IHI) *Triple Aim Framework* (2021), and The Institute of Medicine *Future of Nursing Report* (2010). This framework functions in alignment with the United States National Quality Standards (NQS) (Ahrq.gov 2011) which focuses on six priorities to advance the IHI aims including (1) reducing harm in the delivery of health care; (2) engaging the patient and families as partners in care; (3) providing effective communication and care coordination; (4) promoting the most effective treatment and prevention practices; (5)

partnering with communities to improve health; and (6) developing and implementing new healthcare delivery models to achieve affordable, equitable, quality care (Institute of Medicine 2011).

The Institute of Medicine (IOM) *Future of Nursing Report*, first released in 2010, also guided the development of the NCC (Institute of Medicine 2011). The report release, aligned with the enactment of the Affordable Care Act (IOM 2010), provided the vision for healthcare system transformation including improving accessibility to diverse populations, improving outcomes, focusing on health promotion while managing disease, and creating and implementing a model of interprofessional collaboration and coordination of care. Four key recommendations were made including that nurses should:

- Practice to the full extent of their education and training including removing systematic and regulatory barriers including scope of practice limitations.
- Achieve higher levels of education and training through an improved education system that promotes seamless academic progression.
- Be full partners with physicians and other healthcare professionals, in redesigning US health care, including having a voice in policy development.
- Improve the effectiveness of workforce planning and policy-making require better data collection and an improved information infrastructure so that new care models and policy decisions are guided by the data and best practices evidence (IOM 2010).

While the key intent of the IOM Future of Nursing Report (2010) was to strengthen the capacity, education, and critical role of the nursing workforce, moving forward, future changes to our model integrate the guidance of the newly released *Future of Nursing Report (2020–2030): Charting a Path to Achieve Health Equity* (National Academy of Sciences, Engineering, and Medicine 2021). The framework of the *Future of Nursing Report (2020–2030)* highlights the "importance of nurses as key players in achieving health equity in the United States and globally…working within and across disciplines." The current COVID-19 pandemic has highlighted systematic, disproportionate healthcare inequities associated with multiple etiologic factors including bias, racism, poverty, and the other social determinants of health that threaten the health of both individuals and communities (National Academy of Sciences, Engineering, and Medicine 2021). Key recommendations for nursing include increasing the "size, distribution, diversity, and educational preparation of the nursing workforce" (National Academy of Sciences, Engineering, and Medicine 2021, p. 6). Nationally, more work is required to remove scope of practice restrictions and to design better payment models which recognize care provided by nurse practitioners and RNs. Another recommendation is to expand nursing education to include an additional focus on community and population health learning experiences, thereby expanding an understanding of health equity and improving outcomes and access to care (National Academy of Sciences, Engineering, and Medicine 2021).

To meet these goals, new care delivery models will be required as well as additional infrastructure to expand access to publicly available broadband Internet and telehealth capabilities within diverse community settings to expand universal access. The report also recognized the impact of the current pandemic and social unrest on nursing and the healthcare workforce, recommending more attention be paid to the importance of the care environment on providers' health and well-being (National Academy of Sciences, Engineering, and Medicine 2021), aligning with the IHI Quadruple Aim (Feeley 2017). The IHI Quadruple Aim added a fourth aim which focused on improving the experience of providing care (Sikka et al. 2015). At the core of this revised model is that "all members of the healthcare workforce have a sense of accomplishment and meaning in their contributions" (Sikka et al. 2015, p. 1). In response, our clinic has already begun to address these needs through expansion of our clinic sites to improve access and reduce costs to meet the needs of more communities, including those with less historical access to services. The NCC is also aligned with the Edge Runner initiative developed by the American Academy of Nursing (2011) which "recognizes nurse-designed models of care and interventions that impact cost, improve healthcare quality and enhance consumer satisfaction" in order to lead the way to transform the health system.

Our current model of co-managed care is critical to the successful evolution of the NCC, as it aligns with the high reliability and regulatory frameworks used to guide the development of this clinic (Joint Commission for Transforming Health Care 2020). Our strategies to align clinical co-management of care assure that processes are in place to promote and maintain safe, cost-effective care and improve access. Program-based NPs and urologists routinely collaborate with one another. Through this model, patients and their families have expanded access to high-quality, safe, and culturally sensitive care as validated through ongoing outcome measurement.

Description of the NCC

Organizational Components

A NP is the lead clinical provider within the NCC. The lead clinical NP was a key driver of this care model, actively developing the vision for the clinic in partnership with the Department of Urology physician leaders and senior hospital leaders, creating the policy and procedures, clinic flow, definitive roles within the clinic, screening process, and patient and family educational information. The NP performs the histories, physical examinations, and circumcision procedure within the NCC. Members of the care team include a pediatric urologist, NP, registered nurse (RN) for patient screening, procedural support, discharge education, and post-procedural monitoring, and a clinical assistant to assess vital signs and provide comfort care. The clinic relies upon the Department of Urology patient experience representatives (PERs) who field family phone calls, RNs who screen patients, pharmacists who supply medications and provide medication counseling as needed, and sterile processing department (SPD) technicians for Gomco device sterilization coordination. The clinic performs procedures weekly but is constantly screening patients to identify patients who may be future candidates for the NP-led NCC.

Parent calls inquiring about a newborn circumcision are initially managed by the patient experience representatives (PERs) who capture the initial demographic information. If infants are less than 8 weeks and less than 5.45 kg (12 lb), they are triaged to an RN who further assesses the patient for any potential safety concerns and the rationale for needing the circumcision. The RN screening assessment includes data collection related to patient age, weight, primary care physician, rationale for the need for circumcision, the presence of a diaper rash, known penile anomaly, any known medical issues including a history of bleeding disorders in the family, the primary care physician's name, and a COVID screen. If the rationale for circumcision is concern for penile anatomic anomaly, the patient is scheduled for a separate visit with a pediatric urologist to ensure the anatomy is suitable for Gomco circumcision. Simultaneously, a PER will send a query to the family asking them to forward the patient's birth records, evidence of administration of Vitamin K, and primary care provider (PCP) records. These records are reviewed by both the RN and the NP to assess for any safety concerns which may preclude the patient from having a circumcision performed safely in the NCC. Both the screening process and the record review are documented in the electronic health record. Once records are reviewed, the patient is scheduled for the procedure. If a medical concern is noted, the NP will consult with the appropriate specialist to assess whether the patient meets the criteria for circumcision by either a NP in the NCC or with a urologist in the operating room.

On the day of the procedure, the patient presents to clinic, and vital signs are obtained. The NP completes a full history and physical and obtains procedural consent from the patient's guardian(s). The procedure, administration of a paramedian penile block, and the Gomco circumcision then take place. The median length of the procedure is 20 min, which includes a 10-min clamp time (Williams et al. 2020). After the procedure, the patient is recovered for 1 h. During this time, postprocedural vital signs are obtained, nursing reviews home discharge education regarding care of the patient, and the infant's penis is evaluated prior to discharge to ensure there is no post-procedural bleeding prior to discharge. Follow-up takes place on an as needed basis. We have the ability to integrate telehealth visits, when appropriate, to assess the wound appearance and healing if there are postoperative questions or concerns. The integration of technology supports our patients and families by improving timely care access, reducing travel time, which is often disruptive to the entire family, and by eliminated additional expenses including lost work time.

Clinic supplies required include medications, procedural and post-procedural supplies. Medications include acetaminophen liquid, 24% oral sucrose, topical bacitracin, and 0.5% lidocaine. Oral syringes for oral medications are utilized, as well as a 5/8 in., 27 gauge needle for lidocaine administration. Procedural supplies include sterile gloves, a circumstraint or patient immobilizer, circumcision tray containing curved and straight hemostats, probe, scissors, forceps, sterile drape, fenestrated drape, bacitracin, sterile 4 × 4 gauze, and circumstraint straps. Additional procedural supplies include the Gomco clamps in (sizes 1.1, 1.3, 1.45, 1.6, and 2.1), a #15 blade, Surgilube, chlorhexidine prep swabs, and a skin marker. Post-procedural supplies include bacitracin, Surgilube, and a diaper. We also utilize pacifiers and warm swaddling blankets as non-pharmaceutical comfort measures.

Services Components of the Service Model

The Boston Children's Nursing Interprofessional Practice model provides the framework to guide how nurses practice, communicate, and develop professionally (Hoffart and Woods 1996). The patient and family are always a central focus of our care, aligning with a recognition of patients and families as our partners in care (Kuo et al. 2011). Our practice is defined by our commitment to quality and safety, leadership, cultivation of a healthy work environment, and evidence-based practice. Our professional practice model is guided through an interprofessional team collaboration philosophy and process. This assures the voices of patients, families, nurses, and interprofessional colleagues are heard through their participation within key committees and practice councils.

Our designation as an American Nurses Credentialing Center (ANCC) Magnet® designated organization confirms the values that guide our professional practice, underscoring the importance of a culture of collaboration and excellence. The Synergy Model of Patient Care developed by the American Association of Critical-Care Nurses (AACN 2000) and relationship-based care are the two conceptual models underpinning our Boston Children's nursing and intraprofessional Practice Model (PPM). The core concept of the AACN Synergy Model "…is that the needs or characteristics of patients and families influence and drive the characteristics or competencies of nurses…" (p. 1). The Synergy Model stresses the importance of alignment between patient and family needs with the skills and competency of each nurse. Transformational leadership and attention to improving the health of the work environment promote ethical care as well as caring practices and healing relationships (ANCC 2020). Boston Children's Nursing/Intraprofessional PPM provides a framework to guide how nurses and team members practice, communicate, and develop professionally.

Description of the Services Provided

The NCC provides newborn clamp-style circumcision to male infants who have not had a circumcision in the newborn period. This is a procedure performed on an outpatient basis with a local anesthetic thus eliminating the need for a general anesthetic. Minimizing pain and distress in neonatal circumcision is a priority to providing patient-centered care in our clinic; our standard practice is the implementation of a comprehensive, multi-model evidence-based circumcision pain control plan, the dorsal penile nerve block blunt behavioral and physiological pain response. During the procedure, the circulating nurse is attentive to proactively mitigating pain, delivering holistic comfort measures utilized including swaddling with warm blankets, providing pacifiers with sucrose, as well as medications for pain management. Swaddling promotes self-regulation assisting in modulating physical response; sucrose produces analgesia through endogenous opioid and non-opioid pathways; sucking has a synergistic response with the sucrose which provides additional soothing (Geyer et al. 2002). Patients must be otherwise healthy, less than 8 weeks of age and 12 lb, and have penile anatomy suitable for clamp-style circumcision.

Setting of the Model/Wherein Services Provided

The NCC was initially housed within the Department of Urology at Boston Children's Hospital. We performed the circumcisions within our Procedural Room in the Urodynamics Suite. This space contains multiple procedure rooms, multiple patient examination rooms, and a patient waiting area. As we piloted this clinic, initially, we chose the Boston Children's Hospital main campus with immediate access to multiple operating rooms and emergency personnel in the event of a medical or surgical emergency related to the circumcision.

Patients are first evaluated with a history and physical in the examination rooms and then taken to the procedure rooms for the circumcision. During the circumcision, the family of the patient waits in the waiting room. Once the procedure is complete, the child and family remain in a private examination room, while postprocedure assessments are completed and to facilitate feeding and comfort care during the initial recovery. A final physical examination takes place in this space 1 h after the procedure, and discharge to home most often follows.

After 4 years of hosting the NCC at the primary campus in Boston, we moved the clinic to a suburban satellite location. The clinic was once again housed within the Department of Urology clinic space. The suburban clinical space contains a procedural room and several examination rooms similar to the hospital clinic setting and also contains several operating rooms which could be utilized in the event of a surgical emergency. Moving the NCC to a satellite setting was consistent with organization goal to support less complex procedures being provided in community settings, providing more convenient access for families. Both Boston and other satellite settings have emergency responders, or a code team, available for acute issues. We closely monitored outcomes to assure the procedure was safe as we slowly expanded services incorporating new locations to provide services in alignment with our Enterprise Commitment to High Reliability (Joint Commission for Transforming Healthcare 2020).

Team Member's Roles and Responsibilities

In addition to the providers who perform circumcision, the NCC team is comprised of diverse team members including Patient Experience Representatives (PERS), Clinical Assistants (CAs), Registered Nurses (RNs) in procedural, post-procedural, lead and chart review roles, and a quality improvement (QI) consultant.

Role	Responsibility
Patient experience representative (PER)	Front desk staff
	Obtains medical records, scheduling
Clinical assistant (CA)	Maintains supplies, performs vital signs, soothes patient during procedure
Registered nurse (RN)	Completes patient assessments, administers medications, performs RN role during circumcision, completes family education, performs chart reviews
Quality improvement consultant (QIC)	Performs quality improvement assessments. Provides project management to guide ongoing improvement efforts

The NP is designated as the team leader and coordinator, overseeing the NCC clinic. In this role, the NP creates and refines processes for patient care in collaboration with the operations team. The NP develops policies, procedural guidelines, family educational materials, and opportunities for staff education in collaboration with the interprofessional clinical and leadership teams. Furthermore, the NP collaborates with the quality improvement consultant to identify metrics to monitor satisfaction, safety, and outcomes; develop measurement tools; analyze the data; and monitor quality and satisfaction. In this role, the NP provides a final pre-procedure patient chart reviews after the RN performs an initial review to ensure patients meet the clinical inclusion criteria to maintain appropriate patient selection.

The NP facilitates timely communication with the covering urologist, reviewing the clinical history of patients prior to each NCC clinic, and to ensure the physician has the necessary baseline clinical knowledge of each patient should a physician intervention be required. The NP completes a pre-op history and physical on the day of the circumcision, obtains the procedural consent, and performs the circumcision, ensuring continuity of care. The same NP then performs the post-procedural check and signs off on safe discharge for each patient. The NP clinic note dictation and billing codes for the procedure are then completed by this same NP.

All NPs providing care in the NCC have competencies previously validated through both an initial onboarding process and via ongoing clinical evaluations. The NP must also have experience in complex patient care and care of the newborn, such that they are qualified to perform an adequate assessment of complex patient histories and respond appropriately to an intra-procedural emergency. National Standards for Core NP Competencies created in 2017 by the National Organization of Nurse Practitioner Faculties focus on scientific foundations, quality, practice inquiry, technology and information literacy, health delivery systems, ethics, and independent practice competencies (Thomas et al. 2017). While there are no national standards for competency for Pediatric Urology Nurse Practitioners, Quallich et al. (2015) suggested 24 core competencies for Adult Urology Nurse Practitioners which complement core NP competencies and blend medical and nursing components of this role. The competencies created specific to the NP role within the NCC are assessed and maintained through ongoing educational programs as well as through simulation experiences, including emergency response simulations.

Competency validation is maintained through the credentialing and privileging process. Practice privileges and guidelines for Boston Children's NPs are requested in writing, reviewed and signed by the collaborating physician, chief of service, nursing director, and the System Chief Nursing Officer. The Credentials Committee reviews the privileges requested by NPs, as submitted to the Committee by the system chief nursing officer. This information is then forwarded to Medical Staff Executive Committee, comprised of all physician chiefs and the system chief nursing officer. Once approved, all recommendations for privileges are submitted to the Board of Trustees who provide final approval of privileges.

A pediatric urologist collaborated with the NP to initially develop and implement the NCC. A lead physician serves as the physician director of the clinic. The physician director in turn assigns a designated pediatric urologist to the clinic, who has received a clinical handoff including the history of each patient having a circumcision during their assigned clinic time. This pediatric urologist is then immediately available on site when the circumcisions are being performed if consultation and/or intervention is requested at the discretion of the NP. Pediatric urologists are also fully integrated with NCC quality improvement efforts, collaboratively identifying opportunities for improvement and growth, including increasing access to traditionally underserved communities. We utilize case reviews in morbidity and mortality conferences to review practices and jointly review all safety event reports.

Methods of Evaluation

Review of parent satisfaction surveys is key to enhancing patient experience and outcomes. Originally, these satisfaction surveys were printed and mailed to families. Due to the poor response rate experienced by so many organizations including our own, we transitioned to an electronic version which provided a far clearer understanding of parent experiences and perceptions, resulting in key changes to patient care delivery practices. Embracing patients and families as partners in care is a core value within the organization and the Department of Urology. Patient satisfaction assessments query demographics, referral information, overall satisfaction, satisfaction with post-procedural education, the patient's post-procedural pain, satisfaction with the appearance of the circumcision site, and courtesy and respect demonstrated by the providers. We also include open-ended questions regarding parental commentary and suggestions for improvements to the overall experience. The surveys are sent out 6 weeks after the circumcision procedure, which allows for some time for the healing process to occur. The quality improvement team meets quarterly to trend outcomes and identify and to develop interventions or changes based upon the data.

A retrospective cohort study of the NCC was performed in 2020, which assessed patient satisfaction, clinical outcomes, and cost impact (Williams et al. 2020). This study provided a foundational understanding of both the demographics of the children/families that we serve and patient outcomes. This information gave merit to the concepts and practices within the NCC. This study found that the NCC has a high level of family satisfaction, few adverse outcomes, and a cost benefit as compared to traditional circumcision procedures completed within an operative setting with general anesthesia (Williams et al. 2020). Specific clinical outcomes from our retrospective study revealed that two infants (0.9%) of our cohort had bleeding events post-procedurally requiring a visit to the Emergency Department for application of a pressure dressing (Williams et al. 2020). No documented events were noted in 95.6% of our cohort at the follow-up visit, with penile adhesions noted as the most common concern. Two patients (0.9%) required circumcision revision in the operating room. We are committed to an ongoing program of research and quality improvement to continue to understand and further strengthen clinical outcomes informed through our quality improvement practices.

Challenges and Opportunities

Challenges faced in the development and implementation of this novel NP-led model were identified and addressed by the investment of key stakeholders since the program's inception in 2016. Critical to the success of this model was evidence that performance of a newborn male circumcision was within NP scope of practice within the state of Massachusetts (KFF 2015). Focusing on collaborative practice supported greater access to care by enabling pediatric urologists to focus on patients with more complex care needs.

Significant variation related to NP scope of practice continues to exist throughout the United States (Mark and Patel 2019). Furthermore, privileging and credentialing standards vary from institution to institution. For these reasons, our initial proposal to create the NCC clearly stated the NP performing the procedure would be required to have completed a defined period of practice and demonstrated specific skills prior to being privileged to perform male infant circumcision.

Reimbursement for services rendered is based upon professional practice statutes within Massachusetts and existing institution-specific payor contracts. It is required that the pediatric urologist be on site during the patient's visit and immediately available to provide assistance and direction. Pediatric urologists are physically present within the Urology Clinic and are briefed regarding patients undergoing procedures in the NP circumcision clinic, thus prepared to intervene in a timely manner should the patient's condition warrant emergency medical attention.

Family Feedback Guides Service Delivery Adjustments

Upon initial review of satisfaction data post-inception of the NCC, it was clear there was a lack of demographic data being collected at the point of service. These data are key to better understand the extent to which care provided is equitable and of high quality. The core NCC team worked with operational leaders to enhance education of staff regarding collection of demographic data, including support for appropriate ways to ask specific demographic questions and the importance of collecting this data. This intervention assisted to increase data collection at the point of service.

Open-ended questions in our patient satisfaction survey allowed for responders to comment on various improvement opportunities, including some not previously considered by the NCC team. Parents commented on the ability to hear babies cry during the procedure. Because of this, we moved the location of the procedure room to a treatment room further separated from the family waiting room. Furthermore, we reassessed sound proofing of the clinic space with our engineering team and obtained white noise machines for use in examination rooms and patient waiting areas.

Parents also indicated in the satisfaction survey that they desired a private space for breastfeeding and recovery after the procedure. Patients recovering in the waiting room and shared patient spaces contributed to anxiety for other parents and additionally limited privacy. We created private recovery areas where parents could breastfeed and soothe their infant in a quiet setting. This early work allowed us to quickly resume care when appropriate during the COVID-19 pandemic while also providing needed social distancing consistent with pandemic-related infection control policies.

Parents desired a centralized location to obtain post-procedure education instructions regarding home care and expectations following the procedure. In addition to printed materials made available post-procedure, a website is currently being created to provide direct access to parent education materials in a centralized location. We also email home care instructions to parents upon request for those families cared for in the NCC. We also began to include the Massachusetts Department of Public Health "All Babies Cry" fact sheet for parents of infants which provides tips on how to soothe a crying infant (Massachusetts Health Promotion Clearinghouse 2015). It became clear that many new parents were seeking additional basic infant care educational materials. This content is now also made available to prepare families for how infants may respond to a procedure with a small measure of discomfort when the block is applied and while the surgical area heals. Finally, a tailored patient education tool was developed "A Photographic Guide to Healing after Newborn Circumcision" (Williams et al. 2019). This Atlas was modeled after "A Photographic Guide to Healing after Surgical Circumcision" created by Dr. Caleb Nelson and Rosemary Grant, RN in 2011, which was found to decrease emergency room visits and parent phone calls after surgical circumcision (Nelson et al. 2012). The Atlas contains photos of several patient's circumcisions healing over 21 days to better manage expectations regarding the healing process after circumcision and help parents to understand when they should call the clinic staff with concerns.

Follow-up in-person visits were initially performed 1 week following the circumcision. This in-person visit was transitioned to a telehealth visit, then to a phone call, and now changed to an as needed visit. Our initial research informed this transition by providing outcome data regarding adverse events and unplanned office visits (Williams et al. 2020).

Transitioning the NCC from the Boston location to a satellite setting was carefully contemplated so that safety was balanced with the benefits of this location change. The relocation considerations included continued public transit access, free parking, increased access to specialized urologic facilities, and continued immediate access to an emergency response team as well as an operating room.

Lessons Learned

Feasibility planning and implementation of the NCC were based upon the principles of holistic care of the infant and family, interprofessional collaboration, and the commitment to research and clinical inquiry.

Our holistic approach differentiates the NCC from similar models. As a NP-led clinic, basic concepts of infant comfort and soothing, family-centered support for young and first-time parents, equitable access to care, and utilizing of holistic comfort care measures including sugar water, warm blankets, pacifiers, and lullabies during the procedure itself are unique aspects of the program's child and family-focused care. Furthermore, our parent satisfaction feedback led to improved recovery practices including the provision of private spaces for soothing infants, support of post-procedure breastfeeding, the use of noise cancelling machines, installation of additional sound proofing, and thoughtful placement of recovering patients.

Clinical team members utilize the 1-h recovery time to perform parent education, providing unique teaching materials specifically created for our patient population. Recognizing that for many families English is not their primary language, we partner with our Interpreter Services team to ensure that skilled resources are available to provide interpretation services in person or via tele-interpreter services as needed. Translated materials in a wide range of languages include consents, family education, and email communications—all to assure that care is provided in a fashion consistent with a family's preferred language. Home care sheets for circumcision care, Massachusetts Department of Public Health "All Babies Cry" fact sheet for parents of infants (Massachusetts Health Promotion Clearinghouse 2015), and *Photographic Atlas of Healing after Newborn Circumcision* are integrated within all nurse-led teachings. These resources are also available in several different languages. Finally, we utilize the enterprise practices of Teach-Back for educating families to ensure what is taught is understood (www.ahrq.gov 2015).

Interdisciplinary collaboration between nurses, physicians, support staff, and hospital leaders remains a key component of success of the NCC. From the inception of this clinic, success was contingent upon alignment with Massachusetts nursing scope of practice criteria and engagement with key organizational stakeholders throughout the organization in supporting this NP-led model. The Boston Children's NCC practice model relies upon collaboration of the NP and physician to mutually confirm appropriate patient selection for the procedure and ensure timely surgeon access in the event of unexpected outcomes or emergencies.

As an ANCC Magnet designated institution, the organization has made the commitment to integrate research and inquiry into clinical and operational practices and processes (American Nurses Credentialing Center Magnet Recognition Program 2017, p. 59). The organization's nursing science fellowship (NSF) model pairs nurse researchers with clinical nurses to develop programs of inquiry. This program has proved to be a key enabler to prepare early career RNs and APRNs to integrate inquiry into practice. The NSF has inspired innovation and inquiry, leading to the creation of nurse-led and NP-led models of practice. It has also strengthened the ability of frontline nurses to engage in clinical inquiry to solve professional practice challenges seen in their practice (Connor et al. 2020). Within the NSF, dedicated mentors guide nursing science fellows via didactic content about clinic inquiry and regularly scheduled mentorship sessions. Fellows then frame a clinical inquiry question and create a scholarly project.

Future Implications for Clinical Practice and Research

Future plans for the NCC include expansion to additional satellite locations and expanded hours of operation. Ongoing education, training, and credentialing of NPs to provide this service will continue. Collaboration with other specialties regarding the translation of full practice authority within a team-based care delivery model is ongoing. In order to provide services with increased frequency and in additional satellite locations, continuous training of RNs and support staff is required. Support for inquiries from other disciplines to have shadow experiences within the NCC to observe key team practices is ongoing. Efforts to facilitate similar models are currently being developed and implemented in other specialty practices.

Our research has identified the need to capture and benchmark patient/family satisfaction, assess the impact and clinical outcomes associated with the program, and to capture the cost savings and less tangible value realization associated with this model (Williams et al. 2020). Due to a paucity of research regarding clinical outcomes associated with male newborn circumcision, there is an opportunity to perform further research to better understand the longitudinal clinical outcomes of patients cared for by NPs.

Conclusion

The NP-Led Newborn Circumcision Clinic at Boston Children's Hospital offers male newborn circumcision to infants not circumcised in the immediate newborn period. Nurse practitioners are the primary providers of this service, contributing organizational leadership related to policy and procedure development, evaluation of care, and ongoing quality improvement and research. The NCC's practices align with the American Academy of Nursing (AAN) Edge Runner models of care which optimize the health needs of diverse populations through nurse-led practices. Based upon the collective needs of infants served in the NCC, the framework of care is based upon health that is holistically defined, individualized, family- and community-centric, and relationship-based, a shift from episodic individual care toward improved access and nurse-led practice innovations. This shift in the model of care allows for broadening traditional views of health to include a more responsive, holistic approach to patient-centered care (Mason et al. 2015). Our model will continue to evolve to reflect lessons learned during the COVID-19 pandemic, further expanding our commitment to healthcare equity as a distinguishing characteristic of nurse-led care delivery practices.

Useful Resources

Websites

1. Boston Children's Hospital Department of Urology Website: Homepage for Boston Children's Hospital Department of Urology which outlines service provided and areas of speciality within the field of pediatric urology, staff members, research, and innovation https://www.childrenshospital.org/centers-and-services/departments/urology
2. A Photographic Guide to Healing After Newborn Circumcision & A Photographic Guide to Healing After Surgical Circumcision: Ordering link for Boston Children's Hospital Surgical and Newborn Atlas of Healing https://bch.orders.com/store/catalog/01-07201988-Brochures
3. Massachusetts Department of Public Health "All Babies Cry" Fact Sheet: Fact sheet for parents offering tips for soothing crying infants https://massclearinghouse.ehs.state.ma.us/PROG-INJPREV/SB3101kit.html
4. Pediatric Urology Nurses and Specialists Group: Website for a professional organization dedicated to improving the care of pediatric urology patients through education, research, and evidence based practice https://punsonline.org/

Social media

5. Boston Children's Hospital Department of Urology Facebook Page: https://Facebook.com/BostonChildrensHospitalDepartmentofUrology
6. Boston Children's Hospital Department of Urology Twitter: https://twitter.com/bch_urology

Acknowledgments The authors wish to acknowledge Dr. Carlos Estrada, Dr. Alan B. Retik, Rosemary H. Grant RN, CPN, Karen Conwell, MSN, RN, CPNP, Lynne Hancock, DNP, RN, NE-BC, Herminia Shermont, MSN, RN, NE-BC, Patricia Pratt, BSN, MA, CPHQ, CPN, Julie Campbell, Boston Children's Hospital Urology and Urodynamics Nursing Staff, and Phillip Main.

References

Ahrq.gov. About the National Quality Strategy | Agency for Health Research and Quality. 2011. https://www.ahrq.gov/workingforquality/about/index.html.
American Academy of Nursing. Edge runners—American Academy of Nursing Main Site. 2011. Aannet.org. https://www.aannet.org/initiatives/edge-runners.
American Academy of Pediatrics Task Force on Circumcision. 2012. Male Circumcision. PEDIATRICS, [online] 130(3), pp.e756–e785. https://doi.org/10.1542/peds.2012-1990.
American Association of Critical-Care Nurses. The AACN Synergy Model for patient care basic information about the AACN Synergy Model for patient care assumptions guiding the AACN

Synergy Model for patient care. 2000. https://www.aacn.org/~/media/aacn-website/nursing-excellence/standards/aacnsynergymodelforpatientcare.pdf?la=en.

American Nurses Credentialing Center. About Magnet. ANA. 2020. https://www.nursingworld.org/organizational-programs/magnet/about-magnet/.

American Nurses Credentialing Center. Magnet Recognition Program. 2019 magnet application manual. Silver Spring: American Nurses Credentialing Centre; 2017.

Bill S.2984 191st. An act promoting a resilient health care system that puts patients first, Bill S.2984, 191st; 2019-2020.

Buxton K, Morgan A, Rogers J. Nurse practitioner lead pediatric baclofen pump program: impact on safety and quality of care. J Neurosci Nurs. 2017;49(5):324–9.

CMR 4.0 (n.d.), Bill S.2984 191st (2019-2020).

Connor JA, Mott S, DeGrazia M, Lajoie D, Dwyer P, Reed MP, Porter C, Hickey PA. Nursing science fellowship at Boston Children's Hospital. Appl Nurs Res. 2020;55:151292.

Engineering and Medicine National Academy of Medicine Committee National Academies of Sciences. FUTURE OF NURSING 2020–2030: charting a path to achieve health equity. Washington, DC: National Academies Press; 2021.

Feeley D. The triple aim or the quadruple aim? Four points to help set your strategy. 2017. Ihi.org. http://www.ihi.org/communities/blogs/the-triple-aim-or-the-quadruple-aim-four-points-to-help-set-your-strategy.

Flinter M, Bamrick K. Training the next generation: residency and fellowship programs for nurse practitioners in Community Health Centers. 2017. www.weitzmaninstitute.org. https://www.weitzmaninstitute.org/NPResidencyBook. Accessed 19 Sep 2021.

Gerber J, Borden A, Broda J, Koelewyn S, Balasubramanian A, Tu D, Koh C, Austin P, Roth D, Seth A. Evaluating clinical outcomes of an advanced practice provider-led newborn circumcision clinic. Urology. 2019;127:97–101. https://www.sciencedirect.com/science/article/abs/pii/S0090429519302067. Accessed 9 Sep 2021.

Geyer J, Ellsbury D, Kleiber C, Litwiller D, Hinton A, Yankowitz J. An evidence-based multidisciplinary protocol for neonatal circumcision pain management. J Obstet Gynecol Neonatal Nurs. 2002;31(4):403–10.

Hoffart N, Woods CQ. Elements of a nursing professional practice model. J Prof Nurs. 1996;12(6):354–64.

Horowitz M, Gershbein A. Gomco circumcision: when is it safe? J Pediatr Surg. 2001;36(7):1047–9. https://www.sciencedirect.com/science/article/pii/S0022346801342902. Accessed 9 Sep 2021.

Institute for Healthcare Improvement. The IHI Triple Aim. 2021. Ihi.org. http://www.ihi.org/Engage/Initiatives/TripleAim/Pages/default.aspx.

Institute of Medicine. The future of nursing: leading change, advancing health. Washington, DC: National Academies Press; 2011. https://www.nap.edu/catalog/12956/the-future-of-nursing-leading-change-advancing-health.

Joint Commission for Transforming Health Care. High reliability in health care. 2020. Centerfortransforminghealthcare.org. https://www.centerfortransforminghealthcare.org/high-reliability-in-health-care/.

KFF. Nurse practitioner scope of practice laws. 2015. https://www.kff.org/other/state-indicator/total-nurse-practitioners/?currentTimeframe=0&selectedRows=%7B. Accessed 8 Sep 2021.

Kibby M, Saliba G, Gregg J, Stinson J. Program value realization: a six-part framework for keeping transformations on track. 2015. https://www.strategyand.pwc.com/us/en/reports/2015/program-value-realization.html.

Kim JK, Koyle MA, Chua ME, Ming JM, Lee MJ, Kesavan A, Saunders M, Dos Santos J. Assessment of risk factors for surgical complications in neonatal circumcision clinic. Can Urol Assoc J. 2019;13(4):E108–12. https://www.ncbi.nlm.nih.gov/pmc/articles/PMC6456348/. Accessed 11 May 2021.

Kleinpell RM, Grabenkort WR, Kapu AN, Constantine R, Sicoutris C. Nurse practitioners and physician assistants in acute and critical care. Crit Care Med. 2019;47(10):1442–9.

Kokorowski PJ, Routh JC, Hubert K, Graham DA, Nelson CP. Trends in revision circumcision at pediatric hospitals. Clin Pediatr. 2013;52(8):699–706.

Kuo DZ, Houtrow AJ, Arango P, Kuhlthau KA, Simmons JM, Neff JM. Family-centered care: current applications and future directions in pediatric health care. Matern Child Health J. 2011;16(2):297–305. https://www.ncbi.nlm.nih.gov/pmc/articles/PMC3262132/.

Liu C, Hebert PL, Douglas JH, Neely EL, Sulc CA, Reddy A, Sales AE, Wong ES. Outcomes of primary care delivery by nurse practitioners: utilization, cost, and quality of care. Health Serv Res. 2020;55(2):178–89.

Mark BA, Patel E. Nurse practitioner scope of practice: what do we know and where do we go? West J Nurs Res. 2019;41(4):483–7.

Mason DJ, Jones DA, Roy C, Sullivan CG, Wood LJ. Commonalities of nurse-designed models of health care. Nurs Outlook. 2015;63(5):540–53.

Massachusetts Health Promotion Clearinghouse. All babies cry fact sheet. 2015. https://massclearinghouse.ehs.state.ma.us/PROG-INJPREV/SB3101kit.html. Accessed 10 Sep 2021.

National Academy of Sciences, Engineering, and Medicine. The future of nursing 2020–2030. Washington, DC: National Academies Press; 2021.

Nelson CP, Rosoklija I, Grant R, Retik AB. Development and implementation of a photographic atlas for parental instruction and guidance after outpatient penile surgery. J Pediatr Urol. 2012;8(5):521–6.

Norful AA, Swords K, Marichal M, Cho H, Poghosyan L. Nurse practitioner–physician comanagement of primary care patients. Health Care Manag Rev. 2019;44(3):235–45.

Quallich SA, Bumpus SM, Lajiness S. Competencies for the nurse practitioner working with adult urology patients. Urol Nurs. 2015;35(5):221.

Sikka R, Morath JM, Leape L. The Quadruple Aim: care, health, cost and meaning in work. BMJ Qual Saf. 2015;24(10):608–10. https://qualitysafety.bmj.com/content/qhc/24/10/608.full.pdf.

Task Force on Circumcision. Male circumcision. Pediatrics. 2012;130(3):e756–85. https://pediatrics.aappublications.org/content/130/3/e756. Accessed 18 Jun 2019.

Thomas A, Katherine Crabtree F, Delaney K, Dumas MA, Kleinpell R, Marfell J, Nativio D, Buchholz S, Dileo H, Dontje K, Haber J, Hart A, Reeve K, Ruppert S, Schaffer S. Nurse practitioner Core competencies content A delineation of suggested content specific to the NP core competencies 2017 NP Core Competencies Content Work Group. 2017. https://cdn.ymaws.com/www.nonpf.org/resource/resmgr/competencies/2017_NPCoreComps_with_Curric.pdf.

US News and World Report. Best Children's Hospitals | Top pediatric hospital rankings | US News Best Hospitals. 2021. Usnewscom. https://health.usnews.com/best-hospitals/pediatric-rankings.

Williams V, Nelson C, Estrada C. A photographic guide to healing after newborn circumcision. Boston: Boston Children's Hospital; 2019.

Williams V, Lajoie D, Nelson C, Schenkel SR, Logvinenko T, Tecci K, Porter C, Estrada C. Experience with implementation of a nurse practitioner-led newborn circumcision clinic. J Pediatr Urol. 2020;16(5):651.e1–7. https://www.sciencedirect.com/science/article/pii/S1477513120304976?via%3Dihub. Accessed 13 Jul 2021.

www.ahrq.gov. Use the Teach-Back Method: tool #5. 2015. https://www.ahrq.gov/health-literacy/improve/precautions/tool5.html.

Analysis of Nurse-Led Models Heath Care and Implications for Practice, Research, Education, and Policymaking

Cecily L. Betz

Introduction

This text has provided readers with exemplary models of nurse-led services and programs from throughout the world. Authors from seven countries worldwide have provided examples of models of care that have demonstrated the breadth and scope of nursing practice that arose out of population need and features the unique needs of their population. The countries of authors' origins include Australia, Brazil, Canada, Sierra Leone, Singapore, South Africa, and the United States of America. Each of the chapters has provided the reader with unique nurse-led models of care that are representative of diverse populations of children, adolescents, and their families, in clinical and community-based settings, featuring specialized areas of practice in these global communities.

Responsive to Healthcare Needs

Collectively, the chapters are representative of the entire life span of childhood, adolescence, and young adulthood as presented in Table 1. Nurse-led programs as presented in this text were developed to address diverse healthcare needs as exemplified for neonates transferring out of the neonatal intensive care unit as described by Drs. Sarik and Masuda in the chapter on the *Baby Steps* program in Miami, Florida, in the United States or the infants with tracheostomies discharged home to families with limited resources in the *Breatheasy* program in South Africa. Several

C. L. Betz (✉)
University of Southern California University Center for Excellence in Developmental Disabilties, Children's Hospital Los Angeles, Los Angeles, CA, USA
e-mail: cbetz@chla.usc.edu

© The Author(s), under exclusive license to Springer Nature Switzerland AG 2023
C. L. Betz (ed.), *Worldwide Successful Pediatric Nurse-Led Models of Care*,
https://doi.org/10.1007/978-3-031-22152-1_17

Table 1 Country, population focus and settings of nurse-led services/programs

Nurse-led service/program	Country	Population focus	Setting
Leading a Nurse Practitioner-designed Newborn Circumcision Clinic	USA	Newborns	Outpatient service
Baby Steps: Improving the Transition from Hospital to Home for Neonatal Patients and Caregivers through Nurse-Led Telehealth	USA	Neonates	Transfer of Care Model: hospital to home
Breatheasy: A Nurse-Led "Care Through Family" Service Model	South Africa	Infants	Transfer of Care Model: hospital to home
Evolution of a Complex and Home Care Programme for Children with Chronic Diseases	Singapore	Children with medical complexity (CMC)	Long-term home care services
Caring for Patients on Extracorporeal Membrane Oxygenation (ECMO) in the Pediatric Intensive Care Setting	Singapore	Critically ill neonates and children with severe respiratory and/or cardiac failure	Pediatric intensive care
Canadian Nurse Practitioner-Led Paediatric Rehabilitation Complex Care Program	Canada	Children and youth with medical complexity	Children's rehabilitation hospital
Affirming and Empowering Kids: Creating an Independent and Comprehensive Gender-affirming Healthcare Center	USA	Transgender and gender-diverse children, youth, and adults	Community-based healthcare center
From Patient Studies to a Hospital-Wide Initiative: A Mindfulness Journey	USA	Nurses and interdisciplinary healthcare professionals	Hospital-wide program
Transitioning from Pediatric to Adult Care in Sickle Cell Disease: An Innovative Nurse-led Service Model	USA	Youth and young adults with sickle cell disease	Outpatient clinic of pediatric medical center
Leveraging a Professional Nursing Organization to Create an Anti-Trafficking Care Model	USA	Children at risk for exploitation and abuse in human trafficking	National initiative
Interactional Model of Caring for Families of Children with Chronic Conditions	Brazil	Families of children with chronic conditions	Clinic located on university campus
A Paediatric Eczema Shared Care Model	Australia	Children and youth with eczema	NP-led paediatric eczema service and national initiative
The Social-Ecological Theory of Child Development: A Framework For Nurse-Led Initiatives And Models of Care	USA	Children, youth, and families	Framework of care
The Sierra Leone National ETAT+ Programme: Delivering Nurse-Led Emergency Paediatric Care	Sierra Leone	Acutely unwell children	National Emergency Services Model

chapters describe nurse-led models of care for populations of children and youth whose needs for services have been called to attention over a relatively more recent period of time.

Dallas Ducar describes the recently establish clinical program, *Transhealth Northampton*, which provides primary and specialty care for transgender and gender-diverse individuals including children and youth. Other programs address more diverse age range of children as presented in the chapter entitled *Canadian Nurse Practitioner Led Paediatric Rehabilitation Complex Care Clinic* that provides follow-up services for children with medical complexity and in the chapter *Evolution of a Complex and Home Care Programme for Children with Chronic Diseases* that features the home care program for children with chronic diseases in Singapore, and *NAPNAP Partners for Vulnerable Youth* initiative, *Alliance for Children in Trafficking (ACT)*.

Two chapters describe nurse-led transition programs for youth and young adults with long-term conditions, which is an ever-growing service need as now it is estimated that a million of these youth enter adulthood annually (Cheng and Shaewitz 2021; Child and Adolescent Health Measurement Initiative 2019; Cornell University 2020; U.S. Census Bureau 2019; U.S. Census Bureau, 2020; University of California, San Francisco 2019), whereas two decades ago, the number of those entering adulthood annually was estimated to be about 500,000 (Lotstein et al. 2005). Dr. Speller-Brown in the chapter *Transitioning from Pediatric to Adult Care in Sickle Cell Disease: An Innovative Nurse-Led Service Model* elucidates the healthcare transition program developed for adolescents and young adults with sickle cell disease that facilitates their transfer of care to adult health services. In the chapter *Nurse-Led Service Models: Lessons Learned Over 25 Years*, Dr. Betz describes nurse-led models of care for adolescents with special health care needs/disabilities transitioning to adulthood.

These chapters are representative of not only unmet needs of pediatric populations but the diversity of the nurse-led service models to address their needs as well. The commonality of all the nurse-led models published in this text is the collective acknowledgement of the healthcare needs that are recognized by the nurse clinical leaders and administrators.

Coupled with the diverse age groups associated with each of the programs, the care needs are different as well. Some of the programs address care needs that are managed in primary and community-based settings such as described in the chapter *Pediatric Eczema Shared Care Model* and in the chapter *Evolution of a Complex and Home Care Programme for Children with Chronic Diseases* that describes the home care program for children with chronic diseases located in Singapore.

Other programs were developed to address the needs of critically ill neonates, and children with severe respiratory and cardiac failures were located in critical and neonatal care units as described in the chapter about the ECMO program at KK Women's and Children's Hospital (KKH), the largest pediatric facility in Singapore in the chapter *Caring for Patients on Extracorporeal Membrane Oxygenation (ECMO) in the Pediatric Intensive Care Setting*. Several programs were integrated into clinical settings of pediatric medical centers as described by Dr. Speller-Brown wherein the sickle cell disease transition clinic is affiliated with Children's National

Medical Center. Transfer of care programs to facilitate the discharge from the hospital to home are described in *Baby Steps* program at Nichlaus Children's Hospital in Miami, Florida, and *Breatheasy* program in the Red Cross War Memorial Children's Hospital in Cape Town South Africa.

Other programs were extensions of existing services to address the challenges associated with access to care to ensure care was provided in a timely manner as described in the chapter on the *Newborn Circumcision Clinic* affiliated with Boston's Children's Hospital and *Paediatric Rehabilitation Complex Care Program* in Canada. Diverse as these direct service programs are, their commonality is their innovative nursing response to address unmet needs to better serve the pediatric population and their families.

All of these nurse-led efforts were initiated based upon unmet patient and family needs. These examples of established and emerging nurse-led models of practice were envisioned, formulated, and implemented in a wide range of settings and with diverse pediatric populations. These nurse-led models brought new, innovative, and accessible care to infants, children, youth, and their families that were not previously available. The *Newborn Circumcision Clinic*, a satellite community-based program of the Boston's Children's Hospital Department of Urology, enabled infants who were not circumcised during the immediate newborn period due to medically related issues to access this care that was affordable, safe, accessible, and family-centered. The *Breatheasy program*, affiliated with Red Cross War Memorial Children's Hospital in Cape Town South Africa enabled children with tracheostomies and on ventilation support to be discharged to home including to home settings with limited resources including water and electricity. The *Breatheasy* program has facilitated earlier discharge to home for these children than what would have not been otherwise possible. The *Nurse Practitioner-Led Paediatric Rehabilitation Complex Care Program* in Toronto, Canada, has created improved access for children with long-term complex medical needs to be seen more regularly with improved coordination of care. Previously, the wait time for admitting new patients for services was over 1 year creating problematic service delays for this vulnerable patient group. *Transhealth Northampton*, the independent and comprehensive gender-affirming healthcare center, was established to provide care to a population of transgender and gender-diverse individuals, across the life span who could access that that was affirming and supportive to their range of health and psychosocial needs. Although now characteristically different from the other nurse-led programs that are patient-centered included in this text, the modified *Mindfulness-Based Stress Reduction (MBSR)* program at Children's National Medical Center initially began as a patient-centered program for adolescents with implanted cardiac devices is now focused on addresses the unmet needs of staff, called *Mindful Mentors* (Freedenberg et al. 2020; Freedenberg et al. 2015). The current intent of this train-the-trainer model is to enable greater outreach to other staff, families, and patients by using the mindfulness techniques learned to reduce their distress. As the examples of the programs described here demonstrate, the nurse-led models are uniquely tailored to meet the diverse needs of their patient population.

Theoretical Frameworks

As presented in Table 2, each of these models is based upon theoretical models that serve to guide the development of these nurse-led models. The theoretical frameworks that guided the development of the nurse-led models presented in these chapters originated in a variety of disciplines that encompass nursing and interdisciplinary perspectives. For example, in the *Baby Steps* program and in one of the transition programs referred to in the Betz chapter, the Meleis' Model of Transition was used (Meleis et al. 2000). A health systems framework was applied in the development of the nurse-practitioner-designed *Newborn Circumcision Clinic*. Family-centered and person-centered frameworks were used with the development of programs discussed in the *Breatheasy* program, the *Paediatric Rehabilitation Complex Care Program* in Canada, the gender-affirming services at *Transhealth Northampton,* and the Pediatric Eczema Shared Care Services.

Other models were based on the evidence of population health needs identified in the local community, regionally, and nationally. The *Sierra Leone National ETAT+ Programme* is an example of a model implemented in selected settings nationwide in Sierra Leone. This program was initiated to make needed improvements with the triage system in hospitals throughout Sierra Leone. Emergency Triage Assessment and Treatment+ (ETAT+) framework, developed by the World Health Organization was used to guide the implementation of the ETAT+ program. Although implemented regionally with implications for replication nationally, *Transhealth Northampton* was created to address the needs of an underserved population of transgender and gender-diverse individuals based upon on informed consent and harm reduction. The *Nurse Practitioner-Led Paediatric Rehabilitation Complex Care Program* is based upon a nursing role framework using the *Participatory, Evidence-Based, Patient-Focused Process for Advanced Practice Nursing (PEPPA)* framework (Bryant-Lukosius and Dicenso 2004). The examples of nurse-led models of care as described here are illustrative of the variety of theoretical foundations upon which the nurse-led models were influenced in their development and implementation. Importantly, in each of the chapters, the authors provide the reader with the rationale for its selection and application to practice as these decisions are predicated not only population need but the experience and expertise of those involved with the programmatic development of these nurse-led models of care.

Two of the chapters address theory-driven approaches to care as found in the Dr. Linda Eanes' chapter entitled *The Social-Ecological Theory of Child Development: A Framework for Nurse-Led Initiatives and Models of Care* and in the chapter *Interactional Model of Caring for Families of Children with Chronic Conditions,* authored by a team of Brazilian nurse researchers led by Dr. Lucila Castanheira Nascimento. As exemplified in both of these chapters, the theoretical framework serves to describe and orient the scope of nursing actions, whether it be practice-focused, research-oriented, or educationally directed to address the health-related needs manifested and evident by the children and families who access the healthcare system for services. In particular, Dr. Eanes explicates the application of Uric

Table 2 Theoretical frameworks, methods of evaluation, staffing of nurse-led services/programs

Nurse-led service/program	Theoretical framework	Methods of evaluation	Staffing

Leading a Nurse Practitioner-designed Newborn Circumcision Clinic	Triple Aim Framework; and The Institute of Medicine Future of Nursing Report	• Demographics
		• Parent satisfaction
		• Clinical outcomes
		  – Clinical appearance
		  – Post procedural pain
		• Cost impact
			• Nurse practitioners

Baby Steps: Improving the Transition from Hospital to Home for Neonatal Patients and Caregivers through Nurse-Led Telehealth	Meleis's Theory of Transition	• Demographic measures • Number of infants and families served • Number of encounters • Number of 30-day readmission rates • Number of emergency care use • Caregiver experience measures	• PhD-prepared nurses • Advanced practice nurses • Registered nurses
Breatheasy: A Nurse-Led "Care Through Family" Service Model	Care Through Family Model	• Demographics • Quality of child's life using Paediatric Tracheotomy Health Status Instrument (PTHSI) • Length of hospital stay • Unplanned hospital readmissions • Mortality and cause of death	• Pediatric nurse practitioners • Ward nurses • Doctors • Allied health professions • Ward housekeeper and cleaners

Nurse-led service/program	Theoretical framework	Methods of evaluation	Staffing

Evolution of a Complex and Home Care Program for Children with Chronic Diseases	Integrated Complex Care Model (ICCM)	• Healthcare resource utilization
		  – Number of ED visits
		  – Number of unplanned hospitalizations
		  – Hospitalization LOS
		• Caregiver burden
		  – Patient Health Questionnaire-9 (PHQ-9)
		  – Perceived Stress Scale (PSS)
		• Quality of life
		  – KIDSCREEN
			• Home care nurses
			• Pediatricians Physiotherapists Occupational Therapists Speech and Language Therapists
			• Dieticians
			• Pharmacists
			• Social Workers
			• Care Coordinators

Caring for Patients on Extracorporeal Membrane Oxygenation (ECMO) in the Pediatric Intensive Care Setting	Intensive Care Unit Team Performance Framework	• ELSO registry
		  – Demographics
		  – Pre-Extracorporeal Life Support (ECLS) Assessment
		  – Pre-ECLS Support
		  – ECLS Assessment
		  – Mode and Equipment
		  – Diagnoses
		  – Procedures
		  – Infections
		  – Outcomes
		  – Addenda
		• Setting-specific data
		  – Caseload statistics
		  – Adverse outcomes
			• ECMO specialist nurses
			• Bedside nurse
			• Perfusionists
			• Physicians

(continued)

Table 2 (continued)

Nurse-led service/program	Theoretical framework	Methods of evaluation	Staffing
Canadian Nurse Practitioner-Led Paediatric Rehabilitation Complex Care Program	Participatory, Evidence-Based, Patient-Focused Process for Advanced Practice Nursing (PEPPA)	• Access and efficiency of care – Wait times – Frequency of clinic visits – Minutes of telephone contact points with families • Caregiver satisfaction – Client Satisfaction Questionnaire (CSQ-8) – Family Professional Partnership Scale • Interprofessional collaboration – Provider Collaboration Survey (PCS)	• Nurse practitioners
Affirming and Empowering Kids: Creating an Independent and Comprehensive Gender-affirming Healthcare Center	Gender-affirming philosophy incorporates patient-centered approach based on informed consent and harm reduction	Patient Outcomes • Patient satisfaction • ↓ Mortality • ↓ Morbidity • Quality of care Staff Outcomes • ↑ staff satisfaction • ↑ staff retention Programmatic Outcomes • Gender-affirming protocols • Gender-affirming philosophy • ↑ access to gender-affirming care • ↑ networking with community practices • Development of client-centered outcomes • Meets budgetary projections	• Advanced practice nurses • Registered nurses

Nurse-led service/program	Theoretical framework	Methods of evaluation	Staffing
From Patient Studies to a Hospital-Wide Initiative: A Mindfulness Journey	Mindfulness-Based Stress Reduction (MBSR)	Project Feasibility • Acceptability • Practicality • Recruitment • Attendance • MBSR evaluation; Participant Outcomes • Negative Outcomes – Stress Distress, Burnout, Anxiety • Positive Outcomes – Mindfulness, Self-efficacy, Compassionate Care, Resilience	• PhD prepared nurse • Interdisciplinary professionals
Transitioning from Pediatric to Adult Care in Sickle Cell Disease: An innovative Nurse-led Service Model	Self-Management; Transition Readiness	• Got Transition feedback surveys • Felt prepared for transfer • Follow-up visit with adult provider	• DNP Nurse Practitioner • RN Nurse Coordinator • Social Worker
Leveraging a Professional Nursing Organization to Create an Anti-Trafficking Care Model	Social Ecological Model; Public Health Intervention Wheel; Policy Circle Model	• Number of persons completing training • Number trainings held • Number of ACT Advocates • Number of organizational partner support endorsements	• PhD prepared Pediatric Nurse Practitioners • Pediatric Nurse Practitioners

(continued)

Table 2 (continued)

Nurse-led service/program	Theoretical framework	Methods of evaluation	Staffing
Interactional Model of Caring for Families of Children with Chronic Conditions	Symbolic Interactionism; Family Vulnerability; Family Resilience Model	Family Outcomes	• PhD professors in Nursing with training in Family Nursing
		• Family satisfaction	• Professor of Psychology at UFMS
		• Improved family's ability to resolve problems	• Nursing graduate students
		• Improved family health literacy	• Nursing undergraduate students with teaching supervision
		• Improved family decision-making	• Nurses
		• Improved family's ability to access social supports	
		• Family participation	
		– Meeting attendance	
		– Number of families who abandon care	
		– Involvement in proposed activities (reading, films, diary)	
		Student Learning	
		• Participation in research group activities	
		• ↑ knowledge and skills in family nursing	
		Programmatic Outcomes	
		• Integration of technology into services	
		• Course development for professionals and graduate students	
		• ↑ scholarship and research	

Nurse-led service/program	Theoretical framework	Methods of evaluation	Staffing
A Paediatric Eczema Shared Care Model	National Allergy Strategy (NAS) Shared Care Model for Allergic Conditions; Framework on Integrated People-Centred Health Services	• Patient-Oriented Eczema Measure (POEM) • Infants' Dermatitis Quality of Life Index (IDQOL) • Children's Dermatology Life Quality Index (CDLQI) • Scoring Atopic Dermatitis Index (SCORAD) • Eczema Area and Severity Index (EASI)	• Nurse practitioner • Physicians • Pharmacist • Advanced practice nurse
The Social-Ecological Theory of Child Development: A Framework For Nurse-Led Initiatives And Models of Care	Social-Ecological Theory (SET)		
The Sierra Leone National ETAT+ Programme: Delivering Nurse-Led Emergency Paediatric Care	World Health Organization-approved ETAT guidelines and training materials Task-sharing initiative, building on the evidence of related initiatives in Sierra Leone and other West African countries; knowledge of the signs of critical illness and of clinical deterioration	• Timing of triage and treatment • Adherence to key aspects of the ETAT+ treatment protocols • Hospital mortality	• State-Enrolled Community Health Nurse (SECHN) grade • State-Registered Nurse (SRN) grade

Bronfenbrenner Social-Ecological Theory (SET) (Bronfenbrenner 1977) as the theoretical guidance to assist nurse leaders in pediatric/paediatric and child health with the development of nurse-led models of care with directed focus on the needs of disadvantaged populations of infants, children, and youth and their families. As detailed in this chapter, Dr. Eanes provides a theoretical template that can be applied to the provision of this underserved pediatric/paediatric and child health population.

The authoring team of Drs Lucila Nascimento, Myriam Mandetta, Eliane Neves, Patricia Kuerten, and Fernanda Marques provides the reader with a thorough description of the model of nursing practice, the *Interactional Family Care Model* that was specially formulated to address the needs of Brazilian families whose children have a chronic condition. As the authors assert, although family models of care have been reported in the international literature, a model that culturally and clinically applicable to Brazilian families with their specialized care needs was not available. Therefore, the authors were motivated to develop a model of care for the purpose of "…promoting empowerment to deal with adversities along the trajectory of the child's chronic health condition." The dimensions of the model are described that were formulated to direct nursing practice together with what have been identified as its strengths and limitations for application in the clinics located at the Federal University of Mato Grosso do Sul, which is in the Central-West region of Brazil.

As has been articulated in each chapter is the essential importance of formulating or selecting a theoretical framework upon which and by which a nurse-led service and program is developed. Several of the nurse-led models of care were based upon established theoretical frameworks such as Meleis' Model of Transition (Meleis et al. 2000) and the Mindfulness-Based Stress Reduction (MBSR) program developed by Dr. Jon Kabat-Zinn (1990). In other nurse-led models described in the text, the theoretical framework was developed by the team members for the service implementation as presented in the chapter on the *Interactional Family Care Model* and in the chapter describing the *Transhealth Northampton* model of care. This commonality of theoretical direction, although varied in its evolution for guiding practice is an essential hallmark of nurse-led model development. The authors in each of the chapters have provided their insights with this important phase of model development.

Sustainability

Sustainability is a major consideration for undertaking the effort to start a nurse-led model program. This is a serious if not essential question to grapple with prior to undertaking the development of a new service model and, in particular, a service model that is nurse-led. The fiscal implications for starting any new nurse-led service by necessity need to include the institution's financial analyst. This individual is expected and will have the financial knowledge and expertise to consult with the team about the fiscal viability of the proposed project. It is likely as well that the financial analyst will rely on the expertise of the service team to answer questions about the proposed services and supports to be offered. In the chapter *Nurse-Led Service Models: Lessons Learned over 25 Years*, the financial analyst was a pivotal team members in generating the information needed to activate the *Movin' On Up* program and be sustainable. Likewise, as described in the start-up efforts of the *Newborn Circumcision Clinic*, operations and facility experts were members of the interprofessional stakeholder team that enabled the establishment of the clinic.

Some programs as described in this text are currently reliant in extramural support for the short-term operational expenditures. As described in the *Baby Steps* program, initial funding for the program was obtained with grant funding from the state of Florida. As authors state, extramural funding remains a tenuous option, one which propels the team to actively seek other sources of funding support. The *Sierra Leone National ETAT+ Programme* was initially started as a pilot program which was later rolled out nationwide across Sierra Leone with government funding.

Several of the programs bill the insurance plan for services. The *Sickle Cell Adolescent Team (SCAT)* program charges for their services that are provided by the program staff. Reimbursement for services in the *Newborn Circumcision Clinic* is based upon Massachusetts professional practice statutes and payor contracts with the medical institution. As described in the chapter on the *Nurse Practitioner-Led Paediatric Rehabilitation Complex Care Program*, nurse practitioners function independently and receive reimbursement for their services in the Canadian system of care. The modified MBSR program at Children's National Medical Center initially began as a small pilot project with 10 adolescent patients with pacemakers or ICD implanted cardiac defibrillators then expanded to larger group of 46 adolescents and eventually to a staff support program *Mindful Mentors* (Freedenberg et al. 2015, 2020). The expansion of the *Mindful Mentors* program throughout the institution for hospital staff was possible with committed institutional support. The *Transhealth Northampton* health center was ushered into operation with the initial generous support of a donor. The initial start-up funding enabled the preliminary work needed for this health center, which included a needs assessment and operational planning. Services provided are now reimbursed with public and private insurance.

None of these programs would have been possible without institutional support. Each of the programs provides the reader with an understanding of the deliberate and involved process that was undertaken to create these nurse-led models of care. The *Breatheasy* program, begun in 1989, by Sister Jane Booth is an institutionally supported program whose staff today consists of two pediatric nurse coordinators and the in-house hospital staff that provide the in-patient care. The establishment of the *SCAT* program was made possible with support of the hospital administration and the sickle cell disease administrative/medical support leaders. The process undertaken to develop and implement this model/service required buy-in from the healthcare system at Children's National Hospital, a large urban pediatric medical center in Washington, DC, that manages over 1500 patients with SCD. Buy-in from administration, the SCD Director and Hematology Division Chief, and the willingness and cooperation of the SCAT team members made this possible.

The *Paediatric Eczema Shared Care Model* is an example of collaborative and partnership support from several resources. Intramural support was funded by the

Perth Children's Hospital (PCH), and in-kind support was obtained from interprofessional staff of the Department of Dermatology, Immunology and Allergy at PCH, and partner organizations, National Allergy Strategy (NAS) and Allergy & Anaphylaxis Australia (A&AA). This partnership effort, described in great detail in the chapter, enabled the implementation of other components of the Paediatric Eczema Shared Care Model beyond the establishment of the nurse-led eczema clinic. The other outreach efforts included the development of a paediatric eczema e-training course for health professionals, webinars and seminars on eczema management for a diverse group of learners that included school and primary care nurses, pharmacists, and dietitians in urban and rural areas of Western Australia. Other resources developed through this collaborative effort include a decision-making algorithm for providers and an Eczema School Kit for school personnel and parents.

The chapter authors provide the readers with the complex and, sometimes, convoluted process undertaken to garner the initial support necessary for the visioning of the proposed nurse-led models of care. The proposals that these authors developed were born out of their recognition of not only an unmet service need of the population they served but also their professional acumen that transcended the current care options available for their patients and risk-taking behavior that inspired these innovative nurse leaders. As these authors disclosed, they had a keen understanding of the organizational matrix and leadership that they were able to engage to bring their project eventually to fruition. These advanced practice nurses and nurse leaders were able to communicate their ideas thoughtfully and professionally to the institutional and public health authorities to proceed forward with the planning of their nurse-led models of care. Their processes as described in each of the chapters provide a template for replication in other settings and circumstances.

Research and Quality Improvement Efforts

As has been detailed in many of these chapters, coupled with the service development efforts, the authors have been involved in research and quality improvement efforts that provide an added dimension of ensuring their work is disseminated to a wider audience of professionals. Through dissemination efforts, authors share their knowledge and evidence whether through presentations given at professional conferences and published in professional journals or shared locally with colleagues. As presented in the chapters, the authors generated empirical evidence that contributes to the body of literature to enhance knowledge and skills in their specialized field of practice and research. Importantly as well, the research and quality improvement efforts chronicled by authors were the means by which they tested selected outcomes in terms of effectiveness, efficiency, efficacy, and feasibility of their program and gained additional insights that would serve to modify the programs.

In the early stages of the establishment of the *Paediatric Rehabilitation Complex Care Program*, the team reported conducting a quality improvement project to measure access to care, program efficiency, and satisfaction of caregiver and interprofessional team members, which were considered important outcomes this team wanted to measure. The quality improvement model design was used to assess the feasibility of the *Mindful Mentors* program. Data gathered to assess feasibility of this program was based using the Bowen model's area of focus (Bowen et al. 2009). In this chapter, Dr. Freedenberg provides preliminary findings in answer to the basic question "can it work?"

Immersion in programmatic efforts will inevitability lead to other related venues of research and clinical practice. As demonstrated in these chapters, investigative efforts are born out of the practice challenges and experiences with the provision of services in these nurse-led models of care. Brandon and colleagues identified one of the challenges they encountered in the *Paediatric Rehabilitation Complex Care Program* was healthcare transition planning for transition-age youth and young adults and their families. The challenges associated with facilitating the transfer of care, which authors highlight in the chapter, are expanded upon in their study that explored the perspectives of young adults, parents, and physicians (Brandon et al. 2019).

Dr. Freedenberg's involvement with modified Mindfulness-Based Stress Reduction (MBSR) program demonstrates the evolution with programmatic and research efforts that can occur over the years. As has been described in her chapter and earlier in this chapter, the modified MBSR evolved from an adolescent-centered program to one for hospital staff at Children's National Medical Center. The research findings of her earlier research with adolescents with cardiac diagnosis and the programmatic development associated with *Mindful Mentors* provide colleagues with findings and the maturation of her work (Freedenberg et al. 2015, 2017, 2020).

As described in the chapter *Breatheasy: A Nurse-Led 'Care Through Family' Service Model*, three data-based papers have been published demonstrating the effectiveness of the *Breatheasy* program (Din et al. 2020; Groenendijk et al. 2016; Van der Poel et al. 2017). Complementary to the outcome findings of the *Breatheasy program*, nurse scholars interviewed nurses involved with this African nursing model and others to investigate nursing practices using a qualitative observational case study design (North et al. 2020). One of the outcomes of their research efforts was the development of the conceptual nursing model of care, *Care Through Family*. This model is reflective of the culturally responsive nursing care practice that exists in Africa (North et al. 2019). The authors provide examples of the application of the *Care Through Family* model of care in the *Breatheasy* program. The *Care Through Family* conceptual model has led to the development of self-assessment tool for practice improvements for nursing teams. As authors state, the *Care Through Family* model will serve as the theoretical basis for future research studies investigating African nursing practices with emphasis on nurse-led services.

Unlike the research undertaken in other nurse-led models of care, Dr. Peck shares the challenges associated with conducting studies in the chapter *Leveraging a Professional Nursing Organization to Create an Anti-Trafficking Care Model*. As Dr. Peck notes, the focus of human trafficking has been framed primarily as a criminal justice issue; efforts to enlarge the understanding and attention of human-trafficking as a healthcare issue have been largely rebuffed. In this environment, funding for research exploring the biopsychosocial consequences upon children and their families has been challenging. To date, research generated has been largely unfunded; as Dr. Peck noted, advances in knowledge and intervention models will be hindered with the lack of extramural funding available for these studies. Demonstrative of these issues, chapter *Leveraging a Professional Nursing Organization to Create an Antitrafficking Care Model*, the development of clinical practice guidelines for human trafficking in the chapter, reveals the lack of evidence to support practice recommendations (Peck 2020).

Some of the projects reported in this text are in the early stages of implementation such as the *Transhealth Northampton* health center. However, given the mission, the current public attention, and policy-related initiatives, it is likely that *Transhealth Northampton* will have an important impact and voice on the provision of health services to transgender and gender-affirming individuals. As the authors of the chapter *A Paediatric Eczema Shared Care Model* note, "…we are also keen to be more involved in eczema research and new eczema treatments for children with eczema." As reported in the chapter, efforts have been directed to evaluation outcomes such as examination of key performance indicators.

Unlike other programs reported in this text, as described in the chapter entitled *Interactional Model of Caring for Families of Children with Chronic Conditions*, outcome data have been and are planned to be gathered from families, professionals, and students. Qualitative methods have been employed to gather data on family satisfaction, their ability to resolve problems and conflicts, family health literacy improvements, participation in decision-making, and accessing community-based social support network. Student outcomes include their participation in learning activities and acquisition of skills and knowledge in the provision of care to this group of families. Those pertaining to professionals include metrics associated with presentations, dissemination, research, and service outreach.

Authors and nurse researchers, Drs. Sarik and Matsuda, bring a research-intensive focus unlike the other research projects associated with and generated from the nurse-led models of care in the text in the chapter *Baby Steps: Improving the Transition from Hospital to Home for Neonatal Patients and Caregivers through a Nurse-Led Telehealth Program*. To begin with, these researchers were members of the organizational matrix that envisioned and implemented the *Baby Steps* program. As the authors detail, *Baby Steps* program was organized and coordinated by three teams—the clinical members of the neonatal intensive care unit (NICU) team, the specialists of the telehealth team, and the research team led by Drs. Sarik and Matsuda. Uniquely, the nurse research team of Drs. Sarik and Matsuda represents an academic-clinical partnership as Dr. Sarik is the nurse scientist at Nichlaus Children's Hospital in Miami, Florida, and Dr. Matsuda is faculty member of the University of Miami School of Nursing and Health Sciences. Together, this team has been involved with all aspects of *Baby Steps* including program development, grantsmanship to support *Baby Steps*, involvement with scholarly and research presentations and publications. In their chapter, authors provide readers with 24-month evaluation data on 450 infants enrolled in the *Baby Steps* program. As authors indicate, they are exploring extensions of their work to address mental health concerns of mothers as *Baby Steps* is currently focused on clinical outcomes (Matsude et al. 2021). Additionally, interconnected to the *Baby Steps* program, a telehealth simulation program was developed for nursing students to educate them about telehealth nursing care using *Baby Steps* as an exemplar (Matsuda et al. 2022).

As Speller-Brown reveals in the chapter *Transitioning from Pediatric to Adult Care in Sickle Cell Disease: An Innovative Nurse-Led Model*, quality improvement and research are integral components of this nurse-led transition model of care for adolescents and young adults with sickle cell disease. The team has incorporated in the Sickle Cell Adolescent Team (SCAT) program, a systematic approach to closely track adolescents and young adults (AYA) whose care is transferred to adult providers, which has been highly successful, wherein 90% report having established care with an adult provider. Currently, tracking efforts have been undertaken for 6 years with plans to continue into the foreseeable future. Coupled with tracking their post-outcome efforts, the team is engaged in other research efforts to inform their work. For example, survey findings exploring the AYA and caregivers' healthcare transition experience after their transition are presented in the chapter. Several research papers have been generated by Dr. Speller-Brown and the team on the transition needs/services for AYA with sickle cell disease (Speller-Brown et al. 2015, 2018).

As authors assert in the chapter *Leading a Nurse Practitioner-designed Newborn Circumcision Clinic*, the planning and implementation of this clinic included "… the commitment to research and clinical inquiry." As the program was developed, research and evaluation planning were integrated throughout to monitor and measure the evaluation. Currently, the program is collecting data on patient/family satisfaction, clinical outcomes, cost savings, and realization (Williams et al. 2020).

The importance of sharing research and quality improvement findings cannot be understated. It is vital to the growth of nursing specialty practice, particularly as it pertains to the development, implementation, and testing new models of nursing care. Advances in nursing practice will be enhanced with the collective sharing of practice and research efforts as a means of encouraging others to undertake similar projects, fostering networking among colleagues in areas of mutual interest, and to forge new pathways for innovation and discovery. As has been highlighted, these programs take this responsibility seriously and have and will continue to advance the science of nurse-led models of care.

Evaluation Measures

As presented in Table 2, each of the programs selected methods of evaluations that were predicated on the outcomes selected for measurement, population served, and the resources available to conduct programmatic evaluations. All of the care models collected demographic data; many gathered input on satisfaction and perceptions of the quality of care with services from the recipients of services. Measurements of clinical outcomes included data that was more easily retrievable such as number of emergency department visits and hospitalizations and hospital length of stay. Patient outcomes included morbidity and mortality data and quality-of-life measures.

Evaluation measures included those that were specifically designed by the clinical team and empirically validated tools such as the KIDSCREEN (Bullinger et al. 2002) and Client Satisfaction Questionnaire (CSQ-8) (Larsen et al. 1979) to name a few. Evaluation methods and challenges of selected programs are highlighted below.

As described in the chapter *The Sierra Leone National ETAT+ Programme: Delivering Nurse-Led Emergency Paediatric Care*, the methods of evaluation were systematically conducted according to the plan specified in this national initiative which involved both local and national evaluation reviews. At the local level, evaluation plan consisted of time-intensive data collection efforts as mentor teams conducted pre- and post-implementation measures from the hospitals involved with this national initiative. Data collection involved accessing patient records directly and in some circumstances additionally tracking of the patient's course of care to properly resolve discrepancies in the data reported at the national level. As Hands noted, challenges were encountered with the evaluation process due to inconsistencies with the gathering and reporting of data.

Authors Williams, Wood, and Lajoie noted in their chapter *Leading a Nurse Practitioner-designed Newborn Circumcision Clinic (NCC)* that initially the response rate of patient satisfaction was problematic. Initially, satisfaction surveys were mailed 6 weeks following circumcision which did not produce sufficient evaluation data; response rates were improved when an electronic format was instituted. Survey data are integral to the *NCC*; it is reviewed on a quarterly basis and guides the program's development and changes with interventions.

Several methods of evaluation are used in the KKH's pediatric and neonatal ECMO program. As a member Extracorporeal Life Support Organization (ELSO), ECMO program data are inputted into the ELSO registry, which serves as an international data repository on ECMO patients. The KKH ECMO conducts quarterly audit meetings to monitor caseload and ELSO benchmarks. The KKH home care program for children with chronic conditions gathers both clinical and psychosocial data from the recipients of services. This program tracks healthcare utilization and uses several validated tools to measure parental stress and the child's quality of life as listed in Table 2.

Conclusions

These projects are exemplars of nursing practice that provide new understandings of what is possible for replication elsewhere. As has been demonstrated throughout this text, the projects although diverse in target populations, different in structure, and distinct in its mission reflect the opportunities available for nurses to develop innovation nurse-led models of care for infants, children, youth, and their families. Although regulatory environments differ internationally, full practice authority (FPA) will enable advanced practice nurses to extend their scope of practice to function independently and to the full extent of their practice (ANA 2020; Bosse et al. 2017; Stucky et al. 2020). This is a vision of practice that has yet to be fully realized in the United States and internationally. Nevertheless, as presented in this text, a vast array of nurse-led practice models have been presented, some of which are staffed with nurses with varied nursing degrees. The diversity of nurse-led efforts need not be confined to a prescribed set of professional and health system expectations but rather created based on nursing best practices and the population healthcare needs of the infants, children, youth, and families. The nurse-led models of care presented in this text are shining examples of the possibilities for pediatric/paediatric and child health nursing practice.

References

American Nurses Association. ANA's principles for advanced practice registered nurse (APRN): full practice authority. 2020. https://www.nursingworld.org/~49f695/globalassets/docs/ana/ethics/principles-aprnfullpracticeauthority.pdf. Accessed 12 Nov 2020.

Bosse J, Simmonds K, Hanson C, Pulcini J, Dunphy L, Vanhook P, Poghosyan L. Position statement: full practice authority for advanced practice registered nurses is necessary to transform primary care. Nurs Outlook. 2017;65(6):761–5. https://doi.org/10.1016/j.outlook.2017.10.002.

Bowen DJ, Kreuter M, Spring B, Cofta-Woerpel L, Linnan L, Weiner D, Bakken S, Kaplan CP, Squiers L, Fabrizio C, Fernandez M. How we design feasibility studies. Am J Prev Med. 2009;36(5):452–7.

Brandon E, Ballantyne M, Penner M, Lauzon A, McCarvill E. Accessing primary health care services for transition-ages young adults with cerebral palsy; perspectives of young adults, parents and physicians. J Trans Med. 2019;1(1):20190004.

Bronfenbrenner U. Toward an experimental ecology of human development. Am Psychol. 1977;32:513–31.

Bryant-Lukosius D, Dicenso A. A framework for the introduction and evaluation of advanced practice nursing roles. J Adv Nurs. 2004;48(5):530–40. https://doi.org/10.1111/j.1365-2648.2004.03235.x. PMID: 15533091.

Bullinger M, Schmidt S, Petersen C. Assessing quality of life of children with chronic health conditions and disabilities: a European approach. Int J Rehabil Res. 2002;25(3):197–206.

Cheng L, Shaewitz D. The 2021 youth transition report: outcomes for youth and young adults with disabilities. Washington, DC: Institute for Educational Leadership; 2021.

Child and Adolescent Health Measurement Initiative. National survey of children's health 2016–2017 data query. Baltimore: Data Resource Center for Child and Adolescent Health; 2019.

Cornell University. Estimate of disability statistics for youth and young adults based on analysis of 2019. American Community Survey Public Use Microdata Sample. Special tabulations prepared by William Erickson, Yang-Tan Institute; 2020.

Din TF, McGuire J, Booth J, Lytwynchuk A, Fagan JJ, Peer S. The assessment of quality of life in children with tracheostomies and their families in a low to middle income country (LMIC). Int J Pediatr Otorhinolaryngol. 2020;138:110319. https://doi.org/10.1016/j.ijporl.2020.110319.

Freedenberg VA, Thomas SA, Friedmann E. A pilot study of a mindfulness based stress reduction program in adolescents with implantable cardioverter defibrillators or pacemakers. Pediatr Cardiol. 2015;36(4):786–95.

Freedenberg VA, Hinds PS, Friedmann E. Mindfulness-based stress reduction and group support decrease stress in adolescents with cardiac diagnoses: a randomized two-group study. Pediatr Cardiol. 2017;38(7):1415–25.

Freedenberg VA, Jiang J, Cheatham CA, Sibinga EM, Powell CA, Martin GR, Steinhorn DM, Kemper KJ. Mindful mentors: is a longitudinal mind–body skills training pilot program feasible for pediatric cardiology staff? Glob Adv Health Med. 2020;9:2164956120959272.

Groenendijk I, Booth J, van Dijk M, Argent A, Zampoli M. Paediatric tracheostomy and ventilation home care with challenging socio-economic circumstances in South Africa. Int J Pediatr Otorhinolaryngol. 2016;84:161–5. https://doi.org/10.1016/j.ijporl.2016.03.013.

Kabat-Zinn J. Full catastrophe living: the program of the stress reduction clinic at the. Worcester: University of Massachusetts Medical Center; 1990.

Larsen DL, Attkisson CC, Hargreaves WA, Nguyen TD. Assessment of client/patient satisfaction: development of a general scale. Eval Program Plann. 1979;2(3):197–207.

Lotstein DS, McPherson M, Strickland B, Newacheck PW. Transition planning for youth with special health care needs: results from the National Survey of Children with Special Health Care Needs. Pediatrics. 2005;115(6):1562–8. https://doi.org/10.1542/peds.2004-1262. PMID: 15930217.

Matsude Y, McCabe BE, Behar-Zusman V. Mothering in the context of mental disorder: effect of caregiving load on maternal health in a predominantly Hispanic sample. J Am Psychiatr Nurses Assoc. 2021;27(5):373–82.

Matsuda Y, Valdes B, Salani D, Foronda C, Roman Laporte R, Gamez D, et al. Baby Steps Program: telehealth nursing simulation for undergraduate public health nursing students. Clin Simul Nurs. 2022;65:1–10.

Meleis AI, Sawyer LM, Im EO, Hilfinger Messias DK, Schumacher K. Experiencing transitions: an emerging middle-range theory. ANS Adv Nurs Sci. 2000;23(1):12–28. https://doi.org/10.1097/00012272-200009000-00006. PMID: 10970036.

North N, Sieberhagen S, Bonaconsa C, Leonard A, Coetzee M. Making children's nursing practices visible: using visual and participatory techniques to describe family involvement in the care of hospitalised children in southern African settings. Int J Qual Res Methods. 2019;18:160940691984932. https://doi.org/10.1177/1609406919849324.

North N, Leonard A, Bonaconsa C, Duma T, Coetzee M. Distinctive nursing practices in working with mothers to care for hospitalised children at a district hospital in KwaZulu-Natal, South Africa: a descriptive observational study. BMC Nurs. 2020;19(1):1–12.

Peck JL. Human trafficking of children: nurse practitioner knowledge, beliefs, and experience supporting the development of a practice guideline: part two; 2020. https://doi.org/10.1016/j.pedhc.2019.11.005.

Speller-Brown B, et al. Measuring transition readiness: a correlational study of perceptions of parent and adolescents and young adults with sickle cell disease. J Pediatr Nurs. 2015;30(5):788–96. https://doi.org/10.1016/j.pedn.2015.06.008.

Speller-Brown B, Varty M, Thaniel L, Jacobs M. Assessing disease knowledge and self-management in youth with sickle cell disease. J Pediatr Oncol Nurs. 2018;36(2):143–9.

Stucky CH, Brown WJ, Stucky MG. COVID 19: an unprecedented opportunity for nurse practitioners to reform healthcare and advocate for permanent full practice authority. Nurs Forum. 2020;56:222. https://doi.org/10.1111/nuf.12515.

University of California, San Francisco. Estimate of young adult chronic condition prevalence based on analysis of the 2017 Behavioral Health Risk Surveillance System. Special tabulations prepared by Sally Park; 2019.

US Census Bureau. Annual estimates of the resident population by single year of age and sex for the United States, April 1, 2010 to July 2018. Washington, DC: US Census Bureau, Population Division; 2019.

US Census Bureau. Current population survey, annual social and economic supplement, 2019. Washington, DC: US Census Bureau, Population Division; 2020.

Van der Poel LA, Booth J, Argent A, van Dijk M, Zampoli M. Home ventilation in south African children: do socioeconomic factors matter? Pediatr Allergy Immunol Pulmonol. 2017;30(3):163–70. https://doi.org/10.1089/ped.2016.0727.

Williams V, Lajoie D, Nelson C, Schenkel SR, Logvinenko T, Tecci K, Porter C, Estrada C. Experience with implementation of a nurse practitioner-led newborn circumcision clinic. J Pediatr Urol. 2020;16(5):651.e1–7. https://www.sciencedirect.com/science/article/pii/S1477513120304976?via%3Dihub. Accessed 13 Jul 2021.

Printed in the United States
by Baker & Taylor Publisher Services